ADVANCES IN

Anesthesia

Editor-in-Chief
Laurence C Torsher, MD

Associate Editors
Richard P. Dutton, MD, MBA
Arna Banerjee, MD, MMHC, FCCM
Evan Pivalizza, MBChB, FFA

ELSEVIER

An Imprint of Elsevier, Inc.

PHILADELPHIA   LONDON   TORONTO   MONTREAL   SYDNEY   TOKYO

ADVANCES IN
Anesthesia

VOLUMES 1 THROUGH 38 (OUT OF PRINT)

VOLUME 39

VOLUME 40

Director, Continuity Publishing: Dolores Meloni
Editor: Joanna Gascoine
Developmental Editor: Varun Gopal

Cover images courtesy of James P. Rathmell, MD, Brigham and Women's Hospital, Boston, MA

Editorial Office:
Elsevier
1600 John F. Kennedy Blvd,
Suite 1800
Philadelphia, PA 19103-2899

International Standard Serial Number: 0737-6146
International Standard Book Number-13: 978-0-443-13039-7

ADVANCES IN
Anesthesia

Editors

LAURENCE C. TORSHER, MD

RICHARD P. DUTTON, MD, MBA, FASA

ARNA BANERJEE, MD, MMHC, FCCM

EVAN PIVALIZZA, MBCHB, FFA

Editor-in-Chief

LAURENCE C. TORSHER, MD, Assistant Professor of Anesthesiology and Medical Education, Department of Anesthesiology and Perioperative Medicine, Mayo Clinic, Rochester, Minnesota

Associate Editors

RICHARD P. DUTTON, MD, MBA, FASA, Chair of Anesthesiology, University of Maryland Capital Region Medical Center, Largo, Maryland

ARNA BANERJEE, MD, MMHC, FCCM, Professor of Anesthesiology and Critical Care, Surgery, Medical Education and Administration; Executive Medical Director Critical Care Adult Enterprise; Assistant Vice-Chair Anesthesiology Faculty Affairs, Senior Director, Center for Experiential Learning and Assessment, Vanderbilt University Medical Center, Nashville, Tennessee

EVAN PIVALIZZA, MBCHB, FFA, Distinguished Teaching Professor, Department of Anesthesiology, Critical Care and Pain Medicine, McGovern Medical School at UTHealth, Houston, Texas

ADVANCES IN
Anesthesia

CONTRIBUTORS

ROBIN J. ALDWINCKLE, BMBS, FRCA, Clinical Professor of Anesthesiology, Medical Director of Same Day Surgery Center, Department of Anesthesiology and Pain Medicine, Sacramento, California

KATHERINE W. ARENDT, MD, Department of Anesthesiology and Perioperative Medicine, Mayo Clinic, Rochester, Minnesota

NATHAN E. ASHBY, MD, Associate Professor of Clinical Anesthesiology and Critical Care Medicine, Division of Critical Care Medicine, Department of Anesthesiology, Vanderbilt University Medical Center, Nashville, Tennessee

ADITI BALAKRISHNA, MD, Division of Anesthesiology and Critical Care Medicine, Department of Anesthesiology, Vanderbilt University Medical Center, Nashville, Tennessee

FREDERIC T. BILLINGS IV, MD, MSc, Division of Anesthesiology and Critical Care Medicine, Department of Anesthesiology, Vanderbilt University Medical Center, Nashville, Tennessee

ROBERT BISHOP, B Biomed Sci, B Med, FANZCA, Assistant Professor of Anesthesiology, Department of Anesthesiology and Pain Medicine, University of California, Davis Medical Center, Sacramento, California

ROBERT B. BRYSKIN, MD, Pediatric Anesthesiologist, USAP Florida, Orlando, Florida

AMY CHEN, MD, Assistant Professor, Anesthesiology and Pain Medicine, University of California, Davis, Sacramento, California

IVET T. CORDOBA TORRES, MD, Assistant Professor, Department of Anesthesia, Jackson Memorial Hospital, University of Miami, Miami, Florida

RICHARD P. DUTTON, MD, MBA, FASA, Adjunct Professor, Department of Anesthesiology, Texas A&M College of Medicine, Baylor University Medical Center, Chief Quality Officer, US Anesthesia Partners, Dallas, Texas

ROBYN E. FINNEY, APRN, CRNA, DNAP, Assistant Professor of Anesthesiology, Department of Anesthesiology and Perioperative Medicine, Mayo Clinic, Rochester, Minnesota

ESLAM A. FOUDA, MD, Fellow Transplant Anesthesia, Department of Anesthesia, Jackson Memorial Hospital, University of Miami, Miami, Florida

JULIE FOWLER, MD, Clinical Director, Obstetric Anesthesia, Associate Professor, Anesthesiology and Pain Medicine, University of California, Davis, Sacramento, California

ADAM K. JACOB, MD, Professor of Anesthesiology, Department of Anesthesiology and Perioperative Medicine, Mayo Clinic, Rochester, Minnesota

MICHAEL JUNG, MD, MBA, Assistant Clinical Professor, Associate Program Director, Pain Fellowship, Department of Anesthesiology and Pain Medicine, University of California, Davis Medical Center, Sacramento, California

LARRY R. HUTSON, Jr, MD, FASA, Assistant Professor, Baylor College of Medicine-Temple, Assistant Professor, Texas A&M University School of Medicine-Temple, Department of Anesthesiology, Baylor Scott & White Medical Center-Temple, Temple, Texas

MARIYA KOTOVA, PharmD, Senior Pharmacist, Pain Management, Department of Pharmacy, University of California, Davis Medical Center, Sacramento, California

YAN H. LAI, MD, MPH, FASA, CBA, Associate Professor, Department of Anesthesiology and Perioperative Pain Medicine, Mount Sinai West-Morningside Hospitals, New York, New York

JESSIE LO, MD, Director, Trauma Education Program, Department of Anaesthesia, Cedars-Sinai Medical Center, Los Angeles, California

MARCOS G. LOPEZ, MD, MS, Division of Anesthesiology and Critical Care Medicine, Department of Anesthesiology, Vanderbilt University Medical Center, Nashville, Tennessee

OLIVIA LOUNSBURY, MS, Quality and Safety Department, Johns Hopkins Children's Center

STEPHEN MACRES, MD, PharmD, Clinical Professor of Anesthesiology, Director of Perioperative Pain Services, Department of Anesthesiology and Pain Medicine, University of California, Davis Medical Center, Director, Acute Pain Service, Professor, Anesthesiology and Pain Medicine, The University of California, Davis, Sacramento, California

RUSSELL K. McALLISTER, MD, FASA, Professor, Baylor College of Medicine-Temple, Professor, Texas A&M School of Medicine-Temple, Department of Anesthesiology, Baylor Scott & White Medical Center-Temple, Temple, Texas; Chair of Anesthesiology, Baylor Scott & White Health-Central Texas

ROBERT J. McCUSKER, DO, Anesthesiology, Penn State Health, Hershey, Pennsylvania

TRICIA A. MEYER, PharmD, MS, FASHP, FTSHP, Adjunct Professor, Texas A&M University School of Medicine-Temple, Speaker, Consultant, Eagle Pharmaceuticals, Consultant, Heron Therapeutics

PHILLIP M. MORRIS, MD, Clinical Assistant Professor, Texas A&M University School of Medicine-Temple, Department of Anesthesiology, Baylor Scott & White Medical Center-Temple, Temple, Texas

CONRAD S. MYLER, MD, Assistant Professor of Anesthesiology, Penn State Health, Hershey, Pennsylvania

POONAM PAI B.H., MD, MS, Assistant Professor, Department of Anesthesiology and Perioperative Pain Medicine, Mount Sinai West-Morningside Hospitals, New York, New York

SHIVANI PATEL, MD, MPH, FASA, CBA, LAc, Resident Physician, Department of Anesthesiology and Perioperative Pain Medicine, Mount Sinai West-Morningside Hospitals, New York, New York

RYAN PERLMAN, MSc, MD, FRCPC, Director, Trauma Anesthesia, Department of Anesthesia, Cedars-Sinai Medical Center, Los Angeles, California

SCOTT G. PRITZLAFF, MD, Associate Professor, Division of Pain Medicine, Program Director, Pain Medicine Fellowship, Department of Anesthesiology and Pain Medicine, University of California, Davis Medical Center, Sacramento, California

MYRNA ELIANN REINHARDT, MD, MD Candidate, Albany Medical College, Albany, New York

USHA SALDAHNA, MD, Assistant Professor of Anesthesiology and Pain Medicine, Program Director, Regional Anesthesia Fellowship, Department of Anesthesiology and Pain Medicine, University of California, Davis Medical Center, Sacramento, California

JOSH SANTOS, MD, Assistant Professor of Anesthesiology and Pain Medicine, Director, Pre-Anesthesia Readiness and Education Program, Sacramento, California

EMILY E. SHARPE, MD, Department of Anesthesiology and Perioperative Medicine, Mayo Clinic, Rochester, Minnesota

AESHA S. SHUKLA, MHA, MBA, CPHQ, Vice President, Quality, Analytics and Patient Experience, US Anesthesia Partners

ELIZABETH SINZ, MD, MED, FCCM, FSSH, Professor of Anesthesiology, Penn State Health, Hershey, Pennsylvania

TRAVIS J. SMITH, MD, Anesthesiology, Penn State Health, Hershey, Pennsylvania

FOUAD G. SOUKI, MD, MS, Associate Professor, Department of Anesthesia, Jackson Memorial Hospital, University of Miami, Miami, Florida

MARION 'RED' STARKS, MD, MBA, Pediatric Anesthesiologist, USAP North Texas, Dallas, Texas

KEVIN TSAI, MD, Resident Physician, Department of Anaesthesia, Cedars-Sinai Medical Center, Los Angeles, California

PATRICE A. VINSARD, MD, Department of Anesthesiology and Perioperative Medicine, Mayo Clinic, Minnesota

JEREMY WALCO, MD, Division of Anesthesiology and Critical Care Medicine, Department of Anesthesiology, Vanderbilt University Medical Center, Nashville, Tennessee USA

JONATHAN WHEELWRIGHT, DO, Anesthesiology, Penn State Health, Hershey, Pennsylvania

WILLIAM DEROIS YATES, MD, Assistant Professor, Anesthesiology and Pain Medicine, University of California, Davis, Sacramento, California

ADVANCES IN
Anesthesia

CONTENTS   VOLUME 41 • 2023

> Tranexamic acid is a well-known antifibrinolytic that has
> numerous clinical indications, and it is efficacious and safe
> in many perioperative scenarios including patients with
> some thrombotic risks. However, further studies that
> characterize clinical outcomes concerning dosing, timing,
> and routes in combination are needed in ultra high-risk populations.

> This article's objective is to present the latest evidence and
> information on the management of postoperative nausea

and vomiting (PONV). PONV continues to affect 30% of the surgical population causing patient dissatisfaction, extending length of stay, and increasing overall costs. This review includes the introduction of 2 new intravenous formulations of antiemetics (amisulpride, aprepitant), updates on nontraditional therapies, suggestions for combination prophylaxis, emerging data on rescue treatment, and considerations for special populations and settings. Both of the new antiemetics provide promising options for pharmacologic interventions for PONV with favorable safety profiles.

Peer Support and Second Victim Programs for Anesthesia Professionals Involved in Stressful or Traumatic Clinical Events

Robyn E. Finney and Adam K. Jacob

Modern anesthetic care is very safe, but stressful and traumatic clinical events may occur. When they occur, anesthesia professionals are vulnerable to second victim experiences, resulting in significant and long-lasting psychological and emotional consequences if not addressed. Peer support can help anesthesia professionals cope with the negative effects of second victim experiences.

Care for the Obstetric Patient with Complex Cardiac Disease 53
Patrice A. Vinsard, Katherine W. Arendt, and Emily E. Sharpe

The prevalence of cardiac disease-related maternal morbidity and mortality is on the rise in the United States. To ensure safe management of pregnancy in patients with cardiovascular disease, pre-delivery evaluation by a multidisciplinary Pregnancy Heart Team should occur. Appropriate anesthetic, cardiac, and obstetric care are essential. Risk stratification tools evaluate the etiology and severity of cardiovascular disease to determine the appropriate hospital type and location for delivery and anesthetic management. Intrapartum hemodynamic monitoring may need to be intensified, and neuraxial analgesia and anesthesia are generally appropriate. The anesthesiologist must be prepared for obstetric and cardiac emergencies.

Update and Advances on Post-dural Puncture Headache

Robert Bishop, Amy Chen, William Derois Yates, Julie Fowler,
and Stephen Macres

This document provides an overview of post-dural
puncture headache (PDPH), covering its historical
perspective, anatomy and physiology of cerebrospinal
fluid (CSF), pathophysiology, risk factors, diagnosis, and
treatment options. PDPH is a common complication of
dural puncture, characterized by a postural headache
due to CSF leakage. The understanding of CSF and
dural anatomy has evolved over time, leading to
advancements in diagnosing and managing PDPH.
Treatment options range from conservative measures to
epidural blood patch, intrathecal catheter, and regional
techniques like sphenopalatine ganglion block and
greater occipital nerve block. Further research is needed
to optimize treatment approaches and improve patient outcomes.

Reconceptualizing Acute Pain Management in the 21st Century

Stephen Macres, Robin J. Aldwinckle, Usha Saldahna,
Scott G. Pritzlaff, Michael Jung, Josh Santos, Mariya Kotova,
and Robert Bishop

Acute pain can have many etiologies that include surgical
procedures, trauma (motor vehicle accident),

musculoskeletal injuries (rib fracture) and, burns among others. Valuable components of a multimodal approach to acute pain management include both opioid and non-opioid medications, procedure specific regional anesthesia techniques (peripheral nerve blocks and neuraxial approaches), and interventional approaches (eg, peripheral nerve stimulation and cryo-neurolysis). Overall, successful acute perioperative pain management requires a multimodal, multidisciplinary approach that involves a coordinated effort between the surgical team, the anesthesia team, nursing, and pharmacy staff using Enhanced Recovery After Surgery (ERAS) protocols.

Expert Advice for the Expert Witness

Richard P. Dutton

The malpractice system in the United States provides civil remedies–payment–for patients injured by non–standard-of-care medical practice. Anesthesiologists are not sued often, but one can still expect to be named in a suit at least once in their career. Although many prefer not to be involved in malpractice cases, there is a critical role for anesthesiologist expert witnesses to educate and inform the court regarding the appropriate standard of anesthesia care, and the contribution, if any, of anesthesia clinicians to specific adverse outcomes. This article describes the basic features of malpractice litigation, offering advice for anesthesiologist expert witnesses.

Pediatric Anesthesia in the Community   127
Richard P. Dutton, Robert B. Bryskin, Marion 'Red' Starks,
Aesha S. Shukla, and Olivia Lounsbury

Pediatric anesthesia is a diverse subspecialty practiced at
thousands of hospitals and ambulatory surgery centers
across the country. Most unusual and high-risk cases are
performed in dedicated children's hospitals. However,
the majority of cases and practitioners are based in the
community. We present a review of demographics in
pediatric anesthesia in the United States across 7 years
of data from US Anesthesia Partners, a national
anesthesia practice, which covers the full range of
hospitals and outpatient facilities.

Trauma Anesthesiology Perioperative Management Update   143
Ryan Perlman, Kevin Tsai, and Jessie Lo

Anesthesia for patients with life-threatening injuries is an
essential part of post-accident care. Unfortunately, there
is variability in trauma anesthesia care and numerous
nonstandardized methods of working with patients
remain. Uncertainty exists as to when and how best to
intubate trauma patients, the use of vasopressors, and

the appropriate management of severe traumatic brain injury. Some physicians recommend prehospital rapid sequence intubation, whereas others use bag-mask ventilation at lower pressures with no cricoid pressure and early transport to a trauma center. Overall, the absence of uniformity in trauma anesthesia care underlines the need for continued study and dialogue to define best practices and optimize patient outcomes.

Perioperative Concerns in the Patient with History of Alcohol Use

Ivet T. Cordoba Torres, Eslam A. Fouda,
Myrna Eliann Reinhardt, and Fouad G. Souki

Alcohol use is common in patients presenting for surgery and can result in significant physiologic changes and postoperative complications. Anesthesia providers must be aware of the potential risks associated with alcohol consumption and take steps to minimize them. Perioperative management includes assessing patients for alcohol use, providing alcohol cessation interventions, adjusting the anesthetic plan according to the patient's alcohol use history, providing appropriate pain management strategies, and closely monitoring patients during and after surgery for signs of alcohol withdrawal.

Diagnosis and Treatment of New-Onset Perioperative Atrial Fibrillation

Robert J. McCusker, Jonathan Wheelwright, Travis J. Smith, Conrad S. Myler, and Elizabeth Sinz

This article reviews medical and surgical risk factors for developing atrial fibrillation (AF), the most common sustained dysrhythmia in the United States. Evidence for assessment and management of patients with AF, including AF newly identified in the preoperative clinic, immediately preoperatively, intraoperatively, and unstable AF, is presented. A stepwise approach to guide anesthetic decision-making in the assessment of newly identified preoperative AF is proposed. Anesthetic considerations, including the potential impacts of anesthetic and vasopressor selection, and current evidence related to rate control and rhythm control via pharmacologic or electrical cardioversion as well as anticoagulation strategies are discussed.

Perioperative Acute Kidney Injury: Implications, Approach, Prevention

Aditi Balakrishna, Jeremy Walco, Frederic T. Billings IV, and
Marcos G. Lopez

Acute kidney injury remains a common and significant
contributor to perioperative morbidity. Acute kidney
injury worsens patient outcomes, and anesthesiologists
should make significant efforts to prevent, assess, and
treat perioperative renal injury. The authors discuss the
impact of renal injury on patient outcomes and putative
underlying mechanisms, evidence underlying treatments
for acute kidney injury, and practices that may prevent
the development of perioperative renal injury.

Donation After Cardiac Death: Origins, Current State, and New Directions

Nathan E. Ashby

Donation after cardiac death (DCD) is a growing source of
organs for transplantation. DCD can be challenging to
understand due to variations in practice. DCD also

holds great potential for ethical compromise making it uncomfortable for many practitioners. This article traces the origin of DCD from the beginnings of organ transplant and lays out the general pattern of the process before touching on advances to this rapidly changing field.

Advances in Anesthesia 41 (2023) xxiii–xxiv

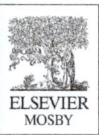

ADVANCES IN ANESTHESIA

PREFACE

Welcome to the 2023 Issue of *Advances in Anesthesia*

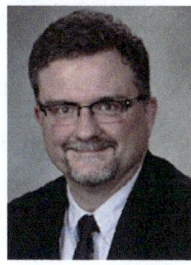

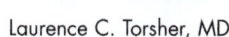

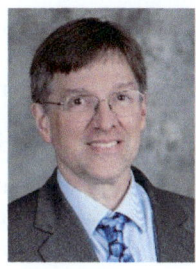

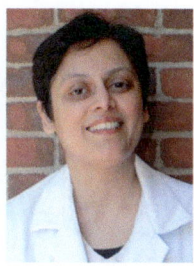

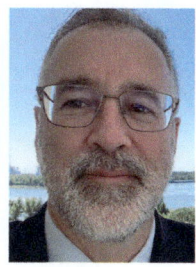

Laurence C. Torsher, MD   Richard P. Dutton, MD, MBA   Arna Banerjee, MD, MMHC   Evan Pivalizza, MBChB, FFA

Editors

With each issue of *Advances in Anesthesia*, we strive to provide articles on new topics to the field of anesthesia as well as updates to subjects in which the field is evolving.

Tranexamic acid use is established in some surgical specialties but is expanding into more clinical venues. An update on postoperative nausea and vomiting is timely, as it remains an ongoing problem and has been suggested as a quality measure by some. As stress and burnout in the workplace continues, we provide an article on peer support and second-victim programs. Additional articles include care of the obstetric patient with complex cardiac disease, updates on the management of postdural puncture headache, new innovative approaches to acute pain management, an understanding of the place of expert witness testimony, the role of the pediatric anesthesiologist in current community practice, updates on trauma care, perioperative concerns in the patient with alcohol use disorder, management of acute onset atrial fibrillation, acute kidney injury and clinical implications, and finally, organ donation after cardiac death.

https://doi.org/10.1016/j.aan.2023.08.001
0737-6146/23/© 2023 Published by Elsevier Inc.

All articles are written by experts in their field from across the nation bringing insightful interpretation and explanation to the topics at hand.

Laurence C. Torsher, MD
Department of Anesthesiology and
Perioperative Medicine
Mayo Clinic Rochester
Rochester, MN 55905, USA

E-mail address: torsher.laurence@mayo.edu

Richard P. Dutton, MD, MBA
University of Maryland
Capital Region Medical Center
Largo, MD 20774, USA

E-mail address: Richard.dutton@usap.com

Arna Banerjee, MD, MMHC
Center for Experiential Learning and Assessment
Vanderbilt University Medical Center
Nashville, TN 37232, USA

E-mail address: arna.banerjee@vumc.org

Evan Pivalizza, MBChB, FFA
Department of Anesthesiology, Critical Care
and Pain Medicine
McGovern Medical School at UTHealth
Houston, TX 77030, USA

E-mail address: Evan.G.Pivalizza@uth.tmc.edu

Advances in Anesthesia 41 (2023) 1–15

ADVANCES IN ANESTHESIA

Updated Clinical Review
Perioperative Use of Tranexamic Acid in Orthopedics and Other Surgeries

Poonam Pai B.H., MD, MS*, Shivani Patel, MD, Yan H. Lai, MD, MPH, FASA, CBA, LAc

Department of Anesthesiology and Perioperative Pain Medicine, Mount Sinai West-Morningside Hospitals, 1000 Tenth Avenue, Suite 1G, New York, NY 10019, USA

Keywords
- Anti-fibrinolytic • Tranexamic acid • Bleeding

Key points
- Perioperative administration of tranexamic acid (TXA) is effective and safe.
- Even in high-risk populations, there is sufficient data to conclude that its use is safe.
- In populations with a risk of thrombosis, topical administration may be considered as an alternative to intravenous TXA in orthopedic surgery.

INTRODUCTION

Tranexamic acid (TXA) or trans-4-amino-methyl-cyclohexane-carbonic acid is a synthetic analog derivative of amino acid lysine that inhibits fibrinolysis by reversibly binding the 5 lysine receptor sites on plasminogen [1]. It competitively inhibits plasminogen activation and prevents it from binding or degrading fibrin thereby preserving the fibrin mesh [2]. TXA suppresses fibrinolysis that has been demonstrated by reduced levels of D-dimer in blood, but it does not affect blood coagulation parameters [2]. Overall, TXA prevents clot breakdown rather than promoting new clot formation. It might have an anti-inflammatory effect by inhibiting plasmin-mediated activation of complement, monocytes, and neutrophils [3]. Since its discovery in 1950 by Utaka Okamoto, TXA has shown to be an effective agent in preventing hemorrhage. In 2009, it was included in the World Health Organization's list of essential medicines [4].

*Corresponding author. E-mail address: poonampaibh@gmail.com

https://doi.org/10.1016/j.aan.2023.05.001
0737-6146/23/© 2023 Elsevier Inc. All rights reserved.

TXA can be administered in oral, intravenous (IV), or topical forms. A dosage of 500 mg to 1g by slow IV injection three times daily or 1 to 1.5 g two to three times daily orally is recommended for fibrinolysis [5]. With a half-life of 3 hours, maximum plasma concentrations are achieved within 3 hours of oral administration. Adverse effects include mild gastrointestinal effects, headaches, hypersensitivity, and postoperative seizures reported with high doses [5,6].

TXA accumulates in tissues and diffuses to synovial fluid and membranes [2,5,6]. It crosses the placenta to reach the fetus [2,5,6] and is excreted in breast milk in concentrations that are 100 times lower than plasma [2,5,6]. No teratogenic effects have been shown in in vitro studies [2,5,6].

Contraindications to TXA include acute venous or arterial thrombosis, history of thromboembolic disease, hereditary thrombophilia, and macroscopic hematuria [7].

Antifibrinolytics have carved a niche in cardiac, trauma, spine, liver transplantation, obstetric, orthopedic surgeries as well as some urologic procedures. TXA is a part of enhanced recovery after surgery (ERAS) protocols and blood conservation strategies in the perioperative setting. Uses outside the operating room include prevention or treatment of bleeding during tooth extraction in hemophilia A/B and some other coagulation disorders such as Von Willebrand disease, hereditary angioedema and hyperfibrinolysis states. They are also used in the management of recurrent epistaxis, upper gastrointestinal bleeding, and primary menorrhagia [7].

The goal of this review is to provide an update on the current use of TXA during the perioperative period in orthopedics, acute trauma, cardiac surgery, vascular surgery, and obstetrics.

Use in orthopedic surgery

Earlier data on orthopedic surgery patients showed an estimated average of 3.2 units of blood loss for primary total hip arthroplasties (THA) and an average of 4 units during revision procedures [8,9]. Total knee arthroplasty (TKA) was found to cause a comparable blood loss of 1000 to 1500 mL on average [10,11]. Since the year 2000, transfusion rates are estimated to be as high as 32.3% in THA and 28% in TKA [12–14].

TXA has reduced the frequency of blood transfusions during these procedures. Gandhi and colleagues conducted a meta-analysis in patients who underwent TKA and THA where TXA was compared with placebo or no treatment. Mean overall blood loss favored the TXA group with reduced transfusion requirements with no increased incidence of deep vein thrombosis (DVT) [15].

Zhang and colleagues conducted a separate meta-analysis in TKA cohorts to evaluate the efficacy and safety of oral TXA administration. Results indicated that the oral TXA group had less total blood loss (-235.5 mL, $P < .001$), lower postoperative hemoglobin decline (-0.80 MD, $P < 0.001$), and lower transfusion rates (odds ratio [OR] $= 0.40$, $P < 0.001$) compared with the control group. No differences were found regarding the rate of thrombotic events and operative time [16].

Wind and Barfield retrospectively reviewed 1494 primary THA patients who received IV, topical or no TXA and assessed the risk of blood transfusion. IV TXA produced a difference in transfusion rate ($P <$ .001) while topical TXA failed to show a difference. The transfusion rate without TXA was 19.86%, 4.39% with TXA IV (odds ratio [OR] = 5.36), and 12.86% (OR = 1.67) with topical TXA [17].

The use of TXA has been evaluated in other orthopedic procedures such as elective total shoulder arthroplasty (TSA), spine, and ankle surgeries. Along with rates of transfusion, there is a reduced rate of hematoma formation, wound complications, and length of hospital stay with no increased rate of thrombotic events.

Anthony and colleagues conducted a population-based study and concluded that TXA was administered in 12.8% of patients with TSA nationwide. TXA reduced transfusion risk by 36% and decreased risk for combined complications by 35%. It also decreased the length of hospital stay by 6.2%. While TXA utilization in TSA is still low, its effectiveness highlights the need for future studies [18]. Carbone and colleagues addressed concerns regarding the administration of TXA during TSA in patients who have a history of thrombotic events. They conducted a meta-analysis and found that TXA did not cause an increase in complication rates in TSA patients with a history of thrombotic events. The study also supported a wider TXA use based on these findings [19].

When Pauzenberger and colleagues used IV TXA in TSA they found lower total blood loss and mean visual analog scale (VAS) pain scores in the IV TXA group. There was a decrease in postoperative pain in the IV TXA group compared with the placebo (mean VAS scores from preoperative 7 to postoperative as well as reduced incidence of hematoma formation; 25.9% in TXA, 59.3% in placebo). Although the rate of hematoma formation was considered mild in the TXA group, it was more likely to be identified as moderate or severe hematomas in the placebo group [20].

A meta-analysis and systematic review was performed by Yerneni and colleagues on topical TXA in spinal surgery to evaluate the efficiency and safety of the blood conservation agent. They recorded a decrease in postoperative blood loss, and length of hospital stay in the topical TXA group compared with the control group [21].

Pai and colleagues aimed to evaluate the potential benefit and role of TXA in foot and ankle surgeries in reducing post-op wound complications and blood loss and concluded that there was no significant difference between the placebo and intervention groups [22].

Use in trauma

Trauma-induced coagulopathy and fibrinolysis, which can occur early at the time of injury, can be multifactorial leading to morbidity and mortality. Early recognition and treatment may improve outcomes in trauma resuscitation [23].

The CRASH II trial is a large multinational randomized placebo-controlled trial carried out in 274 hospitals in 40 countries and enrolled 20,211 adult trauma patients. Patients were randomized within 8 h of injury to either the TXA group (1 g loading dose over 10 min followed by an infusion of 1 g over 8 h) or a matching placebo [24]. TXA reduced all cause of mortality within 28 days and death due to bleeding. The authors concluded that TXA safely reduced the risk of death from bleeding in the hemorrhaging trauma patient. In their opinion, TXA should be considered for administration in bleeding trauma patients. Further exploratory analysis in the study revealed that caution should be taken when administering TXA to patients greater than 3 h out from the time of injury as the patients might be more acidotic, hypothermic, and in a more prothrombotic phase of their traumatic injury [24].

Another landmark trial, MATTERs, was designed to study the efficacy of TXA administration in patients receiving at least one unit of packed red blood cells in combat-related injuries. Despite being more severely injured (mean ISS 25.2 [TXA] versus 22.5 [no TXA] $P < .001$), the TXA group had a lower unadjusted mortality than the no TXA group (17.4 vs 23.9%, $P = .03$). This benefit was greater in the group receiving massive transfusion (14.4 vs 28.1%, $P = .004$). The authors concluded that TXA use results in the improvement of coagulopathy and survival post-combat injury in patients requiring blood transfusion [25].

Use in cardiac/vascular surgery

Long-term outcomes of endovascular abdominal aortic aneurysm repair shrinkage after TXA administration were compared by Aoki and colleagues and found that the TXA group had significantly greater aneurysm shrinkage ($P = .035$). This suggests that coagulation and fibrinolysis play roles in shrinkage and treatment with antifibrinolytics may play a role in successful treatment [26].

Myles and colleagues concluded that among patients undergoing coronary-artery surgery, TXA was associated with a lower risk of bleeding than placebo, without a higher risk of death or thrombotic complications within 30 days after surgery, however, was associated with a higher risk of postoperative seizures [27]. Hasegawa and colleagues opined that TXA reduced operative time, dopamine dose, peak serum lactate, intubation time, chest tube drainage, duration, and hospital stay in children (<20 kg) who underwent bloodless cardiac surgery compared with no TXA group (2014) [28].

Use in obstetrics

The World Maternal ANtifibrinolytic (WOMAN trial) trial was a pragmatic, randomized placebo-controlled multicenter trial that was conducted in 20,060 women with postpartum hemorrhage (PPH) in 21 low- and middle-income countries patients received TXA (1–2 g) or placebo [29].

The main finding was a 19% decrease in death from bleeding in women who were given TXA versus placebo (mortality rate, 1.9% vs 1.5%; relative risk [RR], 0.81; 95% confidence interval [CI], 0.65–1.0; $P = .045$). This was seen especially if TXA was administered within 3 hours of birth [29].

Although this study proved to reduce maternal mortality, it is unclear whether this has an impact on the reduction of maternal morbidity. The WOMAN-2 trial is currently being pursued to understand the impact of TXA on postpartum bleeding in women with moderate or severe anemia. This study will likely shed light on the prevention of PPH in women who deliver vaginally and if the administration of 1 g of TXA within 15 minutes of umbilical cord clamping has an impact [29].

Besides international collaboratives, 2 other multicenter randomized placebo-controlled trials evaluated the efficacy of TXA for PPH prevention. When TXA was administered in women after vaginal delivery versus placebo (Tranexamic Acid for Preventing Postpartum Hemorrhage Following a Vaginal Delivery–TRAAP1 study), the PPH rate was not significantly different in the TXA and placebo groups (8.1% vs 9.8%; RR, 0.83; 95% CI, 0.68–1.01; $P = .07$) [30].

In the TRAAP2 study, when women were administered TXA after cesarean delivery, they had a lower likelihood of PPH compared with placebo (26.7% vs 31.6%; adjusted RR, 0.84; 95% CI, 0.75–0.94; $P = .003$). No thromboembolic events were reported in both studies [31].

Dosing

Depending on the surgical procedure, typical dosing in the perioperative setting is a 10 to 30 mg/kg IV loading dose with or without an infusion. There is no clear consensus and there is significant variability regarding optimal dosing, timing, frequency, or method of administration [32,33].

Maniar and his group studied the most effective TXA dosing regimen in TKA. According to this study, single-dose TXA was not efficacious. The two-dose regimen of preoperative and intraoperative TXA given before tourniquet deflation was the least amount necessary for effective results. The intraoperative dose followed by postoperative was also found to be ineffective. The three-dose regimen of pre-operative, intraoperative, and postoperative TXA produced the maximum effective reduction of drain loss and total blood loss [34]. In another study by Morrison and colleagues using 30 mg/kg maximum of 2.5 g as a single IV dose as a part of the ERAS protocol was associated with a significant reduction in transfusion requirements for both total hip and knee arthroplasty [35].

Poeran and colleagues performed a retrospective study evaluating the effectiveness of perioperative IV TXA dose (none, ≤1000, 2000, and ≥3000 mg) in orthopedic surgery and concluded that patients that received TXA (vs those who did not) showed lower rates of allogeneic or autologous transfusion (7.7% vs 20.1%), thromboembolic complications (0.6% vs 0.8%), acute renal failure (1.2% vs 1.6%), and combined complications (1.9% vs 2.6%); all $P < .01$ [36].

Another study by Zufferey and colleagues provoked the dosing debate further, questioning if additional perioperative administration of tranexamic acid had any effect on reducing blood loss. A meta-analysis from the same authors showed no incremental efficacy of additional perioperative administration of tranexamic acid [37].

Revision THAs are arguably the bloodiest procedure in orthopedics. In this model, a study by Sershon and colleagues provided evidence that there is not a single dosing regimen of TXA that is more effective. The study compared hemoglobin levels, blood loss, and transfusion rates in patients receiving TXA. Four regimens were studied: 1 g IV TXA perioperative, 1 g IV TXA perioperative and followed by 1 g IV after wound closure, a combination of 1 g IV TXA perioperative and 1 g intraoperative topical TXA, and a multidose oral group (3 doses of TXA total). The study concluded that there was no significant difference between hemoglobin, blood loss, and transfusion rates in the 4 regimens studied. The authors concluded that irrespective of the method of TXA administration, all regimens were equivalent [38].

Raman and colleagues investigated the optimal dosing strategy of TXA for adult spinal deformity. The study compared patients who received a high dose of TXA compared with patients who received a low dose of TXA. The high-dosage group (40 mg/kg loading dose with a 1 mg/kg/h maintenance dose, 30 mg/kg loading dose with a 10 mg/kg/h maintenance dose, or 50 mg/kg loading dose with a 5 mg/kg/h maintenance dose), compared with the low-dose group (10 or 20 mg/kg loading dose with a 1 or 2 mg/kg/h maintenance dose), had reduced estimated blood loss (EBL) and transfusion rates. The study concluded that a high-dosage regimen of TXA in spine surgery is more effective than a low dose of TXA [39].

A retrospective cohort study performed by Weissmann and colleagues compared the effectiveness of IV TXA to topical TXA in spinal deformity. The patients were separated into 4 groups: no TXA, IV TXA, topical TXA, and combined TXA. There was reduced postoperative blood loss in the combined TXA group compared with the control group. Patients in the IV TXA group and combined TXA group had their drain taken out 1 day earlier than the control group ($P = .002$). There were no TXA-related complications noted in this study [40].

Other routes
Topical
Topical TXA has provided an attractive alternative for those concerned with safety profile with intravenous administration. TXA directly at the site of bleeding has been considered to have better efficacy and safety profile limiting systemic absorption compared with intravenous [32]. A single topical intra-articular dose of 3 g of TXA signaled non-inferiority to two 15-mg/kg IV TXA doses in a randomized controlled trial conducted by Sabatini [41].

While recent studies on topical TXA report a wide range of dosing between 0.25 and 3 g in a single dose, Xu and colleagues evaluated that 2 to 3 g TXA with 1 to 2 h contact time would yield greater than 60% reduction in the drainage volume in TKA [42–44].

A randomized controlled trial (RCT) conducted to evaluate the optimal dosage of topical TXA in TKA showed a decrease in EBL and frequency of transfusion between the control and intervention groups with a topical dose of 1 g [45]. In addition, Liu and colleagues conducted a separate meta-analysis comparing the efficacy of combined use of intravenous and topical TXA for patients undergoing THA and concluded that the combined use of TXA may reduce the total blood loss compared with intravenous use alone without increasing the risk of postoperative complications [46].

Sun and colleagues conducted a meta-analysis comparing the efficiency of IV, topical, and combined administration of TXA in reducing blood loss and transfusion rates in THA and TKA. The study concluded that there was no significant difference in blood loss between IV and topical TXA and transfusion rates. The single-route TXA group had higher blood loss than the combined TXA group and higher transfusion rates ($P < .05$). IV and topical TXA were adjuncts in efficacy and safety. Overall, the combined TXA group was more efficient than the IV and topical TXA groups alone in blood conservation [47].

Oral

Oral TXA is a cheaper alternative to intravenous. In terms of efficacy, oral TXA was compared with IV in TKA and THA in a meta-analysis, which demonstrated that there were no significant differences in measured endpoints between the oral and IV TXA groups [16].

Another systematic review indicated that oral TXA has a comparable effect with IV TXA and was superior to the control group in reducing blood loss after total joint arthroplasty (TJA) [48]. However, the maximal antifibrinolytic effect of oral TXA occurs approximately 2 hours after ingestion [48]. Its absorption is quick and complete, and they recommended oral TXA 2 hours before surgery for maximum benefit [48].

Yuan and colleagues compared IV, oral, and topical routes of TXA in TKA and found that the 48 h Hb loss and drainage volume with these routes were less than those in the control group. They recommended oral TXA due to the cost-benefit ratio [49].

A meta-analysis studied the efficacy of oral TXA in THA compared with IV TXA and concluded that the odds of receiving a blood transfusion and blood loss were similar in both groups, multiple does of oral TXA was effective in blood conservation, reduced hemoglobin drops, and transfusion rates in THA compared with a single oral dose [50].

As oral routes become increasingly popular due to reduced cost, there is a need for studies evaluating their efficacy in high-risk populations as well.

Use in a high-risk population

Administration of TXA is often debated in patients with history of venous or arterial thromboembolism or active thromboembolic disease, myocardial infarction, stroke, and pulmonary embolism. But recent studies in this high-risk cohort have supported its efficacy and safety [51]. It is worth mentioning that recent studies have included the higher-risk populations as well, especially those with DVT and pulmonary emoblism (PE) as literature reveals no increased thromboembolic events. Novel studies like one by Martin and colleagues on topical TXA conclude safe efficacy profiles in high-risk populations also [52].

In 2015, a large single-center retrospective cohort study in 13,262 elective TKA or THA procedures, showed that the odds of postoperative venous thromboembolism (VTE) (OR = 0.98; 95% CI 0.67–1.45) and 30 day mortality (OR = 0.26, 95% CI 0.04–1.80) were overall unchanged with TXA administration. The study supported the safe use of TXA even in high-risk orthopedic patients [53].

Another retrospective review evaluated patients with risk factors for thromboembolic events and measured 30 day postoperative symptomatic thromboembolic events and postoperative transfusion. There were no significant differences in symptomatic thromboembolic events within 30 days of surgery between patients who received TXA and those who did not. In fact, in the high-risk group, there was a decrease in transfusion rates and no change in thromboembolic events confirming the safe use of TXA even in high-risk patients [54].

A multicenter retrospective study evaluated the safety of TJA in former or current cancer patients. It was concluded that TXA was not associated with an increased risk of venous thromboembolism within 90 days post-op in current or former cancer patients. There were no other complications associated with the use of TXA. The study highlighted the need for future TXA studies to include patients with cancer [55].

A population study by Poeran and colleagues aimed to evaluate the safety and effectiveness of TXA in patients with preexisting comorbidities. TXA administration in high-risk patients receiving lower-extremity arthroplasty resulted in fewer transfusions. There was no association between TXA and venous thromboembolism, myocardial infarction, seizures, ischemic strokes or transient ischemic attacks [56].

Controversies and adverse effects
Apart from the earlier mentioned adverse effects of TXA such as headache, abdominal pain, nausea, diarrhea, fatigue, impaired color vision and anaphylaxis, several case reports of thrombo-embolism have been mentioned in the literature in patients who were administered antifibrinolytic agents but almost all of them had another confounding or associated hypercoagulable conditions (Table 1).

Though the above case reports have an association with TXA use, the direct causal relationship is lacking. Animal studies followed by histochemical specimen examinations in humans after TXA administration have revealed that TXA did not suppress the fibrinolytic activity in the vessel walls [62–64]. Decreased fibrinolytic activity within the wound bed was seen after IV TXA administration but not in peripheral venous blood as measured by assays for fibrinolysis and coagulation [65].

Rivas and colleagues performed a multi-centered, retrospective study to investigate whether there was an association between the use of TXA and

Table 1
Several case reports of thrombo-embolism associated with antifibrinolytic use

Author, year	Case	Duration of antifibrinolytic	Complication	Risk factor for hypercoagulability
Achiron et al [57], 1990	42 year old woman who was on epsilon amino caproic acid (EACA) for menorrhagia	7 mo of 3 g/d of EACA on the days of blood loss	Superior sagittal and left transverse sinus thrombosis	Obese with hyperestrogenism
Rydin & Lundberg [58], 1976	Two women aged 31 and 32 years of age with menorrhagia	1–4.5 g of TXA daily for menorrhagia for a period of 1 y.	Intracranial thrombosis	Thrombocytosis
Davies & Howell [59], 1977	39 year old woman with c1 esterase deficiency	TXA and EACA for 4 y	Death due to stroke	Takayasu's arteritis
Nardi et al [60], 2011	Two women aged 44 and 49 years with uterine bleeding after undergoing curettage	TXA 500 mg/d for 3 d	Occlusion of middle cerebral artery and near occlusion of internal carotid artery	Pregnancy, heterozygous for the methylene-tetrahydrofolate reductase C677 T gene
Taparia et al [61], 2002	29 year old man patient with known history of acquired hemophilia with a high titer Factor VIII inhibitor and recurrent bleeds	TXA prophylaxis	Pulmonary embolism	?

VTE. The study concluded that there was no significant association between the administration of TXA and the incidence of VTE. TXA was associated with reduced transfusion need and mortality rates [66].

While no studies found that the administration of TXA increases the VTE risk in a population, it is important to note that all major studies before 2017 excluded high-risk patients. These major studies lacked control of standard TXA dosing, timing, or route of administration. Most of these studies do not account for rare complications including symptomatic DVT or PE with an incidence range of 0.5%–2%. These studies differ greatly in the method of finding thromboembolic events. These limitations highlight the necessity for studies that focus primarily on thromboembolic risks and high-risk patients.

A systematic review by Taeuber and colleagues investigated whether the administration of IV TXA is associated with thromboembolic events. The systemic review and meta-analysis found a total of 2.1% total thromboembolic events in the patients who received IV TXA and 2.0% total thromboembolic events were found in the control group. It was concluded that IV TXA, irrespective of dosing, is not associated with an increased risk of thromboembolic events [67].

More alarmingly, an acute ST-elevation myocardial infarction due to in-stent thrombosis following TXA administration was reported in a 59 year old patient with a history of anterior wall myocardial infarction (MI) 3 years prior and positive stress 18 months prior. The patient was on aspirin and stopped prasugrel for 5 days. The patient was administered 1 g of IV TXA [68]. An acute coronary artery thrombus was reported in a 71 year old patient with coronary stents following the administration of TXA during TSA is another case reported [69]. Perhaps cardiac stents remain a unique contraindication that should still be respected with caution for TXA administration.

Apart from the controversial risk of thromboembolism, TXA has been associated with catastrophic drug errors. Accidental intrathecal administration has a 50% mortality rate and high incidences of permanent neurologic damage and paraplegia have been reported in patients who have survived spinal TXA [70].

Majority of case reports of TXA-associated seizures have been reported in cardiac surgery patients, where a generalized tonic–clonic activity with some myoclonus has been noted in the post-operative period. TXA binds to glycine receptors resulting in a decrease in inhibitory current, thereby increases central nervous system excitability and seizures. Electroencephalogram monitoring may help in diagnosis. Certain inhalational anesthetics such as isoflurane, sevoflurane, desflurane, and propofol also have an effect of glycine receptors helping in reversing and prevention of TXA-induced seizures [71]. There have been some case reports of color vision abnormalities in patients on TXA without ocular pathology that subsided after cessation of the medication [72].

SUMMARY

To summarize, TXA is a well-known antifibrinolytic that has numerous clinical indications. There seems to be sufficient data in terms of its efficacy and safety in perioperative scenarios through multiple retrospective studies and RCTs; however, further studies that characterize clinical outcomes concerning dosing, timing, and routes in combination are needed even in high-risk populations.

TXA (IV, IA, topical, combination) is beneficial and safe in patients even in the high-risk population and should be considered the centerpiece of blood conservation strategy and ERAS protocol in the perioperative setting.

CLINICS CARE POINTS

- Antifibrinolytics have carved a niche in cardiac surgeries, trauma, spine surgeries, liver transplantation, obstetric surgeries, orthopedic surgeries as well as some urologic procedures.
- TXA is a centerpiece of the ERAS protocol and blood conservation strategies in the perioperative setting. There are sufficient data to conclude that TXA administration is safe in the perioperative setting even in high-risk populations.
- In the ultra high-risk populations (i.e. patients with coronary stents or pre-existing thromboembolic pathologies), we need more outcome data to guide clinical indications, safety, dosing, timing, and routes of administration.

DISCLOSURE
The authors have no conflict of interest.

Acknowledgments
The authors thank Ms Emma Laurence for her help with an updated literature search.

References
[1] Tengborn L, Blombäck M, Berntorp E. Tranexamic acid–an old drug still going strong and making a revival. Thromb Res 2015;135(2):231–42.
[2] Dunn CJ, Goa KL. Tranexamic acid: a review of its use in surgery and other indications. Drugs 1999;57(6):1005–32.
[3] Barrett CD, Moore HB, Kong YW, et al. Tranexamic acid mediates proinflammatory and anti-inflammatory signaling via complement C5a regulation in a plasminogen activator-dependent manner. J Trauma Acute Care Surg 2019 Jan;86(1):101–7, PMID: 30575685.
[4] Okamoto S, Okamoto U. Amino-Methyl-Cyclohexane-Carbolic Acid: AMCHA. A New Potent Inhibitor of Fibrinolysis. Keio J Med 1962;11:105–15.
[5] Mannucci PM. Hemostatic drugs. N Engl J Med 1998;339(4):245–53.
[6] Ker K, Roberts I. Tranexamic acid for surgical bleeding. BMJ 2014;349:g4934.
[7] Mahdy AM, Webster NR. Perioperative systemic haemostatic agents. Br J Anaesth 2004;93(6):842–58.
[8] Spahn DR, Casutt M. Eliminating blood transfusions: new aspects and perspectives. Anesthesiology 2000;93(1):242–55.
[9] Toy PT, Kaplan EB, McVay PA, et al. Blood loss and replacement in total hip arthroplasty: a multicenter study. The Preoperative Autologous Blood Donation Study Group. Transfusion 1992;32(1):63–7.
[10] Keating EM, Meding JB, Faris PM, et al. Predictors of transfusion risk in elective knee surgery. Clin Orthop Relat Res 1998;357:50–9.

[11] Berman AT, Geissele AE, Bosacco SJ. Blood loss with total knee arthroplasty. Clin Orthop Relat Res 1988;234:137–8.

[12] Pedersen AB, Mehnert F, Overgaard S, et al. Allogeneic blood transfusion and prognosis following total hip replacement: a population-based follow up study. BMC Musculoskelet Disord 2009;10:167.

[13] Thomas D, Wareham K, Cohen D, et al. Autologous blood transfusion in total knee replacement surgery. Br J Anaesth 2001;86(5):669–73.

[14] Fafalak, Marc BS*; Cushner, Fred D. MD† Blood Loss in Orthopedic Surgery: A Historical Review, Techniques in Orthopaedics: March 2017.

[15] Gandhi R, Evans HM, Mahomed SR, et al. Tranexamic acid and the reduction of blood loss in total knee and hip arthroplasty: a meta-analysis. BMC Res Notes 2013;6:184.

[16] Zhang LK, Ma JX, Kuang MJ, et al. The efficacy of tranexamic acid using oral administration in total knee arthroplasty: a systematic review and meta-analysis. J Orthop Surg Res 2017;12(1):159.

[17] Wind TC, Barfield WR, Moskal JT. The effect of tranexamic acid on blood loss and transfusion rate in primary total knee arthroplasty. J Arthroplasty 2013;28(7):1080–3.

[18] Anthony SG, Patterson DC, Cagle PJ Jr, et al. Utilization and Real-world Effectiveness of Tranexamic Use in Shoulder Arthroplasty: A Population-based Study. J Am Acad Orthop Surg 2019;27(19):736–42.

[19] Carbone A, Poeran J, Zubizarreta N, et al. Administration of tranexamic acid during total shoulder arthroplasty is not associated with increased risk of complications in patients with a history of thrombotic events. J Shoulder Elbow Surg 2021;30(1):104–12.

[20] Pauzenberger L, Domej MA, Heuberer PR, et al. The effect of intravenous tranexamic acid on blood loss and early post-operative pain in total shoulder arthroplasty. Bone Joint Lett J 2017;99-B(8):1073–9.

[21] Yerneni K, Burke JF, Tuchman A, et al. Topical tranexamic acid in spinal surgery: A systematic review and meta-analysis. J Clin Neurosci 2019;61:114–9.

[22] Pai P, Diskina D, Lin HM, et al. Use of tranexamic acid does not influence perioperative outcomes in ambulatory foot and ankle surgery-a prospective triple blinded randomized controlled trial. Int Orthop 2021;45(9):2277–84.

[23] Simmons J, Sikorski RA, Pittet JF. Tranexamic acid: from trauma to routine perioperative use. Curr Opin Anaesthesiol 2015;28(2):191–200.

[24] Roberts I, Shakur H, Coats T, et al. The CRASH-2 trial: a randomised controlled trial and economic evaluation of the effects of tranexamic acid on death, vascular occlusive events and transfusion requirement in bleeding trauma patients. Health Technol Assess 2013;17(10): 1–79.

[25] Morrison JJ, Dubose JJ, Rasmussen TE, et al. Military Application of Tranexamic Acid in Trauma Emergency Resuscitation (MATTERs) Study. Arch Surg 2012;147(2):113–9.

[26] Aoki A, Suezawa T, Yamamoto S, et al. Effect of antifibrinolytic therapy with tranexamic acid on abdominal aortic aneurysm shrinkage after endovascular repair. J Vasc Surg 2014 May;59(5):1203–8.

[27] Myles PS, Smith JA, Forbes A, et al. ATACAS Investigators of the ANZCA Clinical Trials Network. Tranexamic Acid in Patients Undergoing Coronary-Artery Surgery. N Engl J Med 2017;376(2):136–48, Erratum in: N Engl J Med. 2018 Feb 22;378(8):782. PMID: 27774838.

[28] Hasegawa T, Oshima Y, Maruo A, et al. Intraoperative tranexamic acid in pediatric bloodless cardiac surgery. Asian Cardiovasc Thorac Ann 2014;22(9):1039–45.

[29] Shakur H, Elbourne D, Gülmezoglu M, et al. The WOMAN Trial (World Maternal Antifibrinolytic Trial): tranexamic acid for the treatment of postpartum haemorrhage: an international randomised, double blind placebo controlled trial. Trials 2010;11:40.

[30] Sentilhes L, Daniel V, Darsonval A, et al. Study protocol. TRAAP - TRAnexamic Acid for Preventing postpartum hemorrhage after vaginal delivery: a multicenter randomized, double-blind, placebo-controlled trial. BMC Pregnancy Childbirth 2015;15:135.

[31] Sentilhes L, Daniel V, Deneux-Tharaux C. TRAAP2 Study Group and the Groupe de Re-cherche en Obstétrique et Gynécologie (GROG). TRAAP2 - TRAnexamic Acid for Prevent-ing postpartum hemorrhage after cesarean delivery: a multicenter randomized, doubleblind, placebo- controlled trial - a study protocol. BMC Pregnancy Childbirth 2020;20(1):63.

[32] Panteli M, Papakostidis C, Dahabreh Z, et al. Topical tranexamic acid in total knee replace-ment: a systematic review and meta-analysis. Knee 2013;20(5):300–9.

[33] Lin PC, Hsu CH, Huang CC, et al. The blood-saving effect of tranexamic acid in minimally invasive total knee replacement: is an additional pre-operative injection effective? J Bone Joint Surg Br 2012;94(7):932–6.

[34] Maniar RN, Kumar G, Singhi T, et al. Most effective regimen of tranexamic acid in knee ar-throplasty: a prospective randomized controlled study in 240 patients. Clin Orthop Relat Res 2012;470(9):2605–12.

[35] Morrison RJM, Tsang B, Fishley W, et al. Dose optimisation of intravenous tranexamic acid for elective hip and knee arthroplasty: The effectiveness of a single pre-operative dose. Bone Joint Res 2017;6(8):499–505.

[36] Poeran J, Rasul R, Suzuki S, et al. Tranexamic acid use and postoperative outcomes in pa-tients undergoing total hip or knee arthroplasty in the United States: retrospective analysis of effectiveness and safety. BMJ 2014;349:g4829.

[37] Zufferey PJ, Lanoiselée J, Chapelle C, et al. Intravenous Tranexamic Acid Bolus plus Infusion Is Not More Effective than a Single Bolus in Primary Hip Arthroplasty: A Randomized Controlled Trial. Anesthesiology 2017;127(3):413–22.

[38] Sershon RA, Fillingham YA, Abdel MP, et al. The Optimal Dosing Regimen for Tranexamic Acid in Revision Total Hip Arthroplasty: A Multicenter Randomized Clinical Trial. J Bone Joint Surg Am 2020;102(21):1883–90.

[39] Raman T, Varlotta C, Vasquez-Montes D, et al. The use of tranexamic acid in adult spinal deformity: is there an optimal dosing strategy? Spine J 2019;19(10):1690–7.

[40] Weissmann KA, Lafage V, Barrios Pitaque C, et al. Efficacy of topical versus intravenous tra-nexamic acid in spinal deformity. Eur Spine J 2020;29(12):3044–50.

[41] Sabatini L, Atzori F. Topical intra-articular and intravenous tranexamic acid to reduce blood loss in total knee arthroplasty. Ann Transl Med 2015;3(Suppl 1):S18.

[42] Sarzaeem MM, Razi M, Kazemian G, et al. Comparing efficacy of three methods of tra-nexamic acid administration in reducing hemoglobin drop following total knee arthroplasty. J Arthroplasty 2014;29(8):1521–4.

[43] Sangasoongsong P, Chanplakorn P, Wongsak S, et al. An In Vivo Study of Low-Dose Intra-Articular Tranexamic Acid Application with Prolonged Clamping Drain Method in Total Knee Replacement: Clinical Efficacy and Safety. BioMed Res Int 2015;2015:164206.

[44] Xu R, Shi D, Ge W, et al. Quantitative efficacy of topical administration of tranexamic acid on postoperative bleeding in total knee arthroplasty. Br J Clin Pharmacol 2017;83(11): 2485–93.

[45] Kim JK, Park JY, Lee DY, et al. Optimal dose of topical tranexamic acid considering efficacy and safety in total knee arthroplasty: a randomized controlled study. Knee Surg Sports Trau-matol Arthrosc 2021;29(10):3409–17.

[46] Liu X, Liu J, Sun G. A comparison of combined intravenous and topical administration of tra-nexamic acid with intravenous tranexamic acid alone for blood loss reduction after total hip arthroplasty: A meta-analysis. Int J Surg 2017;41:34–43.

[47] Sun Q, Li J, Chen J, et al. Comparison of intravenous, topical or combined routes of tranexa-mic acid administration in patients undergoing total knee and hip arthroplasty: a meta-analysis of randomized controlled trials. BMJ Open 2019;9(1):e024350.

[48] Li GL, Li YM. Oral tranexamic acid can reduce blood loss after total knee and hip arthro-plasty: A meta-analysis. Int J Surg 2017;46:27–36.

[49] Yuan X, Li B, Wang Q, et al. Comparison of 3 Routes of Administration of Tranexamic Acid on Primary Unilateral Total Knee Arthroplasty: A Prospective, Randomized, Controlled Study. J Arthroplasty 2017;32(9):2738–43.

[50] Xu Y, Sun S, Feng Q, et al. The efficiency and safety of oral tranexamic acid in total hip arthroplasty: A meta-analysis. Medicine (Baltim) 2019;98(46):e17796.

[51] Porter SB, Spaulding AC, Duncan CM, et al. Tranexamic Acid Was Not Associated with Increased Complications in High-Risk Patients with Intertrochanteric Fracture. J Bone Joint Surg Am 2022 Jul 6;104(13):1138–47.

[52] Martin JG, Cassatt KB, Kincaid-Cinnamon KA, et al. Topical administration of tranexamic acid in primary total hip and total knee arthroplasty. J Arthroplasty 2014;29(5): 889–94.

[53] Duncan CM, Gillette BP, Jacob AK, et al. Venous thromboembolism and mortality associated with tranexamic acid use during total hip and knee arthroplasty. J Arthroplasty 2015;30(2): 272–6.

[54] Whiting DR, Gillette BP, Duncan C, Smith H, Pagnano MW, Sierra RJ. Preliminary results suggest tranexamic acid is safe and effective in arthroplasty patients with severe comorbidities. Clin Orthop Relat Res.

[55] Varady NH, Chen AF, Drayer NJ, et al. Tranexamic acid in patients with current or former cancer undergoing hip and knee arthroplasty. J Surg Oncol 2021;123(8): 1811–20.

[56] Poeran Jashvant, Chan Jimmy J, Zubizarreta Nicole, et al. Safety of Tranexamic Acid in Hip and Knee Arthroplasty in High-risk Patients. Anesthesiology 2021;135:57–68.

[57] Achiron A, Gornish M, Melamed E. Cerebral sinus thrombosis as a potential hazard of antifibrinolytic treatment in menorrhagia. Stroke 1990;21(5):817–9.

[58] Rydin E, Lundberg PO. Letter: Tranexamic acid and intracranial thrombosis. Lancet 1976;2(7975):49.

[59] Davies D, Howell DA. Tranexamic acid and arterial thrombosis. Lancet 1977;1(8001):49.

[60] Nardi K, Pelone G, Bartolo M, et al. Ischaemic stroke following tranexamic acid in young patients carrying heterozygosity of MTHFR C677T. Ann Clin Biochem 2011;48(Pt 6): 575–8.

[61] Taparia M, Cordingley FT, Leahy MF. Pulmonary embolism associated with tranexamic acid in severe acquired haemophilia. Eur J Haematol 2002;68(5):307–9.

[62] Astedt B. Fibrinolytic inhibitors in human retroplacental blood. Acta Obstet Gynecol Scand 1974;53(3):227–9.

[63] Astedt B, Nilsson IM. Recurrent abruptio placentae treated with the fibrinolytic inhibitor tranexamic acid. Br Med J 1978;1(6115):756–7.

[64] Whiting DR, Duncan CM, Sierra RJ, et al. Tranexamic Acid Benefits Total Joint Arthroplasty Patients Regardless of Preoperative Hemoglobin Value. J Arthroplasty 2015;30(12): 2098–101.

[65] Benoni G, Fredin H. Fibrinolytic inhibition with tranexamic acid reduces blood loss and blood transfusion after knee arthroplasty: a prospective, randomized, double-blind study of 86 patients. J Bone Joint Surg Br 1996;78(3):434–40.

[66] Rivas L, Estroff J, Sparks A, et al. The incidence of venous thromboembolic events in trauma patients after tranexamic acid administration: an EAST multicenter study. Blood Coagul Fibrinolysis 2021;32(1):37–43.

[67] Taeuber I, Weibel S, Herrmann E, et al. Association of Intravenous Tranexamic Acid With Thromboembolic Events and Mortality: A Systematic Review, Meta-analysis, and Meta-regression. JAMA Surg 2021;156(6):e210884.

[68] Kaptein YE. Acute ST-elevation myocardial infarction due to in-stent thrombosis after administering tranexamic acid in a high cardiac risk patient. BMJ Case Rep 2019;12(4): e227957.

[69] Bridges KH, Wilson SH. Acute Coronary Artery Thrombus After Tranexamic Acid During Total Shoulder Arthroplasty in a Patient With Coronary Stents: A Case Report. In Pract 2018;10(8):212–4.
[70] Palanisamy A, Kinsella SM. Spinal tranexamic acid - a new killer in town. Anaesthesia 2019;74(7):831–3.
[71] Lecker I, Wang DS, Whissell PD, et al. Tranexamic acid-associated seizures: Causes and treatment. Ann Neurol 2016;79(1):18–26.
[72] Kiser AS, Cooper GL, Napier JD, et al. Color vision disturbances secondary to oral tranexamic acid. J Am Coll Emerg Physicians Open 2021;2(3):e12456.

Advances in Anesthesia 41 (2023) 17–38

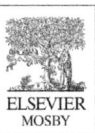

ADVANCES IN ANESTHESIA

A Postoperative Nausea and Vomiting Update
Current information on New Drugs, Old Drugs, Rescue/Treatment, Combination Therapies and Nontraditional Modalities

Tricia A. Meyer, PharmD, MS[a,*], Larry R. Hutson Jr, MD[a,b,c], Phillip M. Morris, MD[a,c], Russell K. McAllister, MD[a,b,c,*]

[a]Texas A&M University-School of Medicine, Temple, TX, USA; [b]Baylor College of Medicine – Temple, TX, USA; [c]Department of Anesthesiology, Baylor Scott & White Medical Center-Temple, 2401 South 31st Street, Temple, TX 76508, USA

Keywords
• Antiemetics • Amisulpride • Aprepitant • Complementary therapies

Key points

- Newer antiemetics have been introduced that may have improved safety profiles, quicker onset of action, longer duration of action, and/or better efficacy.
- Many older drugs are seeing a resurgence of use in an attempt to diversify chemoreceptor targets.
- Complementary and alternative techniques may offer effective and/or cost-effective alternatives but lack the rigorous data behind pharmacologic interventions.
- Emerging data show different drugs and doses may be more effective at rescue treatment than prophylaxis treatment, although prophylaxis remains far better studied.
- Cost-benefit analysis on newer more costly medications comes down to individual hospital system pressures and labor costs versus negotiated drug pricing.

*Corresponding authors. Department of Anesthesiology, Baylor Scott & White Medical Center-Temple, 2401 South 31st Street, Temple, TX 76508. E-mail addresses: triciameyer@tamu.edu (T.A.M.); Russell.McAllister@BSWHealth.org (R.K.M.)

https://doi.org/10.1016/j.aan.2023.05.002

INTRODUCTION

Postoperative nausea and vomiting (PONV) ranks as the primary concern of patients for common complications following surgery. PONV is associated with poor patient satisfaction and can result in serious adverse events in the recovery process. Despite ongoing research, numerous publications, and updated guidelines, 30% of patients will experience PONV. Much remains to be understood about the prevention and treatment/rescue of this familiar condition. However, findings from the past 2 to 3 years have led to advances in the management of PONV including the launch of novel agents, development of alternative/complementary therapies, and increased focus on postdischarge nausea and vomiting (PDNV).

INTRAVENOUS AMISULPRIDE FOR PROPHYLAXIS AND TREATMENT

Amisulpride is a substituted benzamide and shows affinity for both dopamine receptors (D_2 and D_3) and a low affinity for 5-hydroxytryptamine (5-HT_{2B} and 5-HT_7) receptors [1,2]. The approved indication for intravenous (IV) amisulpride is for the prevention and treatment of PONV (prevention: 5 mg dose, alone or in combination with antiemetics from a different therapeutic class; treatment is the recommended 10 mg dose in patients who received prophylactic antiemetics from a different class or who have not received prophylaxis) [3]. Amisulpride has been used in Europe since 1988 as an oral atypical antipsychotic (in higher doses than approved for PONV). Repurposing a drug, such as amisulpride, for a new therapeutic indication provides the advantage of having ample human safety data for the repurposed medication [1,2].

Amisulpride selectively inhibits D_2 and D_3 receptors in the limbic versus the striatal structure, resulting in lower occurrences of extrapyramidal symptoms (EPS) [4,5]. The drug has a terminal half-life of 4 to 5 hours, and, after a 5 to 10 mg dose, the drug has a therapeutic level for approximately 24 hours [1]. Amisulpride's reduced potential for drug interactions is due to minimal metabolism, no inhibition of the cytochrome P450 (CYP 450) enzymes, and low plasma protein binding [1,2]. An exception is to avoid using with dopamine agonists (eg, levodopa), which can cause a reciprocal antagonism of effects of both drugs [3].

A recognized side effect of many of the dopamine antagonist antiemetics is QTc interval prolongation on the electrocardiogram. The QTc interval prolongation is mediated by binding to the potassium ion channel (the human Ether-à-go-go-Related Gene [hERG] channel). Although the prescribing information for IV amisulpride carries a QTc prolongation warning, amisulpride has a weak affinity for binding to the hERG potassium channel. The risk is considered as an inconsequential effect on the QTc interval [1,2,6]. An increase in serum prolactin is a predictable effect of dopaminergic medications [7]. Amisulpride was reported to lead to increased prolactin levels, but they were within normal levels for nonpregnant females [8].

Although amisulpride is indicated for both prevention and treatment of PONV, the emphasis and clinical need is for rescue therapy. In a rescue trial, patients received standard antiemetic prophylaxis (one or more nondopaminergic antiemetics). Patients who experienced PONV within 24 hours after surgery were randomized to receive amisulpride 5 or 10 mg or placebo. The primary end point was a complete response within 24 hours after starting treatment. Significantly more patients treated with amisulpride 10 mg (41.7%) had a complete response compared with placebo (28.5%). Patients receiving 10 mg amisulpride had a 35-minute shorter length of stay in the postanesthesia care unit (PACU). The most common adverse reaction was infusion site pain [9]. A subsequent meta-analysis of 5 randomized controlled trials (RCT) demonstrated similar results compared with placebo [10].

INTRAVENOUS APREPITANT FOR POSTOPERATIVE NAUSEA AND VOMITING PROPHYLAXIS

Neurokinin 1 (NK1) receptor antagonists (aprepitant, fosaprepitant, vestipitant) are some of the newer medications for treatment of nausea and vomiting. Most of the data and US Food and Drug Administration (FDA) indications revolve around treatment of cancer-induced nausea and vomiting rather than PONV. The safety profile is excellent with the most commonly documented side effects being headache, constipation, and drowsiness with this class of medications currently carrying no additional monitoring recommendations for the central nervous system (CNS), cardiac system, or respiratory system. The new IV form of aprepitant (Aponovie) is the only one (IV formulation) currently with an FDA indication for PONV prophylaxis. Vestipitant is not yet approved for the treatment of PONV; however, research has shown promising results, specifically for rescue of established PONV [11]. IV aprepitant is a selective high-affinity antagonist for the human substance P/NK1 receptors and is indicated for the prevention of PONV in adults. Aprepitant has minimal or no affinity for serotonin, dopamine, and corticosteroid receptors [12]. A randomized open-label phase 1 study conducted with 32 healthy volunteers found that IV aprepitant 32 mg administered as a 30-second IV injection is bioequivalent to an oral preparation of aprepitant 40 mg. The study also showed that IV aprepitant was well tolerated and had a similar safety report when compared with oral aprepitant [13]. Aprepitant given IV reaches drug levels associated with a greater than or equal to 97% receptor occupancy in the brain within 5 minutes. The drug maintains therapeutic plasma concentrations for at least 48 hours [14,15]. Aprepitant IV offers the advantage of avoiding an oral dosage form in a patient who is nil per os. Drug interactions related to the CYP 450 enzyme system during hepatic metabolism can occur with NK1 receptor antagonists [15,16]. Despite several pharmacokinetic interactions related to its metabolism, aprepitant remains a safe drug with a low frequency of side effects [17]. Clinical doses of aprepitant have not been associated with significant risk of QTc prolongation [18]. Sedation, a frequent side effect of many of the antiemetics and frequently responsible for delays in discharge from postanesthesia care, was not seen in the clinical trials for aprepitant's approval [12,19,20].

Oral aprepitant has been used for the prevention of PONV since 2006 and is now available in a generic form along with the newer IV formulation. For IV aprepitant approval, the FDA reviewed 2 clinical studies comparing oral aprepitant to ondansetron for the prevention of PONV for a 48-hour period. The studies found aprepitant to be more effective for the prevention of vomiting at 24 and 48 hours compared with ondansetron [19,20].

Weibel and colleagues [21] published a comprehensive Cochrane network meta-analysis comparing available antiemetic prophylactic medications for PONV. The review contains a ranking of antiemetic drugs based on efficacy and safety. The findings showed, with high-certainty evidence, that 5 single drugs (aprepitant, ramosetron, granisetron, dexamethasone, and ondansetron) reduce vomiting. Of these, aprepitant was the most effective and had comparable efficacy to most of the multidrug combinations [21].

OLDER DRUGS

Many older medications from different drug classes are still used as part of the regimen to prevent PONV. Because the consensus guidelines recommend treating at-risk patients with multiple drugs from differing classes, it is important to be familiar with the options available and their reported efficacies.

5-Hydroxytryptamine 3 antagonists

The 5-HT$_3$ antagonists are one of the most common drug classes used to treat PONV and have an excellent safety profile. Ondansetron is the best studied and most commonly used drug in this class and is a standard component of most PONV regimens. This drug is available as a 4 and 8 mg oral disintegrating tablet. Other 5-HT$_3$ antagonists include dolasetron, granisetron, tropisetron, ramosetron, and palonosetron, and all have demonstrated excellent efficacy when used alone or in combination with medications from other drug classes [22]. There is a known risk of QTc prolongation, but it seems to be dose dependent and transient; systematic reviews of ondansetron have shown little risk of malignant arrhythmias at the 4 to 8 mg prophylaxis dose when used in routine patients [23,24]. Other side effects of this class of drugs are generally mild such as headache and constipation. Palonosetron has been shown in meta-analysis to be more effective than ondansetron and confers the unique benefit of a 40-hour half-life for a prolonged duration of action.[25]

Corticosteroids

Corticosteroids have a long history of efficacy for PONV. Dexamethasone is a glucocorticoid that has been used for many years to prevent PONV, typically in doses from 4 to 8 mg IV. Data support the early administration of dexamethasone at the beginning of the case to achieve the best results [26]. Lower doses (4–5 mg) seem to be equally effective as higher doses (8–10 mg) [27]. Although the safety of dexamethasone has been questioned for years with regard to multiple parameters, when used in smaller clinically effective doses, dexamethasone has not been associated with increased risk of wound infection, increased surgical bleeding, delayed wound healing, or clinically significant perioperative hyperglycemia [28,29]. When given to an awake patient it can cause substantial perineal burning sensation and may be better suited for intraoperative administration. Methylprednisolone in varying doses has also exhibited efficacy in preventing PONV, whereas betamethasone demonstrated little to no benefit [30–32].

Antidopaminergics

Many of the antipsychotic medications in the phenothiazine and butyrophenone classes are used for the treatment of PONV and work via blockade of dopaminergic receptors. Before the FDA's black box warning in 2001 related to prolonged QTc and sudden cardiac death in doses higher than 25 mg, droperidol, a butyrophenone antipsychotic, was a commonly used first-line agent for the prevention and treatment of PONV. The utilization of droperidol dropped off significantly in most countries following the FDA's black box warning. However, the drug has been studied more extensively and, in low doses (0.625 mg), is thought to have similar risk of QTc prolongation to ondansetron. A large study of more than 20,000 patients found no increased risk of cardiac rhythm disturbances with low-dose droperidol [33].

Haloperidol is another butyrophenone antipsychotic agent that has been used for PONV, especially following the FDA black box warning against droperidol, even though it has a similar risk profile for QTc prolongation as droperidol and ondansetron. The efficacy of haloperidol as a rescue agent for PONV is similar to that of ondansetron; however, it can also be associated with sedation [34].

Butyrophenone medications have a higher CNS penetration and, therefore, a higher incidence of sedation. Similarly, butyrophenones have a higher affinity for potassium channels resulting in a theoretic higher risk of QTc prolongation, although this has not been shown to be true in studies.

Phenothiazine medications have a high affinity for cholinergic, adrenergic, and histamine receptors and are associated with a higher incidence of EPS, orthostatic hypotension, and sedation [35]. Several phenothiazine antipsychotics have demonstrated efficacy for treatment of and prophylaxis against PONV; these include promethazine, prochlorperazine, and perphenazine. All have been used as effective components of PONV prophylaxis regimens. Promethazine has gotten notable scrutiny in the form of an FDA black box warning for children younger than 2 years due to the sedating properties and risk of respiratory depression. Lower doses of promethazine have been shown to be as effective as higher doses and cause less sedation. Promethazine is also a vesicant, and it has been noted to cause severe tissue injury and ischemia when given through an extravasated IV catheter. To minimize the risk of tissue damage, caution must be used to adequately dilute the drug, use the lowest possible effective dose (typically 6.25 mg), and administer it slowly into a free-flowing IV line under close observation [35].

Benzamides (amisulpride), in contrast to the other dopamine antagonists, are newer second-generation antipsychotics and show lower CNS penetration or potassium receptor affinity. This feature has led to a favorable safety profile with lower incidence of EPS, no meaningful QTc prolongation at 5 to 10 mg PONV doses, and increases with blood prolactin levels with no clinical consequences levels [21].

Metoclopramide in a 10 mg dose has demonstrated mixed efficacy in multiple studies over the years. This drug was initially believed to be ineffective based on a meta-analysis. The knowledge surrounding the efficacy was clouded by the fact that several studies by Fujii and colleagues were found to be fabricated and were then retracted. A more recent meta-analysis that excluded the retracted studies showed that metoclopramide may be effective [36]. Another study showed efficacy only in higher doses (25 or 50 mg), with the downside that the risk of EPS was greater in the high-dose metoclopramide groups [37,38].

Antihistamines

Several antihistamine medications have shown effectiveness for treating patients with a history of motion sickness and PONV. Dimenhydrinate, diphenhydramine, meclizine, cyclizine, and hydroxyzine have all been used effectively in the treatment of PONV. Promethazine also has significant antihistamine properties. This class of drug may be more effective in high-risk patients, such as those who are having middle ear surgery. Drowsiness can be a disadvantageous side effect, especially with diphenhydramine.

Anticholinergics

Transdermal scopolamine is a centrally acting muscarinic anticholinergic agent that has been shown to be effective for PONV prophylaxis. The benefit of this delivery system is long-term coverage of cholinergic chemoreceptors with the slow and sustained release of medication. The delayed onset of action makes it advantageous to place it as much as 6 to 8 hours before surgery, although, anecdotally, many think that, even if placed just before surgery, it can still be quite effective against PDNV. Transdermal scopolamine can be used effectively as a single agent and is as effective as ondansetron alone. Ondansetron combined with transdermal scopolamine is more effective than either agent used alone. The most common side effects are generally mild and include dry mouth or visual disturbances. Transdermal scopolamine is often avoided in the elderly because of the increased risk of confusion, delirium, or oversedation [39]; it can also cause increased intraocular pressure and should be avoided in those with known narrow-angle glaucoma [40].

COMPLEMENTARY AND ALTERNATIVE PROPHYLAXIS AND TREATMENT

Aromatherapy

Aromatherapy perioperatively can be administered in the form of oils applied directly onto the patient's skin in the head and neck area, onto gauze placed on or near the patient, onto sticks that the patient can wave near their own nose, and even adhesive patches with the aroma already embedded into them for an easy way to peel and stick to the patient's gown.

An analysis of 16 clinical trials of aromatherapy for PONV demonstrated a large heterogeneity in outcomes, in part due to the variety of scents used. Most studies found that certain scents were as effective as traditional prophylaxis, in addition to improving patient satisfaction [41].

Ginger essential oil garnered the greatest success. One study demonstrated a 65% reduction in PONV scores compared with a 43% decrease with the placebo [42]. Other trials showed only a slight immediate effect but a significant decrease in PONV at the 6-hour mark after surgery [43,44]. When used in combination with other oils, such as lemon and/or lavender, PONV scores decreased anywhere from 21% to 94%, with the need for antiemetic therapy declining 20% in the treatment groups [45,46]. Other studies found that the use of ginger–either alone or in a mix of scents–was equivalent to receiving one dose of a traditional antiemetic [47].

In contrast, several scents were found to be no better than placebo, including peppermint oil, rose essential oil, and the simple isopropyl alcohol swab [41,42].

Oral ginger
One gram of oral ginger given preoperatively had similar effects as using one traditional antiemetic [47,48]. There are few risks to the healthy patient, but caution should be used in those patients on blood thinners and hypoglycemic medications [49].

Dextrose
Released in response to a need for calories, the hormone ghrelin causes an increase in gastric acid secretion as well as a sense of hunger. The longer the fasting period persists, the more is the amount of ghrelin that is released. Some patients are sensitive to the climbing levels of this hormone, resulting in nausea on top of their hunger [50].

Caloric intake can break the spiraling cycle of increased ghrelin release and perhaps reduce the nausea it causes. Patients at high risk for PONV were provided with a 5% solution of dextrose preoperatively and experienced a 44% reduction in the need for rescue antiemetics when compared with placebo. Length of stay in the recovery room was also shortened by 20% [51]. Another study found no immediate improvement with either oral or IV carbohydrate administration, but at the 6- and 24-hour marks after surgery, patients reported a statistically significant reduction in pain and PONV than the placebo group. Furthermore, blood glucose levels were comparable across the 3 groups [52].

Hydration
Outside of enhanced recovery after surgery (ERAS) protocols, many patients arrive for surgery after prolonged fasting from fluids and, therefore, dehydrated. A study of patients who underwent laparoscopic cholecystectomy revealed that patients who received less than 2 mL/kg/h of crystalloid were at increased risk of PONV [53].

In a review of 41 studies in which primarily healthy outpatients received supplemental fluids during their surgical cases, there was moderate evidence to suggest that improved hydration leads to decreased PONV, cutting the relative risk for both nausea and vomiting approximately in half. In addition, when broken down into early (0–6 hours) and late (6–24 hours) PONV, the beneficial effects persisted well after leaving the recovery room [54].

A meta-analysis of 9 RCTs compared crystalloid and colloid for their effects on PONV. It was only in elective noncardiac surgical cases lasting longer than 3 hours that colloid administration resulted in a slight decrease in PONV over those receiving only crystalloid [55]. Unfortunately, colloids are far more expensive than not only crystalloids but also the currently clinically available antiemetic medications; additionally, some colloids have been shown to cause allergic reactions in patients and negatively affect coagulation [56].

There is also a benefit to simple early oral hydration of patients immediately after surgery. Getting patients to drink water in the recovery room as soon as they are able resulted in lower rates of PONV and greater patient satisfaction [57]. This method is not feasible for all patients, but it is an easily implemented, inexpensive, and well tolerated way to help ease PONV after surgery with minimal deleterious effects.

Acustimulation

Many have advocated for acustimulation of the Pericardium 6 (P6) location for prophylaxis and treatment of PONV. The P6 acupoint site is located on the inner forearm approximately 2 in proximal to the wrist between the palmaris longus and flexor carpi radialis muscle and is typically easy to access perioperatively (Fig. 1) [58].

A Cochrane database study of 59 trials using the stimulation of the P6 acupoint site perioperatively found the evidence for its use in PONV to be of moderate strength. Compared with placebo, acupoint stimulation of P6 resulted in a decreased risk of PONV and was equivalent to administering an antiemetic drug [59]. In a more recent study, all patients received prophylaxis for PONV and half of the participants received acupuncture in addition to the prophylactic medication. Nausea was reduced by almost 60% in the acupuncture group while vomiting episodes were also significantly lower within the first 24 hours [60].

Laser acupuncture involves the use of a relatively low-power laser to provide stimulation. When used in combination with antiemetic drug prophylaxis for PONV, patients immediately after surgery experienced similar rates of PONV whether they received laser stimulation or not. At 6 hours postoperatively, the incidence of nausea and the need for rescue antiemetics were lower in the laser acupuncture stimulation group; the rate of vomiting continued to be the same in both groups [61]. This is a mild improvement for no risk, but requires a piece of equipment that is not typically available in perioperative areas and can be rather expensive.

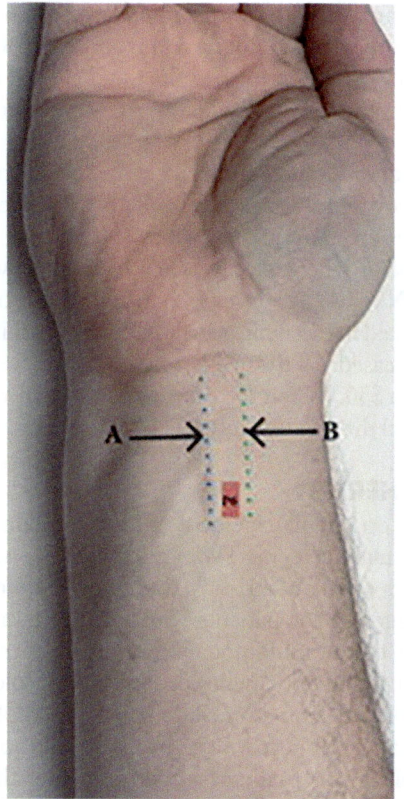

Fig. 1. The P6 acupoint (*red square*) is located 3 finger breadths above the wrist between the palmaris longus tendon (*blue dotted line*, **A**) and the flexor carpi radialis tendon (*green dotted line*, **B**).

Transcutaneous electrical acupoint stimulation (TEAS) applies a small electrical stimulus across a conductive pad. Fourteen RCTs were examined in which TEAS was used in patients undergoing general anesthesia. These trials demonstrated a lower incidence of PONV, the need for antiemetic rescue, and the incidence of dizziness [62]. TEAS has low risk and requires no needles; it does still require additional equipment that is not standard in the perioperative area.

The next question is one of timing. One recent study compared TEAS the day before surgery, 30 minutes before surgery, a combination of both, and a control group that received neither. All 3 treatment groups demonstrated decreased PONV and the need for rescue antiemetics. The patients who received acustimulation the day before surgery and the group that received treatment both the day before surgery and 30 minutes before surgery had similar effective reductions in nausea of 60%. The rate of antiemetic rescue

(4%) was reduced compared with those who only received it 30 minutes before surgery (11%) and those who did not have a treatment (18%) [63]. TEAS has a strong effect on PONV when performed the day before. However, the burden of an additional appointment the day before surgery is problematic for a great number of patients.

The final significant hurdle is reimbursement and patient acceptance. Although an industry-wide survey of insurance companies has not been done, acupuncture and related techniques are reimbursed by many insurance providers (including Medicare) only for pain, whereas only a few have approved it for prevention and treatment of PONV [64]. A survey of patients found that only 68.4% of patients would be interested in receiving acustimulation. Their interest level dropped steeply as the cost increased. Of those interested if it were free, less than half were willing if it cost $20 to $50. When the full reimbursement rate of $175 was proposed, the interest level dropped to only 8.6% [65].

COMBINATION THERAPY

Consensus guidelines on the management of PONV recommend a multimodal approach for PONV management. Two antiemetics are suggested for PONV prophylaxis in patients with 1 to 2 risk factors (mild to moderate risk), and 3 to 4 antiemetics are suggested for patients with greater than 2 risk factors (high risk) (Box 1). A part of the multimodal approach is to reduce baseline risks in addition to administering antiemetics or nonpharmacologic/alternative therapies. Reducing baseline risks may include using propofol for induction, total IV anesthetic, or a background low-dose propofol infusion; perioperative hydration; avoidance of nitrous oxide in surgeries greater than 1 hour; regional anesthesia to avoid volatile anesthetics; minimizing opioids; and the use of sugammadex in place of neostigmine [22]. The management of PONV also involves assessing the right antiemetics for the patient. Antiemetic drugs may have different efficacy, onset, duration, contraindications, metabolism, side effects, and capacity for drug interactions, even within the same pharmacologic class. Selection considerations involve availability of the antiemetics on the drug formulary, institutional restrictions, and cost of the antiemetics.

There is an abundance of literature supporting the combination of antiemetics for prevention of PONV with many showing superiority over

---

Box 1: Risk factors for postoperative nausea and vomiting [22]*

Female gender

Nonsmoker

Hx of PONV/motion sickness

Expected administration of opioids

Hx, history; PONV, postoperative nausea and vomiting. *Three or more risk factors: should consider at least 3 antiemetics from different classes.

monotherapy [21,22]. Use of combination antiemetics for rescue seems to be more efficacious than monotherapy rescue [66]. The most studied combination regimens in RCTs are the serotonin 5-HT$_3$ receptor antagonists with dexamethasone or dopamine receptor antagonists. A recent article described 9 meta-analyses involving 5-HT$_3$ receptor antagonists with 23,000 patients participating from 311 trials. The conclusion was that prophylactic combination therapy was more effective than monotherapy. However, the investigators state that the ideal combination has not been established [67].

Weibel and colleagues [21] found that combining drugs was largely more effective than monotherapy for 29 of 36 drug combinations. The most effective drug combinations based on P scores were (partial list; top 5 combinations are listed)

- Aprepitant-palonosetron
- Dexamethasone-metoclopramide-ondansetron
- Aprepritant-ramosetron
- Metoclopramide-ondansetron
- Aprepitant-dexamethasone

The analysis illuminated several interesting points that may guide the clinician's selection of the optimal combination:

- NK1 receptor antagonists showed favorable antiemetic efficacy, but the antinausea efficacy was less pronounced
- Ramosetron, granisetron, and droperidol all effectively reduce nausea
- Ramosetron, granisetron, or droperidol, when used in combination with NK1 receptor antagonists, confer protection from nausea
- Headache, as a side effect of ondansetron, could be reduced when combined with droperidol

The investigators advise that the certainty of evidence was not assessed for these findings [21]. In addition, providers should consider avoiding antiemetics that have side effects such as sedation, dizziness, EPS, or headache to minimize delays in discharge, especially in susceptible populations such as the elderly.

SELECTING THE RIGHT DRUG CLASS FOR PATIENT POPULATION

The commonly used antiemetic medications have well-documented side effect profiles, and an awareness of these side effects can help guide appropriate prescribing decisions. These considerations can be especially important in the extremes of age (elderly and those younger than two years) or if specific coexisting conditions are present.

SPECIAL CONSIDERATIONS

Outpatient surgery

There is ever-increasing pressure to perform surgeries with same-day discharge and to prevent prolonged PACU stays and unplanned admissions.

In particular, PDNV can decrease patient satisfaction and lead to potential complications from mechanical stress on incisions, tissue damage from excessive retching, and ultimately lead to electrolyte and hydration status abnormalities. With hospital production pressures in mind, the conventional choices of antiemetics with short half-lives may not be the most appropriate medication for a patient leaving the hospital setting. Instead, delayed-release medications, drugs with long half-lives, or agents with downstream mechanisms that propagate past the drug's initial metabolism may better suit the outpatient needs. Transdermal scopolamine with continuous release of medication can provide coverage for several days if the patch is left in place. Dexamethasone's complex mechanism of neurotransmitter modulation seems to provide benefit lasting well past its expected half-life. From the NK1 pathway, aprepitant possesses a long half-life and may provide extended coverage for up to 48 hours following a single dose. Of the 5-HT_3 drugs, palonosetron commands a 40-hour half-life and will remain in the patient's system far longer than the conventional alternative, ondansetron. There is a cost-benefit trade-off to many of these newer drugs relative to older generic options, but with the increased emphasis on PDNV and not just the narrow window of the PACU stay, effective PDNV prophylaxis may justify the use of newer more expensive medications that provide prolonged therapeutic benefits [68].

Elderly

Undoubtedly, an aging population creates an increasing challenge for PONV regimen selection. Increased patient age modifies the pharmacodynamics and pharmacokinetics of our commonly used drugs. There is also an increased risk of drug-drug interactions due to polypharmacy. In particular, medications with anticholinergic or antihistamine mechanisms seem to have increased risk of delirium or prolonged sedation [69]. Some of this can be mitigated by using smaller doses and administering these medications early in the intraoperative phase, but the risk still exists and may be worth prioritizing the more expensive, nonsedating medications in this high-risk group. The dopamine antagonists with high CNS penetration (phenothiazines and butyrophenones) should be used cautiously in elderly patients due to the higher risk of confusion. Amisulpride seems to be tolerated better and has a lower risk for causing confusion in the elderly. All dopamine antagonists should be avoided in patients with Parkinson disease.

POSTANESTHESIA CARE UNIT TREATMENT OF POSTOPERATIVE NAUSEA AND VOMITING

Much of PONV mitigation comes down to appropriate preoperative risk stratification, administration of prophylaxis therapy, and the intraoperative anesthetic technique. Unfortunately, despite increased awareness and focus on PONV prophylaxis, the incidence of PONV in PACU remains as high as 30% [70–72] and may be as high as 80% in high-risk populations [73]. This has been shown to decrease patient satisfaction and has financial implications with an average increased PACU length of stay of 25 minutes [74]. When PONV presents in recovery, there should be a prompt evaluation to rule out reversible causes of nausea such as mechanical bowel obstruction, blood in the throat, or excessive opioid administration [75]. After first ruling out reversible causes of PONV, the next mainstay of therapy is to initiate appropriate pharmacologic intervention.

Postoperative nausea and vomiting after no prophylaxis

If no prophylaxis has been administered, many guidelines currently recommend beginning therapy with a 5-HT$_3$ receptor antagonist. Antiemetics from a different drug class may be equally efficacious for first-line therapy, but the plethora of data on 5-HT$_3$ receptor antagonists are well established with favorable safety profile and it can be considered the gold standard for first-line treatment [75,76]. With improved attention to mitigating PONV, many prophylaxis regimens are becoming more robust and patients have already received a 5-HT$_3$ antagonist such as ondansetron at the end of their anesthetic. This increasingly common scenario requires alternative strategies for rescue therapy to be used in the PACU.

Rescue after prophylaxis fails

The most important principle in deciding which medication to use is initiating therapy from a different pharmacologic category than previously administered medications. There is ample evidence that repeated administration of a drug from the same class within the first 6 hours confers no additional benefit [77]. If a 5-HT$_3$ receptor antagonist has recently been administered, then a drug targeting a different nausea chemoreceptor (eg, antidopaminergic, antihistamine, or NK1 receptor antagonist) should be used.

Just as multimodal treatment is more effective for the prevention of PONV, multimodal therapy may also be more effective for treating established PONV [78,79]. The exception to this trend seems to be NK1 receptor antagonists, which, when used as monotherapy, exceed the performance of many combination therapy treatments in a recent Cochrane meta-analysis [21]. There is also evidence that NK1 receptor antagonists are noninferior to ondansetron, specifically as a rescue modality [11]. The dopamine antagonist amisulpride has recently demonstrated efficacy specifically for the treatment of established PONV with a favorable safety profile and has a recommended 10 mg rescue dose [10,80,81]. In addition, the use of regional anesthesia in the recovery room can improve pain control and minimize opioid consumption. Therefore, effective regional anesthesia can be considered an indirect pharmacologic adjunct to the treatment of PONV [82–84].

More focus is being placed on nonpharmacologic interventions that can be used for rescue therapy. These interventions are addressed in more detail in the complementary and alternative prophylaxis and treatment but include interventions such as oxygen, aromatherapy, acupressure, chewing gum, and more. These interventions are relatively cheap, quick to use, and offer minimal adverse safety implications. In a busy clinical environment with many periop-erative obligations, this can help expedite initiation of rescue treatment by bedside nursing during the period while waiting for physician orders and veri-fication by pharmacy for pharmacologic intervention.

Dosing medications for rescue

Broadly, the question of appropriate dosing for every potential rescue medica-tion is still being actively researched and is less well described compared with PONV prophylaxis dosing. Designing studies to tease out specific dosing re-sponses is hard to perform and often has many confounding variables by the time a patient has arrived to the PACU, failed initial prophylaxis, and then re-ceives one or more rescue agents. Newer data are pointing toward many drugs requiring higher dosing for rescue of established PONV when compared with the effective prophylaxis dose. For example, droperidol is more effective for rescue at a 1.25 mg dose compared with the smaller prophylactic dose of 0.625 mg or amisulpride's 5 mg prophylaxis dose compared the 10 mg rescue dose recommendation [68]. In the absence of concrete rescue dosing data, many are currently starting treatment with the lower, but established, prophy-laxis dosing.

Lack of universal algorithm

Many attempts to protocolize PONV treatment and rescue therapy have been implemented in the form of quality improvement projects, ERAS bundles, and increased anesthesia team education. Most of these efforts show demon-strable improvement in PONV rates, but long-term success is limited by waning compliance with these interventions [85]. There are currently no in-ternational or standard-of-care treatment algorithms for rescue therapy, given the variability in drug availability and pricing structures between different in-stitutions. In addition, patient comorbidities change the appropriateness of the various antiemetics given their known side effect profiles. A recent systematic review provides an algorithm for the approach to rescue PONV including ex-amples of specific recommended medications and evidence-based doses, but this may not be applicable for every institution's drug availability or every in-dividual patient [68]. Ultimately, every patient should be individually as-sessed for suitability of the available pharmaceutical therapies possible taking into account their unique medical history while following the guiding principle of diversifying drug classes to target different chemoreceptor pathways.

ENHANCED RECOVERY AFTER SURGERY PROTOCOLS

ERAS protocols are multidisciplinary evidence-based initiatives with a goal of expediting recovery and decreasing length of stay in the hospital. The preven-tion of PONV is a major component of these protocols. The protocols typically emphasize carbohydrate loading in the preoperative period, minimizing perioperative opioids, and consideration of regional anesthesia and nonopioid

Table 1
Postoperative antiemetic drug characteristics by class/agent [3,12,86–98]

Medication	QT Prolongation	Sedation	EPS	Long Acting	Costly	Use in Elderly	Restless	Hypotension	Use in Parkinson
Dopamine antagonists									
Benzamides									
Amisulpride	-(a)	-			+	+			
Metoclopramide	-(b)	+	+			Beers criteria (c)	+		
Butyrophenones Droperidol	+	+	+			Beers criteria (c)	+	+	
Haloperidol	+	+	+			Beers criteria (c)	+	+	
Phenothiazines									
Prochlorperazine	+		+			Beers criteria (c)			
5-HT$_3$ antagonists									
Ondansetron	+					+		+	+(d)
Palonosetron	-(a)			+	+	+		+	+
Antihistamines									
Diphenhydramine	-	+		+		Beers criteria (oral) (c)		+	+(e)
Promethazine	-	+	+			Beers criteria (c)		+	
NK1 antagonists									
Aprepitant		-			+	+			+
Anticholinergics									
Scopolamine		+		+		Beers criteria (c)	+	+	+(e)
Corticosteroids									
Dexamethasone	-	-		+		+(f)			+

Abbreviations: 5-HT$_3$, 5-hydroxytryptamine; AGS American Geriatrics Society; Ccardiac; EPS, extrapyramidal symptoms; NK1, neurokinin 1; PI, package insert.
Guide: -, avoid use; (a) = listed in PI but less than threshold for regulatory concern; (b) = C case reports; (c) = avoid or consider with caution (see AGS Beers Criteria for specific drug); (d) = do not use if patient is on apomorphine; (e) = possible other side effects; (f) = lowest dose.

analgesics to decrease the incidence of PONV. In addition, the protocols use risk-stratified PONV prophylaxis based on the patient's risk factors.

ANTIEMETICS AND POSTANESTHESIA CARE UNIT PERSONNEL COSTS

It seems logical that the use of inexpensive PONV prophylaxis and antiemetics would confer cost savings by allowing patients to spend less time in the recovery room and instead move on to the next phase of recovery or to their waiting hospital beds while improving their overall satisfaction.

The analysis becomes more complex as the medications used become more expensive. Medication contracts mean different institutions pay differing amounts for the medications they want to use, resulting in variances in medication costs across the nation, with an even greater discrepancy when compared with other countries.

The second part of the equation for cost is personnel, where the variance may be even greater. Nursing hourly rates are not the same within a hospital, often differing between shifts, or regular pay versus overtime, incentive or premium pay, or contracted/traveler nurses from outside agencies earning higher rates. As a result, the calculations of whether a particular antiemetic leads to an overall cost-effectiveness depend on the individual institution and their specific circumstances at that moment.

Even then, the math continues to change as the staffing costs and potential impacts to the surgical schedule vary throughout the day or week. It may make sense to use an expensive antiemetic early in the day when the space is needed in the recovery room to keep the operative schedule running, yet the nursing costs might be the lowest at that time of day. Meanwhile, in the evening nursing costs could be higher, yet getting a patient out of the recovery room would have no effect on the dwindling or even completed remaining operative schedule. After all, there is no cost benefit if the last patient in the recovery room leaves an hour before the last nurse is ending their shift versus the patient being discharged just as they end their shift.

It is therefore up to each institution to determine under which set of conditions the use of costlier antiemetics would provide cost savings, when it would be break even, and when it would not be financially beneficial. All these factors make the cost analysis complex.

SUMMARY

There are many factors that play a role in the management of the complex issue of PONV and PDNV. New medications can be helpful, but costs and benefits as well as the potential side effects must also be considered (Table 1.). Nonpharmacologic techniques may also play a role in some circumstances, and special circumstances have been outlined. In the end, it is important for all to consider patient risk factors, adequate PONV prophylaxis, and the impact of PONV on our patients with regard to efficacy, safety, side effects, costs, and overall patient satisfaction.

CLINICS CARE POINTS

- Amisulpride is the only antiemetic approved for rescue treatment of PONV despite prophylaxis.
- A recent Cochrane network meta-analysis ranked aprepitant as the most effective medication for PONV prophylaxis with comparabe efficacy to most multidrug combinations.
- The American Geriatrics Society Beers Criteria lists medications to avoid in the elderly which include some of the antiemetics.
- Anesthesia professionals should consider the use of long acting antiemetics such as aprepitant, transdermal scopolamine, dexamethasone, or palonosetron when appropriate, particulalry for use in outpatient surgical cases for the extended antiemetic coverage post discharge.
- Use of antiemetics with the side effect of sedation may cause possible delays in discharge.

DISCLOSURE

T.A. Meyer: Speaker and consultant: Eagle Pharmaceuticals, and consultant: Heron Therapeutics. L.R. Hutson, P.M. Morris, and R.K. McAllister: Nothing to disclose.

References

[1] Fox G, Kranke P. A pharmacological profile of intravenous amisulpride for the treatment of postoperative nausea and vomiting. Expet Rev Clin Pharmacol 2020;13(4):331–40.

[2] Smyla N, Koch T, Eberhart LH, et al. An overview of intravenous amisulpride as a new therapeutic option for the prophylaxis and treatment of postoperative nausea and vomiting. Expert Opin Pharmacother 2020;21(5):517–22.

[3] Barhemsys® Amisulpride. Indianapolis, Indiana: Acacia Pharma; 2022.

[4] Schoemaker H, Claustre Y, Fage D, et al. Neurochemical characteristics of amisulpride, an atypical dopamine D2/D3 receptor antagonist with both presynaptic and limbic selectivity. J Pharmacol Exp Ther 1997;280(1):83–97.

[5] Möller HJ. Amisulpride: limbic specificity and the mechanism of antipsychotic atypicality. Prog Neuro Psychopharmacol Biol Psychiatr 2003;27(7):1101–11.

[6] Täubel J, Ferber G, Fox G, et al. Thorough QT study of the effect of intravenous amisulpride on QTc interval in Caucasian and Japanese healthy subjects Br J Clin Pharmacol 2017;83: 339–48.

[7] Besser GM, Delitala G, Grossman A, et al. Chlorpromazine, haloperidol, metoclopramide and domperidone release prolactin through dopamine antagonism at low concentrations but paradoxically inhibit prolactin release at high concentrations. Br J Pharmacol 1980;71(2):569–73.

[8] Gan TJ, Kranke P, Minkowitz HS, et al. Intravenous Amisulpride for the Prevention of Postoperative Nausea and Vomiting: Two Concurrent, Randomized, Double-blind, Placebo-controlled Trials. Anesthesiology 2017;126(2):268–75.

[9] Habib AS, Kranke P, Bergese SD, et al. Amisulpride for the Rescue Treatment of Postoperative Nausea or Vomiting in Patients Failing Prophylaxis: A Randomized, Placebo-controlled Phase III Trial. Anesthesiology 2019;130(2):203–12.

[10] Zhang LF, Zhang CF, Tang WX, et al. Efficacy of amisulpride on postoperative nausea and vomiting: a systematic review and meta-analysis. Eur J Clin Pharmacol 2020;76:903–12.

[11] Kranke P, Thompson JP, Dalby PL, et al. Comparison of vestipitant with ondansetron for the treatment of breakthrough postoperative nausea and vomiting after failed prophylaxis with ondansetron. Br J Anaesth 2015;114:423–9.

[12] Aponvie®IV aprepitant. San Diego (CA): Heron Therapeutics Inc; 2022.

[13] Yamamoto A, Stogard C, Yuan N, Ottoboni T. Phase 1 bioavailability study of HTX-019 intravenous injection compared with aprepitant oral capsules. Presented at: The American Society of Anesthesiologists Annual Meeting, October 21-25, 2022, New Orleans, LA.

[14] Heron Therapeutics. Press release; Heron Therapeutics Announces U.S. FDA Approval of APONVIE™ (HTX-019) for the Prevention of Postoperative Nausea and Vomiting(PONV) September 16, 2022. Available at: https://ir.herontx.com/node/15806/pdf. Accessed February 14, 2023.

[15] Okafor D, Kaye AD, Kaye RJ, et al. The role of neurokinin-1 (substance P) antagonists in the prevention of postoperative nausea and vomiting. J Anaesthesiol Clin Pharmacol 2017;33(4):441–5.

[16] Navari RM, Schwartzberg LS. Evolving role of neurokinin 1-receptor antagonists for chemotherapy-induced nausea and vomiting. OncoTargets Ther 2018;11:6459–78.

[17] Aapro MS, Walko CM. Aprepitant: drug-drug interactions in perspective. Ann Oncol 2010;21(12):2316–23.

[18] Marbury TC, Jin B, Panebianco D, et al. Lack of effect of aprepitant or its prodrug fosaprepitant on QTc intervals in healthy subjects. Anesth Analg 2009;109(2):418–25.

[19] Gan TJ, Apfel CC, Kovac A, et al. A randomized, double-blind comparison of the NK1 antagonist, aprepitant, versus ondansetron for the prevention of postoperative nausea and vomiting. Anesth Analg 2007;104(5):1082–9, tables of contents.

[20] Diemunsch P, Gan TJ, Philip BK, et al. Single-dose aprepitant vs ondansetron for the prevention of postoperative nausea and vomiting: a randomized, double-blind phase III trial in patients undergoing open abdominal surgery. Br J Anaesth 2007;99(2):202–11.

[21] Weibel S, Rücker G, Eberhart LH, et al. Drugs for preventing postoperative nausea and vomiting in adults after general anaesthesia: A network meta-analysis. Cochrane Database Syst Rev 2020;10(10):CD012859.

[22] Gan TJ, Belani KG, Bergese S, et al. Fourth Consensus Guidelines for the Management of Postoperative Nausea and Vomiting. Anesth Analg 2020;131(2):411–48 [Erratum in: Anesth Analg. 2020 Nov;131(5):e241].

[23] Charbit B, Albaladejo P, Funck-Brentano C, et al. Prolongation of QTc interval after postoperative nausea and vomiting treatment by droperidol or ondansetron. Anesthesiology 2005;102(6):1094–100.

[24] Tricco AC, Soobiah C, Blondal E, et al. Comparative safety of serotonin (5-HT3) receptor antagonists in patients undergoing surgery: a systematic review and network meta-analysis. BMC Med 2015;13:142.

[25] Singh PM, Borle A, Gouda D, et al. Efficacy of palonosetron in postoperative nausea and vomiting (PONV)-a meta-analysis. J Clin Anesth 2016;34:459–82.

[26] Zou Z, Jiang Y, Xiao M, et al. The impact of prophylactic dexamethasone on nausea and vomiting after thyroidectomy: a systematic review and meta-analysis. PLoS One 2014;9:e109582.

[27] De Oliveira GS Jr, Castro-Alves LJ, Ahmad S, et al. Dexamethasone to prevent postoperative nausea and vomiting: an updated meta-analysis of randomized controlled trials. Anesth Analg 2013;116:58–74.

[28] Toner AJ, Ganeshanathan V, Chan MT, et al. Safety of perioperative glucocorticoids in elective noncardiac surgery: a systematic review and meta-analysis. Anesthesiology 2017;126:234–48.

[29] Tien M, Gan TJ, Dhakal I, et al. The effect of anti-emetic doses of dexamethasone on postoperative blood glucose levels in non-diabetic and diabetic patients: a prospective randomised controlled study. Anaesthesia 2016;71:1037–43.

[30] Weren M, Demeere JL. Methylprednisolone vs dexamethasone in the prevention of postoperative nausea and vomiting: a prospective, randomised, double-blind, placebo-controlled trial. Acta Anaesthesiol Belg 2008;59:1–5.

[31] Hasan MR, Hamilton TW, Stickland L, et al. Perioperative adjuvant corticosteroids for postoperative analgesia in knee arthroplasty. Acta Orthop 2018;89:71–6.

[32] Olanders KJ, Lundgren GA, Johansson AM. Betamethasone in prevention of postoperative nausea and vomiting following breast surgery. J Clin Anesth 2014;26:461–5.

[33] Nuttall GA, Malone AM, Michels CA, et al. Does low-dose droperidol increase the risk of polymorphic ventricular tachycardia or death in the surgical patient? Anesthesiology 2013;118:382–6.

[34] Yazbeck-Karam VG, Siddik-Sayyid SM, Barakat HB, et al. Haloperidol versus ondansetron for treatment of established nausea and vomiting following general anesthesia: a randomized clinical trial. Anesth Analg 2017;124:438–44.

[35] Meyer TA, McAllister RK. Pharmacology of Histamine, Muscarine and Dopamine Antagonists. In: Gan T, Habib A, editors. Postoperative nausea and vomiting: a practical guide. Cambridge: Cambridge University Press; 2016. p. 66.

[36] De Oliveira GS Jr, Castro-Alves LJ, Chang R, et al. Systemic metoclopramide to prevent postoperative nausea and vomiting: a meta-analysis without Fujii's studies. Br J Anaesth 2012;109:688–97.

[37] Wallenborn J, Gelbrich G, Bulst D, et al. Prevention of postoperative nausea and vomiting by metoclopramide combined with dexamethasone: randomised double blind multicentre trial. BMJ 2006;333:324.

[38] Apfel CC, Zhang K, George E, et al. Transdermal scopolamine for the prevention of postoperative nausea and vomiting: a systematic review and meta-analysis. Clin Ther 2010;32(12):1987–2002.

[39] Knuf KM, Spaulding FM, Stevens GJ. Scopolamine Toxicity in an Elderly Patient. Mil Med 2019;184(11–12):937–8.

[40] Hamill MB, Suelflow JA, Smith JA. Transdermal scopolamine delivery system (TRANSDERM-V) and acute angle-closure glaucoma. Ann Ophthalmol 1983;15(11):1011–2.

[41] Hines S, Steels E, Chang A, et al. Aromatherapy for treatment of postoperative nausea and vomiting. Cochrane Database Syst Rev 2018;3(3):CD007598.

[42] Karaman S, Karaman T, Tapar H, et al. A randomized placebo-controlled study of aromatherapy for the treatment of postoperative nausea and vomiting. Complement Ther Med 2019;42:417–21.

[43] Lee YR, Shin HS. Effectiveness of Ginger Essential Oil on Postoperative Nausea and Vomiting in Abdominal Surgery Patients. J Altern Complement Med 2017;23(3):196–200.

[44] Adib-Hajbaghery M, Hosseini FS. Investigating the effects of inhaling ginger essence on post-nephrectomy nausea and vomiting. Complement Ther Med 2015;23(6):827–31.

[45] Trandel-Korenchuk SC, Gujral H, Bode C, et al. Aromatherapy Blend for Postoperative Nausea in Ambulatory Surgery Patients. J Perianesth Nurs 2022;37(1):19–23.

[46] Hunt R, Dienemann J, Norton HJ, et al. Aromatherapy as treatment for postoperative nausea: a randomized trial. Anesth Analg 2013;117(3):597–604.

[47] Ernst E, Pittler MH. Efficacy of ginger for nausea and vomiting: a systematic review of randomized clinical trials. Br J Anaesth 2000;84(3):367–71.

[48] Naemi AR, Kashanitabar V, Kamali A, et al. Comparison of the Effects of Haloperidol, Metoclopramide, Dexmedetomidine and Ginger on Postoperative Nausea and Vomiting After Laparoscopic Cholecystectomy. J Med Life 2020;13(2):206–10.

[49] Ginger – Uses, Side Effects, and More. webmd.com/vitamins/ai/ingredientmono-961/ginger. Available at: https://www.webmd.com/vitamins/ai/ingredientmono-961/ginger. Accessed March 26, 2023.

[50] Pradhan G, Samson SL, Sun Y. Ghrelin: much more than a hunger hormone. Curr Opin Clin Nutr Metab Care 2013;16(6):619–24.

[51] Dabu-Bondoc S, Vadivelu N, Shimono C, et al. Intravenous dextrose administration reduces postoperative antiemetic rescue treatment requirements and postanesthesia care unit length of stay. Anesth Analg 2013;117(3):591–6.

[52] Mousavie SH, Negahi A, Hosseinpour P, et al. The Effect of Preoperative Oral Versus Parenteral Dextrose Supplementation on Pain, Nausea, and Quality of Recovery After Laparoscopic Cholecystectomy. J Perianesth Nurs 2021;36(2):153–6.

[53] Hsieh CY, Poon YY, Ke TY, et al. Postoperative Vomiting Following Laparoscopic Cholecystectomy Is Associated with Intraoperative Fluid Administration: A Retrospective Cohort Study. Int J Environ Res Public Health 2021;18(10):5305.

[54] Jewer JK, Wong MJ, Bird SJ, et al. Supplemental perioperative intravenous crystalloids for postoperative nausea and vomiting. Cochrane Database Syst Rev 2019;3(3):CD012212.

[55] Lee MJ, Lee C, Kang H, et al. The impact of crystalloid versus colloid fluids on postoperative nausea and vomiting: A systematic review and meta-analysis of randomized controlled trials. J Clin Anesth 2020;62:109695.

[56] Lewis SR, Pritchard MW, Evans DJ, et al. Colloids versus crystalloids for fluid resuscitation in critically ill people. Cochrane Database Syst Rev 2018;8(8):CD000567.

[57] Wu M, Yang L, Zeng X, et al. Safety and Feasibility of Early Oral Hydration in the Postanesthesia Care Unit After Laparoscopic Cholecystectomy: A Prospective, Randomized, and Controlled Study. J Perianesth Nurs 2019;34(2):425–30.

[58] Acupressure. Available at: https://www.mdanderson.org/cancerwise/4-acupressure-points-to-relieve-headache–nausea-and-anxiety.h00-159463212.html. Accessed March 26, 2023.

[59] Lee A, Chan SK, Fan LT. Stimulation of the wrist acupuncture point PC6 for preventing postoperative nausea and vomiting. Cochrane Database Syst Rev 2015;2015(11): CD003281.

[60] Honca M, Honca T, Babayigit M, et al. The Impact of Acupuncture on Postoperative Nausea and Vomiting in Obese Adult Patients Undergoing Laparoscopic Sleeve Gastrectomy: A Randomized Controlled Trial. J Laparoendosc Adv Surg Tech 2022;32(7):775–80.

[61] Unsal N, Akcaboy ZN, Soyal OB, et al. Effectiveness of Intraoperative Laser Acupuncture Combined with Antiemetic Drugs for Prevention of Postoperative Nausea and Vomiting. J Altern Complement Med 2020;26(1):67–71.

[62] Chen J, Tu Q, Miao S, et al. Transcutaneous electrical acupoint stimulation for preventing postoperative nausea and vomiting after general anesthesia: A meta-analysis of randomized controlled trials. Int J Surg 2020;73:57–64.

[63] Zhu J, Li S, Wu W, et al. Preoperative electroacupuncture for postoperative nausea and vomiting in laparoscopic gynecological surgery: a randomized controlled trial. Acupunct Med 2022;40(5):415–24.

[64] Acupuncture. Available at: https://www.medicare.gov/coverage/acupuncture. Accessed March 26, 2023.

[65] Harbell MW, Barendrick LN, Mi L, et al. Patient Attitudes Toward Acupuncture in the Perioperative Setting. J Integr Complement Med 2022;28(4):349–54.

[66] Gan TJ, Jin Z, Meyer TA. Rescue Treatment of Postoperative Nausea and Vomiting: A Systematic Review of Current Clinical Evidence. Anesth Analg 2022;135(5):986–1000.

[67] Uribe A, Bergese SA. What is the ideal combination antiemetic regimen? Best Pract Res Clin Anaesthesiol 2020;34(4):701–12.

[68] Elvir-Lazo OL, White PF, Yumul R, et al. Management strategies for the treatment and prevention of postoperative/postdischarge nausea and vomiting: an updated review. F1000Res. 2020;9:F1000 Faculty Rev-983.

[69] Yang R, Wolfson M, Lewis MC. Unique Aspects of the Elderly Surgical Population: An Anesthesiologist's Perspective. Geriatr Orthop Surg Rehabil 2011;2(2):56–64.

[70] Apfel CC, Heidrich FM, Jukar-Rao S, et al. Evidence-based analysis of risk factors for postoperative nausea and vomiting. Br J Anaesth 2012;109(5):742–53.

[71] Franck M, Radtke FM, Apfel CC, et al. Documentation of post-operative nausea and vomiting in routine clinical practice. J Int Med Res 2010;38:1034–41.
[72] Johansson E, Hultin M, Myrberg T, et al. Early post-operative nausea and vomiting: A retrospective observational study of 2030 patients. Acta Anaesthesiol Scand 2021;65:1229–39.
[73] Halliday TA, Sundqvist J, Hultin M, et al. Post-operative nausea and vomiting in bariatric surgery patients: an observational study. Acta Anaesthesiol Scand 2017;61(5):471–9.
[74] Habib AS, Chen YT, Taguchi A, et al. Postoperative nausea and vomiting following inpatient surgeries in a teaching hospital: a retrospective database analysis. Curr Med Res Opin 2006;22(6):1093–9.
[75] Gan TJ, Diemunsch P, Habib AS, et al. Society for Ambulatory Anesthesia. Consensus guidelines for the management of postoperative nausea and vomiting. Anesth Analg 2014;118:85–113.
[76] Kazemi-Kjellberg F, Henzi I, Tramèr MR. Treatment of established postoperative nausea and vomiting: a quantitative systemic review. BMC Anesthesiol 2001;1:2.
[77] Kovac AL, O'Connor TA, Pearman MH, et al. Efficacy of repeat intravenous dosing of ondansetron in controlling postoperative nausea and vomiting: a randomized, double-blind, placebo-controlled multicenter trial. J Clin Anesth 1999;11:453–9.
[78] Cho E, Kim DH, Shin S, et al. Efficacy of palonosetron-dexamethasone combination versus palonosetron alone for preventing nausea and vomiting related to opioid-based analgesia: a prospective, randomized, double-blind trial. Int J Med Sci 2018;15:961–8.
[79] Ormel G, Romundstad L, Lambert-Jensen P, et al. Dexamethasone has additive effect when combined with ondansetron and droperidol for treatment of established PONV. Acta Anaesthesiol Scand 2011;55:1196–205.
[80] Candiotti KA, Kranke P, Bergese SD, et al. Randomized, Double-Blind, Placebo-Controlled Study of Intravenous Amisulpride as Treatment of Established Postoperative Nausea and Vomiting in Patients Who Have Had No Prior Prophylaxis. Anesth Analg 2019;128(6):1098–105.
[81] Fox GM, Albayaty M, Walker JL, et al. Intravenous amisulpride does not meaningfully prolong the QTc interval at doses effective for the management of postoperative nausea and vomiting. Anesth Analg 2021;132(1):150–9.
[82] Roberts GW, Bekker TB, Carlsen HH, et al. Postoperative nausea and vomiting are strongly influenced by postoperative opioid use in a dose-related manner. Anesth Analg 2005;101(5):1343–8.
[83] Mansoor A, Ellwood S, Hoffman G, et al. The efficacy and safety of transversus abdominis plane blocks after open cholecystectomy in low- and middle-income countries. J Surg Res 2020;256:136–42.
[84] Najeeb HN, Mehdi SR, Siddiqui AM, et al. Pectoral nerves I, II and serratus plane blocks in multimodal analgesia for mastectomy: A Randomised Clinical Trial. J Coll Physicians Surg Pak 2019;29(10):910–4.
[85] Thomas JS, Maple IK, Norcross W, et al. Preoperative risk assessment to guide prophylaxis and reduce the incidence of postoperative nausea and vomiting. Journal of Perianesthesia Nursing. Official Journal of the American Society of PeriAnesthesia Nurses 2019;34(1):74–85.
[86] Metoclopramide. Package Insert. Hospira Inc. Lake Forest Il. 60045.
[87] American Parkinson's Disease Association. Medications to be avoided or used with caution in Parkinson's Disease. Revised March 2018. Available at: https://www.apdaparkinson.org/wp-content/uploads/2018/05/APDA-Meds_to_Avoid.pdf. Accessed on April 14, 2023.
[88] Okun M. Parkinson's Treatment Tips on the Worst Drugs for Parkinson's Disease. Univ. of Florida Movement Disorder & Neurorestoration Program Blog. Sept. 22, 2011. Available at: https://movementdisorders.ufhealth.org/2011/09/22/parkinsons-treatment-tips-on-the-worst-drugs-for-parkinsons-disease/. Accessed April 14, 2023.

[89] Rumore MM. Cardiovascular adverse effects of metoclopramide: Review of literature. Int J Case Rep Images 2012;3(5):1–10.

[90] American Geriatrics Society. 2019 Updated AGS Beers Criteria® for Potentially Inappropriate Medication Use in Older Adults. J Am Geriatr Soc 2019;67:674–94.

[91] Lexicomp Online, Droperidol Online. Waltham, MA: UpToDate, Inc.; July 30, 2021. Updated 2-23-23 Available at: https://online-lexi-com.srv-proxy1.library.tamu.edu. Accessed April 9, 2023.

[92] Lexicomp Online, Haloperidol Online. Waltham, MA: UpToDate, Inc.; July 30, 2021. Updated 4-12-2023. Available at: https://online-lexi-com.srv-proxy1.library.tamu.edu. Accessed April 9, 2023.

[93] Lexicomp Online, Prochlorperazine Online. Waltham, MA: UpToDate, Inc.; July 30, 2021. Updated 4-4-2023. Available at: https://online-lexi-com.srv-proxy1.library.tamu.edu. Accessed April 9, 2023.

[94] Lexicomp Online, Diphenhydramine Online. Waltham, MA: UpToDate, Inc.; July 30, 2021. Updated 4-15-2023. Available at: https://online-lexi-com.srv-proxy1.library.tamu.edu. Accessed April 9, 2023.

[95] Lexicomp Online, Promethazine Online. Waltham, MA: UpToDate, Inc.; 2021. Updated 4-8-2023. Available at: https://online-lexi-com.srv-proxy1.library.tamu.edu. Accessed April 15, 2023.

[96] Lexicomp Online, Scopolamine Online. Waltham, MA: UpToDate, Inc.; July 30, 2021. Updated 4-15-2023. Available at: https://online-lexi-com.srv-proxy1.library.tamu.edu. Accessed April 15, 2023.

[97] Zofran (ondansetron). Package insert. Research Triangle (NC): GlaxoSmithKline; 2010.

[98] Dexamethasone sodium phosphate Inj. Package insert. Hikma Pharmaceuticals, USA Inc; 2019.

Advances in Anesthesia 41 (2023) 39–52

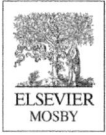

ADVANCES IN ANESTHESIA

ELSEVIER
MOSBY

Peer Support and Second Victim Programs for Anesthesia Professionals Involved in Stressful or Traumatic Clinical Events

Robyn E. Finney, APRN, CRNA, DNAP*, Adam K. Jacob, MD

Department of Anesthesiology and Perioperative Medicine, Mayo Clinic, 200 1st Street Southwest, Rochester, MN 55905, USA

Keywords
- Second victim • Peer support • Health care • CRNA • Anesthetist
- Anesthesiologist

Key points
- Anesthesia professionals are involved in stressful and traumatic clinical events that may evoke emotional responses and lead to second victim experiences.
- High-risk events likely to trigger second victim experiences include intraoperative patient demise, intraoperative cardiac arrest, and adverse events involving pediatric patients.
- Peer support is the most desired form of support by anesthesia professionals involved in such events.
- Second victim peer support programs offer a means for anesthesia professionals to offload and normalize the associated emotional labor and learn about additional supportive resources.
- Developing second victim peer support programs can help reduce departmental and institutional turnover, enhance employee perceptions of support, and foster a culture of safety.

INTRODUCTION

Imagine one of the following scenarios: you inadvertently give an incorrect medication resulting in patient harm, vascular injury occurs in your patient during a routine procedure resulting in resuscitation and massive transfusion,

*Corresponding author. E-mail address: finney.robyn@mayo.edu

https://doi.org/10.1016/j.aan.2023.05.003

or your patient dies after an unexpected intraoperative cardiac arrest. These perioperative scenarios may evoke negative feelings or emotions within any member of the health care team involved in the care of those patients. The patient is the victim of the error or adverse event, but those caring for the patient can also be negatively affected by the experience. Any (or all) members of those health care teams become a second victim (SV).

ADVERSE EVENTS IN ACUTE CARE SETTINGS

It is estimated that 8% to 12% of hospitalized patients experience an adverse event, approximately half of these events are considered preventable [1] and the mortality rate may reach 8% [2]. Most adverse events in hospitalized patients are related to surgical care, medications and fluids, or health care-acquired infection. Approximately 14% of surgical patients experience an adverse event; fortunately, most events are minor–moderate in severity [3]. Adverse events, even minor, can be mentally and emotionally taxing for health care team members involved in the patient's care.

SECOND VICTIMS IN HEALTH CARE

The term SV is commonly defined as a health care professional who is emotionally traumatized following an unexpected adverse event, such as a medical error or patient-related injury or death. In these situations, health care professionals may experience a wide range of negative feelings and emotions such as guilt, shame, anxiety, fear of judgment, or isolation [4].

No one in health care is immune from SV experiences. The prevalence of SVs after an adverse event varies from 10.4% to 43.3% [5]. Nearly half of clinicians involved in these events report moderately or severely negative impact on their lives [6].

SECOND VICTIMS IN ANESTHESIA

Anesthesia professionals, including Certified Registered Nurse Anesthetists (CRNAs) and anesthesiologists, can be profoundly affected by these events. Surveys have estimated that 60% to 80% of anesthesia professionals have been involved in an adverse event during their career that negatively affected them emotionally or physically [7,8], and the majority report compromised well-being. According to a survey conducted within our large, academic anesthesiology department [7], the most frequent feelings or emotions reported by staff include:

- Reliving the event (78%)
- Guilt (72%)
- Anxiety (71%)
- Professional self-doubt (56%)
- Depression (54%)
- Sleeplessness (54%)

During the same departmental survey, the most common perioperative events (ranked most common to least common) that triggered SV experiences among anesthesia professionals include:

- Intraoperative cardiac arrest and/or patient demise
- Event involving a child
- Multiple difficult events over brief time
- Prolonged resuscitation
- Medication error
- Patient known/familiar to staff
- Organ donation case
- Violent patient and/or staff
- Unanticipated difficult airway
- Intraoperative awareness

These results, particularly the most common reason (ie, intraoperative cardiac arrest or death), were similar to a 2012 survey of American Society of Anesthesiologists members [8].

SUPPORTING SECOND VICTIMS

Whether the SV is an anesthesia professional or any member of the health care team, SV experiences can have long-lasting physical and psychosocial consequences. As one surgeon stated "We all hide our grief, suffer in silence. The pain can be close to debilitating" [9]. In rare cases, SV experiences may result in impaired job performance, absenteeism, maladaptive behaviors such as drug or alcohol abuse, job or career change, or even suicidal ideation [4,10,11]. Given the negative impact of adverse events on the well-being of health care professionals, providing easy access to psychological support is crucial.

Most hospitals have an employee assistance program (EAP), but after a patient is harmed, involved staff members may be reluctant to contact EAP. This may be because they worry that the EAP will report back to their supervisor, or because they do not believe that the counselors have the clinical perspective to understand the event. In general, many health care professionals suffer alone [12,13].

Studies have indicated anesthesia professionals most desire talking to peers after involvement in such traumatic events [7,8,14], which is similar among other health care specialties [15–20]. Peer support offers empathy, normalization, and immediacy in provision of support unlike other supportive resources such as an EAP or counseling services. Numerous institutions across the country have developed peer support programs to help SVs process the associated sequelae [8,15–23].

CREATING A PEER SUPPORT PROGRAM

Developing peer support programs takes time, resources, patience, and planning. Numerous SV champions have described the process of creating and launching peer support programs [7,11,15,18,20,23,24,25]. The general process is similar across groups and institutions and involves the following key steps.

- Conduct a needs assessment—*understand the "why"*
- Obtain leadership endorsement—*secure time and resources*
- Create logistical framework—*establish who, what, when, how*
- Recruit and train peer supporters—*ready an army of Trained Peer Supporters*
- Communicate and socialize the program—*ensure the program is known*
- Monitor and maintain—*track program success, continuously review*

Our program began from the interest and discretionary effort of a single champion, who gradually developed the program over 3 years. Within our large anesthesiology department, an SV peer support program called Healing Emotional Lives of Peers (HELP) was officially activated in July 2018 [7].

The HELP Program consists of a three-tiered escalating system of support, modeled after the Scott Three-Tiered Interventional Model of Second Victim support (Fig. 1) [20]. The first tier includes support from supervisors and peers at the local level where the event occurred. The second tier is one-on-one support offered by an anesthesia colleague who has completed specialized training and voluntarily serves as aTPS. The third tier includes supportive resources beyond peers, including the EAP, chaplaincy, and patient safety. The key hallmarks of an SV peer support program include:

- Immediacy of support
- Credibility of peers
- Confidentiality
- Voluntary access
- Emotional support and guidance rather than rehashing event details
- Facilitation of support to resources beyond that of peers
- Proactive rather than reactive outreach

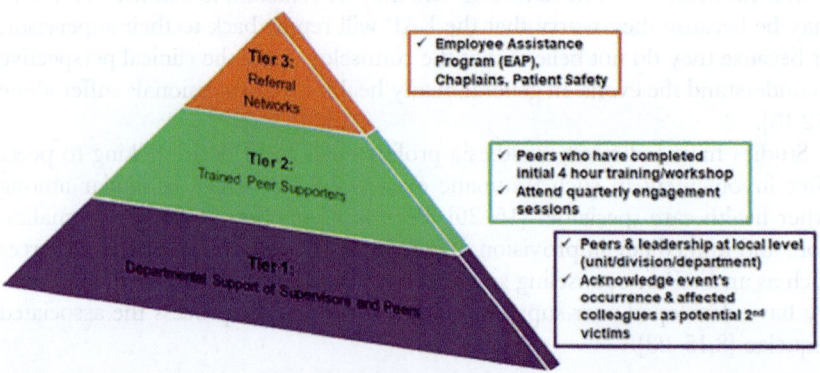

Fig. 1. Three-tiered system of support. (*From* Finney RE, Jacob A, Johnson J, Messner H, Pulos B, Sviggum H. Implementation of a Second Victim Peer Support Program in a Large Anesthesia Department. AANA J. 2021;89(3):235-244.)

Needs assessment and leadership endorsement

To begin, the champion conducted literature reviews, attended workshops, and consulted with subject matter experts (SME) from established peer support programs to become an SME herself. Then, a departmental needs assessment was conducted examining the impact of perioperative adverse events on anesthesia professionals along with their desired support. Sixty-five percent of the department believed that there were inadequate supportive resources available and the most desired form of post-event support was talking to a peer [7]. From this, leadership endorsement was obtained and resources dedicated to augment support for anesthesia professionals as SVs.

Create logistical framework

A leadership/advisory team was created consisting of four CRNAs and five anesthesiologists. These team members, hand-picked and invited to participate, were respected and trustworthy members of the department, held leadership positions, possessed effective communication skills, worked in various clinical areas across the practice, and conveyed passion for the subject matter. The advisory team met monthly, provided guidance for program logistics, and served as champions for the program.

Relationships were established with counselors from the EAP, chaplains, and patient safety/risk managers. These resources agreed to be available for any affected colleague expressing interest in support beyond that of peers. A communication plan was created to disseminate information about the HELP Program across the department. Program brochures and fliers were created and dispersed in clinical work rooms. Presentations were made at departmental grand rounds, divisional meetings, and residency and nurse anesthesia graduate training programs. The program was also featured in departmental newsletters.

An example program format is illustrated in Fig. 2. A program intranet Web site was developed on the departmental homepage and served as the main mechanism to request support from a peer. Requests could be made on behalf of colleagues involved in stressful clinical events or self-referrals could be initiated. Once an online request for support was submitted, it was routed to a dedicated shared electronic mailbox, accessible only by the HELP leadership/advisory team. Members of this team rotate monitoring the inbox for new requests and matching the affected colleagues (ACs) to TPSs. If feasible, the colleague is matched to a TPS in the same clinical division to optimize shared experiences and timely, in-person outreaches due to geographic proximity.

Recruit and train peer supporters

Establishing a group of colleagues to serve as TPSs is crucial for program success. Selecting TPSs can be done with a nomination or volunteer process. Nomination can be done by departmental leadership or by the entire department. We chose to use a volunteer process, and all members within the department were invited to participate in the HELP Program workshop. Our goal was to have a minimum of 5% to 10% of the department serve as TPSs with

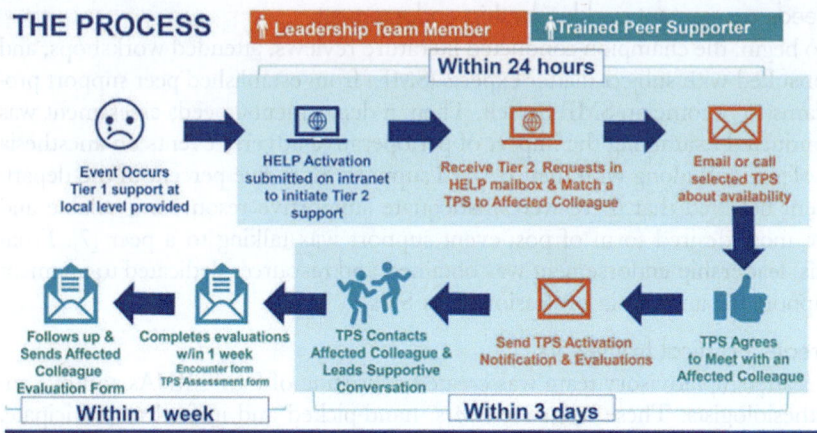

Fig. 2. Example of peer support program process. (*From* Finney RE, Jacob A, Johnson J, Messner H, Pulos B, Sviggum H. Implementation of a Second Victim Peer Support Program in a Large Anesthesia Department. AANA J. 2021;89(3):235-244.)

balanced representation of clinical specialties, sex, age, leadership positions, and educational programs. Having departmental, graduate medical and allied health graduate program leaders attend was important to have them aware of the resource and serve as advocates for the HELP Program. Ideally, anesthesia professionals who serve as a TPS possess emotional intelligence, effective communication, active listening, respect for others, and approachability.

After identifying staff members interested in serving as TPSs, education needs to be provided to ensure that these individuals feel competent and comfortable supporting colleagues as SVs. At our institution, a 4-hour workshop was developed to increase awareness of the SV phenomenon and HELP Program logistics and to equip participants with the knowledge and skills to effectively support colleagues as SVs. Workshop content included recommendations from reputable peer support programs, evidence-based literature on SV educational curriculums [25], and the "Second Victim Train the Trainer" workshop sponsored by the University of Missouri's forYOU Program and the Center for Patient Safety in St Louis, Missouri [20]. An example workshop curriculum is shown in Table 1. TPSs are taught important "Do and Don't" aspects of providing peer support [7,24].

DO

- Provide an empathetic, reassuring, and nonjudgmental presence
- Focus on the emotional implication; how involvement in the event made the affected colleague feel
- Allow for silence; provide space and time for the affected peer to reflect and think
- Actively listen
- Be aware of your nonverbal communication

Table 1
Workshop curriculum

Topic	Objectives
Defining the Second Victim Phenomenon	• Discuss the concept of "Second Victim" • Discuss high-risk situations which lead to second victim phenomenon • Review signs and symptoms
Predictable Recovery Trajectory of Second Victim	• Describe tool for enhancing peer support and understanding second victim experiences • Define the six stages of recovery • Discuss supportive interventions associated with each stage
Peer Support Interventions	• Discuss challenges with seeking and/or providing support • Discuss critical messages for leadership and peers • Define psychological first aid • Discuss characteristics of one-on-one peer interactions • Explain four-step approach to providing peer support (Introduction/Exploration/Normalization/Follow-up)
Caring in Action: Skill Building	• Identify techniques to facilitate supportive interactions with second victims • Practice roles of peer supporter and second victim using four-step approach
SV Peer Support Program Logistics	• Describe three tiers of support • Discuss how peer support program is activated or requested • Discuss resources available beyond peer support • Discuss metrics to monitor and iterate the program

- Reflect on what you heard and paraphrase
- Discuss available support resources and how to access them
- Use informational brochures on SVs
- Keep strictly confidential

DON'T

- Try to fix the situation
- Assume your past experiences are the same
- Insist on a supportive conversation if affected colleague declines
- Fill silence with unnecessary words
- Discuss event details
- Critique what happened in the event
- Tell affected colleague what to do
- Take notes
- Break confidentiality

The workshop was conducted twice by a SME, with provision of protected time and continuing educational credits. Instructional methods included didactic lecture, review of relevant literature, video analysis of anesthesia professionals' SV experiences, round table discussions, skill-building activities, and role-playing exercises [7]. If a local SME is not available to do the training, qualified instructors can be used from external sources at an expense.

Communicate and socialize the program

Once program logistics and a group of TPSs were established, an awareness campaign was conducted to communicate and socialize the HELP Program. Presentations were done at Anesthesia Grand Rounds, divisional meetings, departmental journal clubs, and within the residency and nurse anesthesia educational programs. Informational brochures and fliers were disseminated throughout clinical workrooms.

Monitor and maintain

Efforts are needed to ensure program sustainability. Program evaluation consisted of brief electronic surveys for TPSs and ACs to complete after any supportive outreach/interaction. These surveys evaluated TPSs' experiences in supporting colleagues as SVs and ACs' experiences in receiving support. Program usage was also tracked to assess what types of clinical events triggered requests for peer support, demographic variables of program users, and number of activations requesting peer support. To ensure TPSs remain confident and comfortable in their role, quarterly engagement sessions are offered. These consist of program updates, education on skills, and dedicated time to support each other. Program sustainability should incorporate opportunities for TPSs to stay engaged.

Plans to expand the program should be considered to deal with natural attrition, departmental growth, or desire for peer support outside of a single department. Subsequent workshops were offered on a quarterly basis to onboard additional TPSs and to increase awareness of the SV phenomenon and the HELP Program within the large anesthesiology department. Additional TPSs were recruited from educational programs and high-risk areas such as cardiac, pediatrics, obstetrics, and trauma. Having more TPSs in these clinical specialties made it easier to find available TPSs with shared experiences to do timely outreaches. Related education was built into the curriculums of anesthesia residents and student registered nurse anesthetists, and ongoing educational offerings were conducted at regional and national conferences for anesthesia professionals.

The final aspect of sustainability is having a program that offers support in a proactive manner. Anesthesia professionals are unlikely to seek help for themselves. Successful SV peer support programs won't wait for affected colleagues to show signs of distress. They assume that involved colleagues will benefit from a supportive outreach from a colleague. They start to make supportive outreaches part of the norm within the departmental culture. Peer support is integrated into current clinical processes to make it an automatic referral for colleagues involved in high-risk events. Automated processes should be established for health care professionals involved in cases discussed at morbidity and mortality conferences or root cause analyses. Those in leadership positions can also create a culture where acknowledging events and referral of involved staff to the SV peer support program is the normal situation. Peer support programs should not rely on anesthesia professionals asking for help or manifesting signs of distress, but rather as soon as an event occurs, clinicians are identified and contacted as potential SVs who may benefit from peer support.

OUTCOMES OF DEPARTMENTAL PEER SUPPORT PROGRAM

Over the first 2 years of the HELP Program, 91 requests for peer support were submitted on the program's intranet Web site for 179 anesthesia professionals. Of these, 122 supportive encounters were documented. From these encounters, 85 TPS self-assessments were completed with 84 (98.8%) feeling they were able to provide helpful support and 80 (94.1%) feeling comfortable with their knowledge and skills when supporting colleagues. In addition, 31 evaluations were received from anesthesia professionals that received peer support [7]; 25 (80.6%) indicated the support they received was "extremely" or "very beneficial," and 28 (90.3%) were "extremely" or "very satisfied" with the experience overall. The majority (96.8%) said they would recommend the HELP Program to a colleague in the future [7].

The impact of the HELP Program was assessed 2 years after implementation [26]. Nearly all respondents (227/231; 98.3%) indicated awareness of the SV peer support program. Most (81.7%) agreed that the program contributed to fostering a culture of safety. Other SV peer support programs had similar outcomes related to having positive influence on the department's culture of safety [24].

Besides surveying department members about awareness and impact of a peer support program, an alternative validated instrument (Second Victim Experience and Support [SVEST] Tool) exists that can help groups track the performance of SV support resources [27]. We used the SVEST to compare anesthesia professionals' SV experiences pre-implementation and 2 years post-implementation of the HELP program [26]. A higher proportion of respondents indicated SV-related psychological distress pre-implementation versus post-implementation (24.3% vs 16.4%). This suggests that having a SV peer support program may help mitigate psychological sequalae related to SV experiences. Higher levels of perceived coworker support have been correlated to lower levels of SV-related anxiety and depression [19]. More anesthesia professionals indicated feeling that institutional support was inadequate before HELP Program implementation (23.1% vs 3.7%). Having a peer support program available at the departmental level may positively influence anesthesia professionals' perceptions of support available at the institutional level.

SVs may report feelings of wanting to change jobs or avoid work. Turnover intentions and absenteeism are costly to departments and institutions. At both time periods (pre-implementation and post-implementation), a small number of department members reported SV-related turnover intentions (7.6% pre vs

6.8% post) and absenteeism (5.7% pre vs 9.3% post) [26]. In a study looking at the impact of a SV peer support program on health care professionals in our children's hospital, fewer respondents agreed with having SV-related turnover intentions 1-year post-implementation compared with pre-implementation of the SV peer support program (18.2% vs 9.2%) [16]. This suggests that having an SV peer support program may help SVs work through the associated distress and mitigate SV-related turnover intentions. A cost–benefit analysis indicated that having an SV peer support program may help reduce turnover intentions [28].

Finally, outcomes related to the internal aspect of the HELP Program were assessed by surveying TPSs on their perspective of serving colleagues. The majority (92.5%) agreed that serving as a TPS has been a positive experience, which resonates with other studies looking at retention of peer supporters for SV peer support programs [29]. The best part of serving as a voluntary TPS was reported as:

- Supporting colleagues (93%)
- Increasing awareness of the SV phenomenon (68%)
- Breaking down walls of silence (68%)
- Professional growth (50%)
- Personal growth (48%)

EXPANDING PEER SUPPORT BEYOND ANESTHESIA

When developing a peer support program at the departmental level, plans to expand the program should be considered. Within 6 months of implementing the HELP Program, demand for access to the program came from other disciplines and specialties including surgery, pediatrics, obstetrics, and emergency care. The HELP Program expanded into the affiliated Children's Center, six hospitals and clinics in the health systems, and obstetrics within 18 months. Individual training sessions were conducted with each of these groups to develop TPSs among these specialties and regional areas. Additional requests from other disciplines and groups continued, but volunteer time was exhausted. To ease the burden, a health system engineer was supported by institutional leadership to facilitate program expansion and scalability. Expanding the program throughout the hospital and beyond takes additional time and resources.

Establishing institutional buy-in for SV peer support programs can be challenging. In response to COVID-19, the HELP Program was acknowledged as a silo of excellence and resources were mobilized to ensure that the SV peer support program was available to all employees.[30] Dedicated time and financial resources were provided to expand the program across the organization. Hospital leadership endorsed an operational home and advisory team within employee well-being, along with dedicated administrative support. Key roles were established, including dedicated time (0.4 full time equivalent [FTE]) for an administrative assistant to match new requests to TPSs within 24 to 72 hours of receiving the request. This individual also invites ACs and TPSs to voluntarily complete program evaluations 2 weeks after the initial request via email communication. HELP Program ambassadors were selected from each enterprise site to serve as volunteer champions for the program. The SME was granted administrative time (0.1 FTE) to help with program logistics and ongoing educational needs. The educational training quickly converted from in-person settings to an interactive virtual format, allowing multidisciplinary professionals to attend from various time zones. This format also allowed the same SME, along with a physician colleague, to deliver the content rather than using resources to develop a train-the-trainer curriculum.

A robust marketing campaign was essential for program success across the enterprise. An enterprise-wide HELP Program intranet Web site was established within the protected firewall. This Web site is accessible to all employees and serves as the hub for requesting peer support. SharePoint was used to organize program logistics, lists of TPSs, and new requests for peer support. Presentations were delivered at medical grand rounds, divisional meetings, and new employee orientations. The organization's committee and communications structures were used to share program information via numerous newsletters. Partnerships were developed with high-risk clinical divisions and violent patient workgroups to allow for timely and proactive supportive outreaches. Employees shared their experiences with the HELP Program on the enterprise news center to demystify the resource and to personalize peer support.

OUTCOMES OF ENTERPRISE PEER SUPPORT PROGRAM
Since going live across the institutional enterprise, the HELP Program has been used regularly [7,16,26,30,31]. Between April 2020 and December 2021, 827 employees attended one of the 22 virtual workshops to train TPSs and augment awareness of the HELP Program. After these workshops, 522 employees voluntarily serve as TPSs for the HELP Program.[30]

During this timeframe, a total of 247 activations were submitted through the HELP Program's intranet Web site and peer support was requested for 649 employees. Three-fourths of peer support requests were made on behalf of affected colleagues, whereas one-fourth were self-referrals.[30] The most common events leading to using the HELP Program across the enterprise included:

- Unexpected patient demise (33%)
- Adverse event with pediatric patient (23%)
- Unexpected patient decline (16%)

The program received 268 self-assessments from TPSs who had provided support to affected colleagues as SVs, and 226 (84.3%) believed they provided helpful support. One hundred affected colleagues who received support completed evaluations; 93% indicated being "extremely" or "very satisfied" with the program overall, and 100% indicated they would recommend the HELP Program to a colleague.[30]

The HELP Program has worked closely with high-risk clinical specialties and educational programs to automate referrals for peer support after root cause analyses, morbidity and mortality conferences, violent patient encounters, and other high-risk situations. HELP has also expanded support to all learners in our institutions' allied health programs, graduate medical education, and medical school. In addition, HELP recently welcomed employees involved in acts of racism or discrimination in the workplace, and currently has 20 TPSs with specialty training to support employees as victims of discrimination.

SUMMARY

Modern anesthetic care is very safe, and serious adverse events occur rarely. When they do, anesthesia professionals are vulnerable to SV phenomena. SV experiences can result in significant and long-lasting psychological and emotional consequences if not addressed. Peer support can help anesthesia professionals cope with the negative sequelae of SV experiences. Peer support programs take time and resources to create, but offer great benefit to health care professionals, departments, and institutions once established.

CLINICS CARE POINTS

- Anesthesia professionals will be involved in perioperative adverse events that may lead to emotional or physiological implications, or second victim experiences.
- SV experiences of anesthesia professionals should be acknowledged; proactive support should be offered, focusing on the emotional implications rather than on event details.
- Key interventions when supporting colleagues as second victims include active listening and validation of shared emotions.
- Second victim peer support programs allow for timely support, normalization through shared experiences, minimization of suffering in silence, and connection to resources beyond support from peers.

DISCLOSURE

The authors have no funding sources and no relevant commercial or financial conflicts of interest.

References

[1] Rafter N, Hickey A, Condell S, et al. Adverse events in healthcare: learning from mistakes. QJM 2015;108(4):273-7.

[2] Schwendimann R, Blatter C, Dhaini S, et al. The occurrence, types, consequences and preventability of in-hospital adverse events - a scoping review. BMC Health Serv Res 2018;18(1):521.

[3] Anderson O, Davis R, Hanna GB, et al. Surgical adverse events: a systematic review. Am J Surg 2013;206(2):253-62.

[4] Scott SD, Hirschinger LE, Cox KR, et al. The natural history of recovery for the healthcare provider "second victim" after adverse patient events. Qual Saf Health Care 2009;18(5): 325-30.

[5] Seys D, Wu AW, Van Gerven E, et al. Health care professionals as second victims after adverse events: a systematic review. Eval Health Prof 2013;36(2):135–62.

[6] de Wit ME, Marks CM, Natterman JP, et al. Supporting second victims of patient safety events: shouldn't these communications be covered by legal privilege? J Law Med Ethics 2013;41(4):852–8, Table of Contents.

[7] Finney RE, Jacob A, Johnson J, et al. Implementation of a Second Victim Peer Support Program in a Large Anesthesia Department. AANA J (Am Assoc Nurse Anesth) 2021;89(3): 235–44.

[8] Gazoni FM, Amato PE, Malik ZM, et al. The impact of perioperative catastrophes on anesthesiologists: results of a national survey. Anesth Analg 2012;114(3):596–603.

[9] Han K, Bohnen JD, Peponis T, et al. The Surgeon as the Second Victim? Results of the Boston Intraoperative Adverse Events Surgeons' Attitude (BISA) Study. J Am Coll Surg 2017;224(6):1048–56.

[10] Busch IM, Moretti F, Campagna I, et al. Promoting the Psychological Well-Being of Healthcare Providers Facing the Burden of Adverse Events: A Systematic Review of Second Victim Support Resources. Int J Environ Res Public Health 2021;18(10); https://doi.org/10. 3390/ijerph18105080.

[11] Merandi J, Liao N, Lewe D, et al. Deployment of a Second Victim Peer Support Program: A Replication Study. Pediatr Qual Saf 2017;2(4):e031.

[12] Ullstrom S, Andreen Sachs M, Hansson J, et al. Suffering in silence: a qualitative study of second victims of adverse events. BMJ Qual Saf 2014;23(4):325–31.

[13] Joint Commission. Supporting Second Victims. Quick Safety 2018;39:1–3.

[14] Dhillon AKRD, Stiegler MP. Catastrophic Events in the Perioperative Setting: A Survey of U.S. Anesthesiologists. Int J Emerg Ment Health 2015;17(3):661–3.

[15] Edrees H, Connors C, Paine L, et al. Implementing the RISE second victim support programme at the Johns Hopkins Hospital: a case study. BMJ Open 2016;6(9):e011708.

[16] Finney RE, Czinski S, Fjerstad K, et al. Evaluation of a Second Victim Peer Support Program on Perceptions of Second Victim Experiences and Supportive Resources in Pediatric Clinical Specialties Using the Second Victim Experience and Support Tool (SVEST). J Pediatr Nurs 2021;61:312–7.

[17] Finney RE, Torbenson VE, Riggan KA, et al. Second victim experiences of nurses in obstetrics and gynaecology: A Second Victim Experience and Support Tool Survey. J Nurs Manag 2021;29(4):642–52.

[18] Klatt TE, Sachs JF, Huang CC, et al. Building a Program of Expanded Peer Support for the Entire Health Care Team: No One Left Behind. Jt Comm J Qual Patient Saf 2021;47(12): 759–67.

[19] Merandi JWA, Liao N, Rogers E, et al. Implementation of a second victim program in the neonatal intensive care unit: an interim analysis of employee satisfaction. J Patient Saf Risk Manag 2018;23(6):231–8.

[20] Scott SD, Hirschinger LE, Cox KR, et al. Caring for our own: deploying a systemwide second victim rapid response team. Jt Comm J Qual Patient Saf 2010;36(5):233–40.

[21] Krzan KD, Merandi J, Morvay S, et al. Implementation of a "second victim" program in a pediatric hospital. Am J Health Syst Pharm 2015;72(7):563–7.

[22] Lane MA, Newman BM, Taylor MZ, et al. Supporting Clinicians After Adverse Events: Development of a Clinician Peer Support Program. J Patient Saf 2018;14(3):e56–60.

[23] Thompson M, Hunnicutt R, Broadhead M, et al. Implementation of a Certified Registered Nurse Anesthetist Second Victim Peer Support Program. J Perianesth Nurs 2022;37(2): 167–173 e1.

[24] El Hechi MW, Bohnen JD, Westfal M, et al. Design and Impact of a Novel Surgery-Specific Second Victim Peer Support Program. J Am Coll Surg 2020;230(6):926–33.

[25] Daniels RG, McCorkle R. Design of an Evidence-Based "Second Victim" Curriculum for Nurse Anesthetists. AANA J (Am Assoc Nurse Anesth) 2016;84(2):107–13.

[26] Pelikan M, Finney R, Jacob A. Use of the Second Victim Experience and Support Tool (SVEST) to Assess the Impact of a Departmental Peer Support Program on Anesthesia Providers' SVEs and Perceptions of Support Two Years After Implementation. *AANA J (Am Assoc Nurse Anesth)*, in press.

[27] Burlison JD, Scott SD, Browne EK, et al. The Second Victim Experience and Support Tool: Validation of an Organizational Resource for Assessing Second Victim Effects and the Quality of Support Resources. J Patient Saf 2017;13(2):93–102.

[28] Moran D, Wu AW, Connors C, et al. Cost-Benefit Analysis of a Support Program for Nursing Staff. J Patient Saf 2020;16(4):e250–4.

[29] Connors CA, Dukhanin V, Norvell M, et al. RISE: Exploring Volunteer Retention and Sustainability of a Second Victim Support Program. J Healthc Manag 2021;66(1):19–32.

[30] Rivera-Chiauzzi EY, Huang, L, Osborne, AK et al. Rapid Expansion of the Healing Emotional Lives of Peers (HELP) Program During COVID-19: A Second Victim Peer Support Program for Healthcare Professionals, *J Patient Saf*, in press.

[31] Rivera-Chiauzzi E, Finney RE, Riggan KA, et al. Understanding the Second Victim Experience Among Multidisciplinary Providers in Obstetrics and Gynecology. J Patient Saf 2022;18(2):e463–9.

Advances in Anesthesia 41 (2023) 53–69

ADVANCES IN ANESTHESIA

Care for the Obstetric Patient with Complex Cardiac Disease

Patrice A. Vinsard, MD, Katherine W. Arendt, MD, Emily E. Sharpe, MD*

Department of Anesthesiology and Perioperative Medicine, Mayo Clinic, 200 First Street Southwest, Rochester, MN 55905, USA

Keywords
- Cardiac disease • Congenital heart • Pregnancy • Obstetric anesthesia
- Cardiovascular • Neuraxial analgesia

Key points
- Cardiovascular disease is a leading cause of maternal morbidity and mortality in the United States and the prevalence of cardiac disease in pregnancy is increasing.
- Pregnant patients with cardiovascular disease should be evaluated by a multidisciplinary Pregnancy Heart Team, including an anesthesiologist, in the antepartum period.
- Risk stratification tools such as the ZAHARA, CARPREG II, and the modified World Health Organization Classification of Cardiovascular Disease in Pregnancy guide delivery locale and strategies.
- Anesthesiologists play a crucial role in caring for patients with cardiovascular disease by providing effective labor analgesia and surgical anesthesia, preventing adverse cardiac events, and leading rapid resuscitations.

INTRODUCTION

The maternal mortality rate in the United States in 2020 was 23.8/100,000, which is higher than any other industrialized nation [1]. Death from pregnancy or childbirth disproportionately affects Black and non-Hispanic American Indian or Alaska Native patients [1]. Cardiovascular diseases (CVDs) are the leading cause of maternal mortality in the United States. According to the Centers for Disease Control and Prevention, 28% of pregnancy-related deaths are attributed to various forms of cardiovascular conditions, with 12.5% due to cardiomyopathy alone [1].

*Corresponding author. E-mail address: sharpe.emily@mayo.edu

https://doi.org/10.1016/j.aan.2023.05.004
0737-6146/23/© 2023 Elsevier Inc. All rights reserved.

Experts believe that heart disease has become the leading cause of death in the obstetric population due to an increase in cardiovascular risk factors [2–6]. Over the past few decades, the number of pregnancies in women with congenital heart disease has increased globally and is expected to grow in the future [2,3]. Moreover, in comparison to the past, pregnant people are older and are more likely to have preexisting comorbidities such as diabetes mellitus, hypertension, obesity, and sleep apnea, among other cardiovascular risk factors [4–7].

Numerous organizations have recognized this issue as a crisis and have published national and international statements emphasizing the importance of diagnosing and managing CVDs during all stages of pregnancy and postpartum [5,8–10]. The anesthesiology team plays a critical role in optimizing a patient's hemodynamics and safely guiding a pregnant patient with CVD through delivery and the immediate postpartum period.

The largest available data set is the Registry of Pregnancy and Cardiac Disease cohort that includes 6000 pregnant patients with heart disease from over 60 countries [11]. These data indicate that most patients with CVDs do well when appropriate care is given including preconception counseling, risk stratification, multidisciplinary coordination, and planning. This review will focus on one essential aspect of the multidisciplinary care: the anesthetic management of women with known cardiac disease during delivery.

ANTEPARTUM

Consults/risk stratification

Women with CVD should be evaluated by a multidisciplinary Pregnancy Heart Team before delivery [5]. The American College of Obstetricians and Gynecologists (ACOG) recommends that the team, at a minimum, should consist of cardiologists, maternal–fetal medicine specialists, obstetric providers, and an anesthesiologist [5]. Depending on the underlying problem, other specialties may provide additional care and counseling (eg, neonatologists, geneticists, electrophysiologists, interventional cardiologists, cardiac surgeons, and heart failure specialists).

Individualized assessment by the Pregnancy Heart Team includes preconception counseling, risk stratification, education, and multidisciplinary coordination [12]. After a detailed history, physical examination, and appropriate testing, patients should be risk stratified to facilitate appropriate delivery location and planning. Several risk stratification tools have been published including the CARPEG II, ZAHARA, and the modified World Health Organization Classification of Cardiovascular Disease in Pregnancy (mWHO) (Fig. 1) to guide delivery strategies and support transfer to higher levels of care [13–15]. These tools should be used as a *starting point* to guide planning, but the team should individualize a plan for safe delivery and follow up, taking into account individual components of CVD, such as severity of valvular gradients, life-threatening events requiring hospitalization, or the need for early delivery [12,14,16].

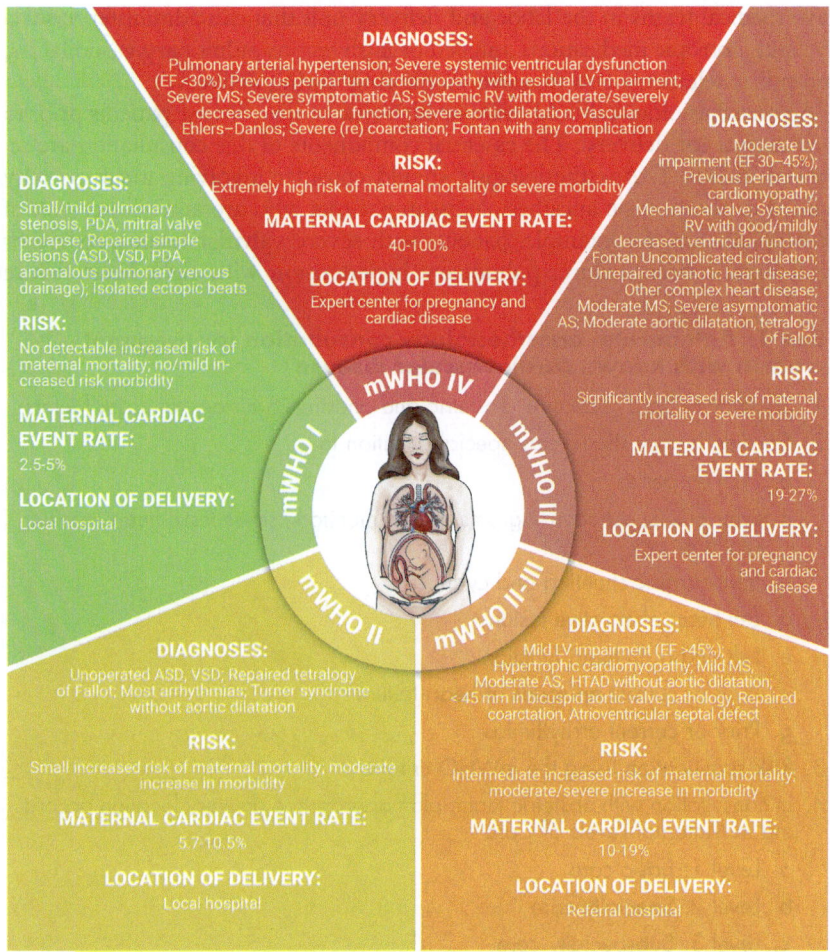

Fig. 1. Modified World Health Organization classifications of cardiovascular disease in pregnancy.[5,9]

Once risk stratified, delivery location should be decided with input from all members of the Pregnancy Heart Team. In 2019, ACOG updated the 2015 consensus on levels of maternal care in the United States. Hospitals are categorized level I to level IV and respectively defined as basic, specialty, subspecialty, and regional perinatal health care centers [17]. In general, women classified as mWHO risk class I may receive care at a maternal level I hospital (or higher) and this includes prepregnancy/pregnancy counseling, delivery and follow up (see Fig. 1) [5,9]. Higher risk patients such as class III and IV should be monitored in a maternal level IV care center where advanced therapies such as extracorporeal membrane oxygenation (ECMO), cardiac surgery, intensive care, and transplant services are available [5,9,12]. Higher levels of care should have medical teams in the labor and delivery unit that can administer vasoactive and inotropic medications, inhaled or intravenous pulmonary vasodilators, and utilize telemetry and invasive monitoring during delivery.

An anesthesiologist should evaluate high-risk cardiac disease patients prior to their arrival for delivery. The essential components of this consultation are reviewed in Box 1. Anesthesiologists should consider involving a subspecialty trained cardiothoracic anesthesiologist in patients who are at a greater risk of decompensation, for example, patients with severe valvular lesions, severe or symptomatic heart failure, pulmonary hypertension with right heart failure

---

Box 1: Antepartum anesthesiology consultation for pregnant women with known cardiovascular disease

1. Summarize cardiovascular, obstetric and anesthesia history, and risk factors
2. Cardiac history should pay special attention to
   a. Prior surgeries
   b. Prior ECGs, echocardiograms, Holter monitors, stress tests, heart catheterizations, etc.
   c. Intra-cardiac shunting and cyanosis
   d. Left heart obstructive lesions
   e. Left and right heart function
   f. Prior or current episodes of heart failure
   g. Prior or current arrhythmias
3. Risk stratification using the mWHO criteria
4. In consultation with obstetric team, plan appropriate delivery location according to Maternal Levels of Care
   a. Level 1: Basic care
   b. Level 2: Specialty care
   c. Level 3: Subspecialty care
   d. Level 4: Regional perinatal health care centers
5. Partner with Pregnancy Heart Team for anticoagulation regimen to optimize ability to perform neuraxial analgesia and anesthesia
6. Clarify in the consultation note plan for pacemaker or defibrillator
   a. Keep AICD "on" during labor
   b. Plan to keep AICD active for cesarean delivery (surgery is below umbilicus)
7. Clarify which obstetric drugs could cause hemodynamic instability
8. Partner with the Pregnancy Heart Team to clarify post-delivery plans for monitoring

Abbreviations: AICD, automatic implantable cardioverter defibrillator; ECG, electrocardiogram; mWHO, the modified World Health Organization Classification of Cardiovascular Disease in Pregnancy.
Adapted from Meng, M.L. and K.W. Arendt, Obstetric Anesthesia and Heart Disease: Practical Clinical Considerations. Anesthesiology, 2021. 135(1): p. 164-183.

or cyanosis, or any patient who may need a combined delivery and cardiac procedure. In addition, cardiothoracic anesthesiologists can provide support with echocardiography, pulmonary pressure monitoring, pulmonary vasodilator titration and ECMO initiation.

Special consideration: termination of pregnancy in high-risk patients

Patients who are categorized as mWHO IV have a high risk of mortality, and there is a general consensus that pregnancy should be discouraged [10]. Termination of pregnancy may be offered to these patients if they are in their first or early second trimester [10]. Termination in these patients can be high-risk and should be performed in a Level IV regional perinatal health care center. In patients up to 9 weeks gestation, an antiprogestin compound like mifepristone can be offered for chemically induced termination of pregnancy [10]. Even for medical abortions, mWHO IV patients should be admitted for monitoring.

For surgical management (eg,: dilation and curettage or evacuation), the choice of anesthesia depends on the severity of the disease and the hemodynamic behavior of the lesion. Neuraxial anesthesia, general anesthesia, and deep sedation with and without paracervical block may all be options; however, deep sedation may be the least optimal choice, considering the elevation of carbon dioxide, respiratory acidosis, and secondary elevation of pulmonary artery pressures. For some, a single injection spinal anesthetic with a dermatomal block to T10 may be an option [18], although rapid identification and treatment of hypotension is necessary and intraarterial blood pressure should be considered with vasopressor/inotropic support.

General anesthesia should be considered, especially for mWHO IV patients with gestational age beyond first trimester or ossification of the fetus (thereby requiring greater cervical dilation for evacuation), increased likelihood of blood loss (eg,: molar or scar pregnancy) [18], or if a patient is unable to lie flat secondary to heart failure [9]. These authors recommend that surgical terminations for mWHO IV patients occur in the cardiovascular operating room suite.

INTRAPARTUM

Vaginal delivery

Vaginal delivery is recommended for most patients with cardiac disease due to the higher risk of obstetric complications with cesarean delivery such as blood loss, infection, and venous thromboembolism [5,9,16,19]. Valsalva maneuver during vaginal delivery is believed a reasonable option for most patients with cardiovascular conditions [16]. There may be instances where assistance with the second stage of labor is recommended to avoid a forceful, prolonged, and repeated Valsalva. Because avoiding Valsalva may result in a greater risk for obstetric complications, there is a spectrum of practice. Maternal fetal medicine subspecialists may recommend assisted second stage in patients with significant ventricular dysfunction, Fontan circulation, aortic root aneurysm and severe pulmonary hypertension [20,21]. In cases where women have enlarged aortic aneurysms, a modified Valsalva maneuver with an open glottis has been described to theoretically reduce shear stress from changes in preload during repeated closed-glottis Valsalva maneuvers [21].

Monitoring during vaginal delivery

The American Society of Anesthesiologists (ASA) guidelines recommend a parturient' s vital signs and fetal heart rate be monitored and documented during neuraxial labor analgesia. Basic maternal monitoring includes heart rate, pulse oximetry, and non-invasive blood pressure measurements [21,22]. These minimum requirements may not be enough for patients with CVD to rapidly recognize cardiac, obstetric, or anesthetic emergencies. The most common cardiac complications in labor include pulmonary edema and arrhythmias. Continuous pulse oximetry with a visible waveform, 5 lead electrocardiographic monitoring, and intra-arterial blood pressure monitoring may need to be considered for patients at increased risk [5,9,14]. Audible alarms should be activated to alert for maternal arrhythmias and desaturations.

Invasive blood pressure monitoring can be considered even before the placement of neuraxial analgesia to maintain maternal blood pressure. It can be especially useful in cardiac, anesthetic, or obstetric emergencies. Consideration should be given to arterial line placement in severe left-sided outflow tract obstructions, mitral stenosis, cardiomyopathy with reduced ejection fraction, right heart dysfunction, pulmonary hypertension, or any form of CVD with concurrent preeclampsia [9].

Intravenous access must be ensured in cardiac patients although central venous access is typically reserved for the sickest patient who may need vasoactive medications or if pulmonary artery catheter pressures are needed to monitor the response of pulmonary vasodilator therapy. Transthoracic echocardiography, or if under general anesthesia transesophageal echocardiography, is useful tool for assessing heart function and can be employed if there are signs of hemodynamic instability [9].

Labor analgesia

During labor, cardiac output increases likely secondary to increased circulating plasma catecholamines, mainly norepinephrine and epinephrine, and an increase in preload during uterine contraction from autotransfusion [22]. Epidural labor analgesia is thought to reduce circulating plasma catecholamines, thereby reducing the risk of cardiovascular events, especially arrhythmias [9,23].

Consideration should be given to anticoagulation regimens in patients with cardiac disease. Communication with the different team members is key to appropriately hold peripartum anticoagulation to facilitate neuraxial procedures and reduce the risk of postpartum hemorrhage (PPH). Guidelines from The American Society of Regional Anesthesia and Society for Obstetric Anesthesia and Perinatology are readily available and help guide decision making regarding holding anticoagulation before and after neuraxial procedures [24,25].

A fluid bolus before neuraxial techniques can worsen pulmonary edema in patients with heart failure. Small fluid boluses (eg,: 200 mL) might be helpful alongside direct vasoactive medications such as phenylephrine to control blood pressure during and after a neuraxial block. If contractility is needed to increase heart rate and systemic vascular resistance (SVR), ephedrine can be a good agent to use in small doses (eg,: 5–10 mg IV). Another example is a norepinephrine infusion at 0.02 to 0.08 mcg/kg/min (or 1–6 mcg/min) to achieve inotropic support and increase SVR. This can be safely administered through a peripheral IV [26]. Other examples of medications that could be required during labor and delivery in cardiac patients include dobutamine, dopamine, and milrinone [9].

Different epidural techniques may be used to initiate labor analgesia, including a combined spinal epidural (CSE), a dural puncture epidural (DPE), or an epidural catheter. Regardless of the technique, the most important aspect is to provide safe and effective analgesia that provides pain relief and can be used for emergent cesarean delivery [9]. A DPE or CSE technique can help confirm catheter placement and facilitate sacral nerve root coverage [27]. Some reviews suggest using a loss of resistance technique with saline (not air) in patients with intracardiac shunting to decrease the chance of a paradoxical air embolism due to inadvertent intravascular puncture [28,29].

Test dose strategies to ensure proper placement of the catheter in the epidural space require special consideration in patients with CVD. A combined test dose with an epinephrine-containing local anesthetic solution (eg, 1.5% lidocaine with 1:200,000 epinephrine) is commonly used to test for intrathecal and intravascular catheter placement. However, an intravascular catheter may cause harm in patients with arrhythmias, stenotic heart lesions, or aortic pathology [9]. Alternative test dose options include a divided test dose (45–60 mg lidocaine to test for potential intrathecal placement followed by 100 mg lidocaine to test for intravascular placement), fentanyl (administer 50–100 mcg of fentanyl and monitor for intrathecal and systemic opioid effects) [30,31], or gradual titration of a dilute solution of local anesthetic in 5 mL aliquots (eg, bupivacaine 0.0625%–0.125% with 1–2 mcg/mL of fentanyl and assess for any signs or symptoms of intrathecal or intravascular placement) [32].

Labor analgesia can be maintained with a continuous epidural infusion or programmed intermittent epidural boluses using a standard local anesthetic infusion combined with opioid (eg, bupivacaine 0.0625%–0.125% with fentanyl 1–2 mcg/mL) [9,16]. During an assisted vaginal delivery, such as with vacuum or forceps, the labor epidural may require increased sacral coverage to decrease pain. Further, the epidural can be converted to a surgical block for cesarean delivery. Either assisted vaginal or cesarean delivery can be facilitated with 5 to 20 mL of epidural lidocaine 2% or chloroprocaine 3% with continued hemodynamic monitoring throughout the procedure and immediately postpartum [9].

Labor analgesia considerations (summary)
- The most common cardiac complications in labor include pulmonary edema and arrhythmias. Appropriate monitoring should be employed for patients at increased risk.

- Anticoagulation is important for patients with CVD; appropriate holding times should be discussed with the Pregnancy Heart Team to facilitate neuraxial analgesia for labor.
- In patients with heart disease, prevent, identify, and rapidly respond to pulmonary edema. Routine fluid boluses should be withheld or cautiously administered before a neuraxial technique.
- Test dose strategies should be carefully selected. Epinephrine containing solutions should be considered carefully in patients with heart disease who could decompensate from the inotropy (eg, HOCM) or arrhythmogenesis (eg, prior history of tachyarrhythmia).
- Vasoactive and inotropic medications to support blood pressure during labor should consider the patient's specific cardiovascular status. Norepinephrine is safe to give peripherally.
- Early placement of an epidural catheter allows time for trouble shooting and replacement if needed.

Cesarean delivery

Cesarean deliveries are typically reserved for obstetric indications [5]. Exceptions include patients who are actively decompensating before delivery or anticipated to acutely deteriorate at the time of delivery. Examples include decompensated severe or critical obstructive lesions, decompensated pulmonary hypertension, or any patient needing tracheal intubation for acute heart failure [9,16]. Cesarean delivery is also considered for cardiovascular indications in patients with significant aortopathy [16]. The repeated fluctuations of cardiac output associated with labor and vaginal delivery may result in an increase in the aortic wall's shear stress and an increased risk of dissection [16]. Another indication for cesarean delivery includes a patient recently anticoagulated with warfarin, as warfarin crosses the placenta while reversal agents do not, increasing the anticoagulated fetus's risk for cerebral hemorrhage during vaginal birth [10].

Cesarean anesthesia

Depending on the lesion and risk stratification, patients with high-risk lesions (such as mWHO III or IV) may benefit from a gradual onset of the neuraxial sympathectomy. This can be achieved by an epidural technique, a CSE technique with intrathecal opioids and epidural local anesthetic, or a sequential CSE in which intrathecal opioids and low-dose bupivacaine (2.5–5 mg) are administered, followed by a slow epidural 2% lidocaine titration to T4–T6 level [33,34]. Other options that have been described include intrathecal catheters [35], and continuous epidural anesthesia with double catheters to ensure slow onset of anesthesia [36]. At the time of block placement, initiation of a prophylactic vasopressor infusion to maintain blood pressure and SVR should occur with either phenylephrine (eg, starting titration at 0.5–0.75 $\mu g\ kg^{-1} \cdot min^{-1}$) or norepinephrine (eg, starting titration at 0.05–0.075 $\mu g\ kg^{-1} \cdot min^{-1}$). We typically use the sequential CSE technique in patients with cardiac disease for planned cesarean delivery. Patients deemed low risk for cardiovascular complications (eg, mWHO I-II) can often tolerate a traditional spinal dose with 10 to 15 mg of hyperbaric bupivacaine and a prophylactic vasopressor infusion [16].

In patients with heart failure who have difficulty tolerating the supine position, general anesthesia is a reasonable option because these patients may further decompensate after delivery due to autotransfusion and aortocaval decompression from uterine involution [16]. During general anesthesia for cesarean delivery in CVD, induction should focus on maintaining hemodynamic stability. Pre-induction intra-arterial blood pressure monitoring and prioritizing hemodynamic stability (over aspiration risk, and newborn sedation) should be considered with a potential slow titration of induction agents such as propofol (1–2 mg/kg) or etomidate (0.1–0.3 mg/kg). Premedication should be considered including medications that are often avoided in obstetrics (eg, lidocaine, fentanyl) or remifentanil (infusion 0.2–0.5 mcg/kg/min for 5–10 minutes or boluses 2–4 mcg/kg) which could theoretically cause less newborn sedation due to its rapid metabolism [37–39]. Vasopressors should be in-line and oxytocin should be infused via an infusion pump immediately after delivery without bolus dosing.

Monitoring during cesarean delivery
Monitoring during cesarean delivery includes standard ASA monitors and a low threshold for intraarterial blood pressure monitoring [40]. Beat-to-beat blood pressure measurements assist with titration of vasopressors like phenylephrine, norepinephrine, and ephedrine during neuraxial or general anesthesia. In cases of right ventricular failure or acute decompensation that requires vasopressors and pulmonary vasculature dilators, central venous catheter and pulmonary artery pressure monitoring should be considered [9]. Point-of-care transthoracic echocardiography can be used to assess volume status, ventricular function, regional wall motion abnormalities, pericardial effusion, valvular function, and changes in the proximal aorta [41,42]. In the case of general anesthesia, transesophageal echocardiography can be also considered.

EMERGENCIES
Identification and response
According to the National Partnership for Maternal Safety, there are several early warning signs and symptoms to rapidly identify women with undiagnosed cardiac disease, or those with known cardiac disease who may be decompensating: shortness of breath, orthopnea, lung crackles or wheezing, resting heart rate lesser than 120 beats/min, resting respiratory rate greater than 30, oxygen saturation less than 95% on room air without a history of CVD (Table 1) [5,12,43]. These signs can be suggestive of heart failure, arrhythmias, or coronary artery disease and should lead to a high clinical suspicion of impending decompensation that would need prompt intervention.

Cardiac ultrasound
A focused cardiac ultrasound can be performed at the bedside to assist in treatment of cardiac-related complications. This tool is easily accessible, safe, and may help reduce the time to diagnosis and treatment [41,42]. Ultrasound can help assess volume status to guide fluid administration, left and right ventricular global function and regional wall abnormalities, pericardial effusions,

Table 1
Maternal early warning signs and symptoms

Vital signs and physical exam signs	Symptoms
Heart rate > 120 or < 50 beats/min	Chest pain at rest or with minimal exertion
Systolic blood pressure > 160 mm Hg or < 90 mm Hg	Shortness of breath at rest, orthopnea, paroxysmal nocturnal dyspnea
Diastolic blood pressure > 100 mm Hg	Extreme fatigue
Respiratory rate > 30 breaths/min	Agitation, confusion, unresponsiveness
Oxygen saturation < 95% on room air without a history of cardiovascular disease	Patient with preeclampsia with headache or shortness of breath
Oliguria < 35 mL/h	Unprovoked or exertional syncope
Wheezing, crackles	
Loud systolic murmur or S4, jugular venous pressure visible 2 cm above clavicle at 45°	
Marked peripheral edema	

valvular regurgitation or stenosis, and changes in the proximal aorta. Uterine displacement of the heart upwards and laterally helps to obtain a parasternal and apical views more easily. The subcostal views may be more challenging to achieve in pregnancy [16].

Cardiac ultrasound can also be useful in cases of maternal arrest as it can help narrow the differential diagnosis in undifferentiated shock or cardiac arrest. In hemorrhage, the heart will be hyperdynamic and the inferior vena cava collapsible. In cardiogenic shock, the ventricular function will be decreased, and B lines can be present as a sign of alveolar fluid accumulation. In obstructive shock, the right ventricle will be dilated, and the inferior vena cava will be non-collapsible. In sepsis, the heart may be hyperdynamic or display decreased function [9].

Fetal distress and emergency cesarean delivery
A plan for emergency cesarean delivery must be delineated with the obstetric team before delivery. All laboring women, including those with CVD, are at risk for placental abruption, umbilical cord prolapse, uterine rupture, or persistent uteroplacental insufficiency that can necessitate emergent cesarean delivery resulting in the need for rapid conversion of preexisting neuraxial labor analgesia to surgical anesthesia. The maternal state and fetal status will dictate how rapidly the epidural medications can be titrated to effect. The anesthesiologist must keep in mind that a rapid conversion to general anesthesia may be required for any laboring patients with CVD and have an emergent general anesthesia induction plan formulated [9]. During labor, the team should be a step ahead of such possible obstetric emergencies with redundant intravenous access as well as additional monitors such as an intra-arterial line and 5 lead ECG in patients categorized as mWHO III or IV.

Medications used in obstetrics have a particular pharmacologic profile that can adversely affect a patient with CVD. For example, terbutaline is used as a uterine relaxing agent due to its beta 2 agonistic effects to improve uteroplacental perfusion. It is administered in the setting of fetal bradycardia caused by uterine tachysystole. It causes vasodilation and tachycardia that could result in hemodynamic collapse in specific patients such as those with hypertrophic cardiomyopathy, severe aortic stenosis, or history of tachyarrhythmias. Nitroglycerin acts as a uterine relaxant and is administered either IV or sublingually. This agent can also cause a rapid decrease in SVR. The entire team should be aware that such drugs, need to be used especially carefully, or in some cases even avoided, in specific cardiac patients [9].

Postpartum hemorrhage

PPH is twice as common in patients with CVD [44,45]. Early recognition of PPH and rapid treatment is important in every postpartum woman, especially in those with CVD disease. Oxytocin is the most effective uterotonic agent. In patients with CVD, oxytocin should be titrated via an infusion pump. Bolus dosing should be avoided because of a potential rapid decrease in SVR that could lead to cardiovascular collapse [46]. For cesarean delivery, the estimated effective dose of oxytocin infusion to obtain satisfactory tone in 90% of parturients in non-laboring patients was 16.2 IU/h and in laboring patients was 44.2 U/h [47–49]. Higher doses are associated with greater side effects. As hypotension occurs from oxytocin, counteraction with a vasoconstrictor is suggested.

Conversely, methylergonovine can increase SVR and pulmonary vascular resistance due to alpha-adrenergic agonism. This increase in blood pressure can result in hypertensive crisis, stroke, or coronary vasospasm that could result in myocardial ischemia and death [47,50,51]. This agent should be avoided in patient with hypertension, preeclampsia, ischemic heart disease, vascular dissection (eg, history of spontaneous coronary artery dissection), intracardiac shunts, and aortic pathology [47,50–52].

Carboprost is a prostaglandin F2-alpha that increases pulmonary artery pressure by 125% and pulmonary vascular resistance by more than 100% [53]. It can also precipitate bronchospasm, hypoxemia, increased intrapulmonary shunt fraction, and death [54–56]. Consideration should be given to avoiding this medication in patients with Fontan circulation, intracardiac shunt, pulmonary hypertension, and preexisting asthma.

Finally, misoprostol is a drug that is well tolerated in this patient population as it has no cardiopulmonary effects, unfortunately it is the least effective uterotonic agent [9]. It is reasonable for this drug to be administered prophylactically in patients with CVD as an adjunct to oxytocin to prevent PPH.

Arrhythmias

Patients with a history of tachyarrhythmias are at increased risk of experiencing arrhythmia during the peripartum period. This can lead to maternal hemodynamic instability and fetal compromise [57,58]. These patients should be monitored with 5 lead electrocardiography during labor with central telemetric monitoring if available [9]. The most common arrhythmias found in pregnancy and delivery are atrial fibrillation and paroxysmal supraventricular tachycardia [58]. Other entities like heart block, ventricular fibrillation, and ventricular tachycardia are rare. If the patient presents with a pacemaker or an implantable cardioverter-defibrillator, these should be left "on" during labor. If an emergency cesarean delivery is needed, it is reasonable to proceed without disabling the defibrillation function according to the most recent guidelines as the incision for a cesarean is below the umbilicus [9,59]. Note that in the setting of elective cesarean delivery an anesthesiologist may choose to have this device interrogated and the defibrillation function turned off and replaced with external pads to reduce the risk of accidental shock. However, in a recent systematic review, no appropriate or inappropriate ICD shocks during delivery were reported in the literature [60].

Management of arrhythmias in pregnancy is the same as for the non-pregnant patient [61]. Chemical and electric cardioversion can be performed in pregnancy [62]. Adenosine can be used for paroxysmal supraventricular tachycardia. Beta blockers and calcium channel blockers can be used for rate control in atrial fibrillation [10,61]. If the patient becomes unstable, immediate cardioversion should occur [61]. If the patient is not in cardiac arrest, then during an arryhthmia episode the fetus should be monitored. Fetal distress can also be an indication for cardioversion. According to the American Heart Association (AHA), application of defibrillation and cardioversion shocks to the maternal chest would be expected to pass minimal energy to the fetus and is considered safe in all stages of pregnancy [61]. Defibrillation would be unlikely to cause electric arcing to fetal monitors, and the presence of fetal monitors should not deter providers from the use of rapid electricity administration when indicated [61].

Cardiovascular surgery
In the case of dissection of a major vessel or other cardiovascular emergency requiring emergent surgery, the presence of a pregnancy should not delay life-saving cardiac surgery. A cesarean delivery may be performed concurrent with the vascular or cardiac surgery in a term pregnancy or for signs of fetal distress in a viable fetus [9]. The risk of prematurity must be weighed with the benefits of delivery on a case-by-case basis. If the decision is made to maintain the pregnancy through a surgery requiring cardiopulmonary bypass, optimizing uteroplacental perfusion with high flow normothermic perfusion is recommended.

Maternal cardiac arrest
In the United States, maternal arrest occurs in about 1 of every 9000 (13.4 per 100,000) hospitalizations for delivery from 2017 to 2018 with the most common etiologies being hemorrhage, heart failure, amniotic fluid embolism, and sepsis [63,64]. According to the AHA and the Society for Obstetric Anesthesiology and Perinatology, cardiopulmonary resuscitation should occur at the site

of the cardiac arrest; chest compressions should be performed at a rate of 100 per minute; with the patient positioned supine with a second provider performing manual left uterine displacement to remove aortocaval compression [61,65,66]. Defibrillation should occur and Advanced Cardiac Life Support medications are dosed as indicated in nonpregnancy patients [61,65,66]. A resuscitative hysterotomy (also called a perimortem cesarean delivery) at the site of arrest is prioritized if return of spontaneous circulation does not occur within 4 minutes [67]. The goal for delivery is 5 minutes after arrest which will release aortocaval compression resulting in improved maternal hemodynamics, reduced maternal oxygen demand, and improved survival of the mother and fetus [65,66]. Maternal cardiac arrest code teams should include a typical hospital code team along with obstetric and neonatal teams. If available, resources to perform transesophageal or transthoracic echocardiography, as well as an ECMO team should be mobilized early in the code [68].

SUMMARY

The anesthesiologist is an essential member of the Pregnancy Heart Team as they are immediately available in labor and delivery, and they have extensive training in caring for patients in acute settings with cardiac disease. Anesthesiologists should embrace the role of the peri-delivery physician leader and provide excellent labor analgesia and surgical anesthesia, prevent adverse cardiac events, rapidly recognize cardiovascular instability, and lead rapid and precise resuscitation in patients with CVD.

CLINICS CARE POINTS

- To ensure safe management of pregnancy in patients with cardiovascular disease, pre-delivery evaluation by a multidisciplinary Pregnancy Heart Team should occur.
- Risk stratification tools evaluate the etiology and severity of cardiovascular disease to determine the appropriate hospital type and location for delivery and anesthetic management.
- Intrapartum hemodynamic monitoring may need to be intensified for patients at increased risk.
- Anticoagulation is important for patients with CVD. Appropriate holding times should be discussed with the Pregnancy Heart Team to facilitate neuraxial blockade for labor analgesia or surgical anesthesia.
- Vasoactive and inotropic medications to support blood pressure during labor should consider the patient's specific cardiovascular status.
- Early placement of an epidural catheter allows time for trouble shooting and replacement if needed and reduces circulating plasma catecholamines.
- The anesthesiologist must be prepared for both obstetric and cardiac emergencies.

DISCLOSURE

The authors have nothing to disclose.

References

[1] Centers for Disease Control, National Center for Chronic Disease Prevention and Health Promotion, Division of Reproductive Health: Pregnancy mortality surveillance system. 2023. Available at https://www.cdc.gov/reproductivehealth/maternal-mortality/pregnancy-mortality-surveillance-system.htm. Accessed 4/27/2023.

[2] van Hagen IM, Roos-Hesselink JW. Pregnancy in congenital heart disease: risk prediction and counselling. Heart 2020;106(23):1853.

[3] Bottega N, Malhamé I, Guo L, et al. Secular trends in pregnancy rates, delivery outcomes, and related health care utilization among women with congenital heart disease. Congenit Heart Dis 2019;14(5):735–44.

[4] Deputy NP KS, Conrey EJ, Bullard KM. Prevalence and Changes in Preexisting Diabetes and Gestational Diabetes Among Women Who Had a Live Birth — United States, 2012–2016. MMWR Morb Mortal Wkly Rep 2018;(67):1201–7.

[5] ACOG Practice Bulletin No. 212. Pregnancy and Heart Disease. Obstet Gynecol 2019;133(5).

[6] Wang MC, Freaney PM, Perak AM, et al. Trends in Prepregnancy Obesity and Association With Adverse Pregnancy Outcomes in the United States, 2013 to 2018. J Am Heart Assoc 2021;10(17):e020717; https://doi.org/10.1161/JAHA.120.020717.

[7] Louis JM, Mogos MF, Salemi JL, et al. Obstructive sleep apnea and severe maternal-infant morbidity/mortality in the United States, 1998-2009. Sleep 2014;37(5):843–9.

[8] Mehta LS, Warnes CA, Bradley E, et al. Cardiovascular Considerations in Caring for Pregnant Patients: A Scientific Statement From the American Heart Association. Circulation 2020;141(23):e884–903.

[9] Meng ML, Arendt KW. Obstetric Anesthesia and Heart Disease: Practical Clinical Considerations. Anesthesiology 2021;135(1):164–83.

[10] Regitz-Zagrosek V, Roos-Hesselink JW, Bauersachs J, et al. ESC Guidelines for the management of cardiovascular diseases during pregnancy. Eur Heart J 2018;39(34):3165–241.

[11] Roos-Hesselink J., Baris L., Johnson M., et al., Pregnancy outcomes in women with cardiovascular disease: evolving trends over 10 years in the ESC Registry Of Pregnancy And Cardiac disease (ROPAC), Eur Heart J, 40 (47), 2019, 3848–3855.

[12] Wolfe D.S., Hameed A.B., Taub C.C., et al., Addressing maternal mortality: the pregnant cardiac patient, Am J Obstet Gynecol, 220 (2), 2019, 167.e1-167.e8.

[13] Silversides C.K., Grewal J., Mason J., et al., Pregnancy Outcomes in Women With Heart Disease: The CARPREG II Study, J Am Coll Cardiol, 71 (21), 2018, 2419–2430.

[14] Drenthen W, Boersma E, Balci A, et al. Predictors of pregnancy complications in women with congenital heart disease. Eur Heart J 2010;31(17):2124–32.

[15] Thorne S, MacGregor A, Nelson-Piercy C. Risks of contraception and pregnancy in heart disease. Heart 2006;92(10):1520.

[16] Meng M.-L., Arendt K.W., Banayan J.M., et al., Anesthetic Care of the Pregnant Patient With Cardiovascular Disease: A Scientific Statement From the American Heart Association, Circulation, 147 (11), 2023, e657–e673.

[17] Levels of Maternal Care: Obstetric Care Consensus No, 9. Obstet Gynecol 2019;134(2): e41–55.

[18] Arendt KW, Long ME. Problems of early pregnancy. In: DH C, editor. Chestnut's obstetric anesthesia: principles and practice. Philadelphia: Elsevier; 2020. p. 350–67.

[19] Ruys TP, Roos-Hesselink JW, Pijuan-Domenech A, et al. Is a planned caesarean section in women with cardiac disease beneficial? Heart 2015;101(7):530–6.

[20] Easter S.R., Rouse C.E., Duarte V., et al., Planned vaginal delivery and cardiovascular morbidity in pregnant women with heart disease, Am J Obstet Gynecol, 222 (1), 2020, 77.e1-77.e11.

[21] Nishimura RA, Tajik AJ. The Valsalva maneuver-3 centuries later. Mayo Clin Proc 2004;79(4):577–8.

[22] Robson S.C., Dunlop W., Boys R.J., et al., Cardiac output during labour, Br Med J, 295 (6607), 1987, 1169–1172.

[23] Tanaka H., Kamiya C., Katsuragi S., et al., Effect of epidural anesthesia in labor; pregnancy with cardiovascular disease, Taiwan J Obstet Gynecol, 57 (2), 2018, 190–193.

[24] Leffert L., Butwick A., Carvalho B., et al., The Society for Obstetric Anesthesia and Perinatology Consensus Statement on the Anesthetic Management of Pregnant and Postpartum Women Receiving Thromboprophylaxis or Higher Dose Anticoagulants, Anesth Analg, 126 (3), 2018, 928–944.

[25] Horlocker T.T., Vandermeuelen E., Kopp S.L., et al., Regional Anesthesia in the Patient Receiving Antithrombotic or Thrombolytic Therapy: American Society of Regional Anesthesia and Pain Medicine Evidence-Based Guidelines (Fourth Edition), Reg Anesth Pain Med, 43 (3), 2018, 263–309.

[26] Ngan Kee WD, Lee SWY, Ng FF, et al. Prophylactic Norepinephrine Infusion for Preventing Hypotension During Spinal Anesthesia for Cesarean Delivery. Anesth Analg 2018;126(6): 1989–94.

[27] Chau A, Bibbo C, Huang C, et al. Dural Puncture Epidural Technique Improves Labor Analgesia Quality With Fewer Side Effects Compared With Epidural and Combined Spinal Epidural Techniques: A Randomized Clinical Trial. Anesth Analg 2017;124(2):560–9.

[28] Jaffe RA, Siegel LC, Schnittger I, et al. Epidural air injection assessed by transesophageal echocardiography. Reg Anesth 1995;20(2):152–5.

[29] Saberski LR, Kondamuri S, Osinubi OY. Identification of the epidural space: is loss of resistance to air a safe technique? A review of the complications related to the use of air. Reg Anesth 1997;22(1):3–15.

[30] Yoshii WY, Miller M, Rottman RL, et al. Fentanyl for epidural intravascular test dose in obstetrics. Reg Anesth 1993;18(5):296–9.

[31] Guay J. The epidural test dose: a review. Anesth Analg 2006;102(3):921–9.

[32] Norris MC, Fogel ST, Dalman H, et al. Labor epidural analgesia without an intravascular "test dose. Anesthesiology 1998;88(6):1495–501.

[33] Arendt KW, Muehlschlegel JD, Tsen LC. Cardiovascular alterations in the parturient undergoing cesarean delivery with neuraxial anesthesia. Expet Rev Obstet Gynecol 2012;7(1): 59–75.

[34] Hamlyn EL, Douglass CA, Plaat F, et al. Low-dose sequential combined spinal-epidural: an anaesthetic technique for caesarean section in patients with significant cardiac disease. Int J Obstet Anesth 2005;14(4):355–61.

[35] El Aidouni G, Merbouh M, El Haddid IA, et al. Caesarean section under continuous spinal anaesthesia in a parturient with pulmonary hypertension: A case report. Ann Med Surg (Lond) 2021;71:102923.

[36] Wang P., Chen X., Zhang J., et al., Continuous epidural anesthesia with double catheters for cesarean section in a patient with severe pulmonary hypertension: A case report, Medicine (Baltim), 100 (47), 2021, e27979.

[37] Orme R.M.L.E., Grange C.S., Ainsrwoth Q.P., et al., General anaesthesia using remifentanil for caesarean section in parturients with critical aortic stenosis: a series of four cases, Int J Obstet Anesth, 13 (3), 2004, 183–187.

[38] Wadsworth R, Greer R, MacDonald JMS, et al. The use of remifentanil during general anaesthesia for caesarean delivery in two patients with severe heart dysfunction. Int J Obstet Anesth 2002;11(1):38–43.

[39] Arendt KW, Lindley KJ. Obstetric anesthesia management of the patient with cardiac disease. Int J Obstet Anesth 2019;37:73–85.

[40] American Society of Anesthesiologists, Committee on Standards and Practice Parameters (CSPP): Standards for Basic Anesthetic Monitoring. Available at: https://

www.asahq.org/standards-and-guidelines/standards-for-basic-anesthetic-monitoring. Accessed April 27, 2023.

[41] Zieleskiewicz L., Bouvet L., Einav S., et al., Diagnostic point-of-care ultrasound: applications in obstetric anaesthetic management, *Anaesthesia*, 73 (10), 2018, 1265–1279.

[42] Laursen CB, Sloth E, Lassen AT, et al. Point-of-care ultrasonography in patients admitted with respiratory symptoms: a single-blind, randomised controlled trial, Lancet Respir Med 2014;2(8):638–46.

[43] Mhyre JM, D'Oria R, Hameed AB, et al. The maternal early warning criteria: a proposal from the national partnership for maternal safety. Obstet Gynecol 2014;124(4):782–6.

[44] Practice Bulletin No. 183. Postpartum Hemorrhage. Obstet Gynecol 2017;130(4): e168–86.

[45] Cauldwell M, Von Klemperer K, Uebing A, et al. Why is post-partum haemorrhage more common in women with congenital heart disease? Int J Cardiol 2016;218:285–90.

[46] Rosseland LA, Hauge TH, Gindheim G, et al. Changes in blood pressure and cardiac output during cesarean delivery: the effects of oxytocin and carbetocin compared with placebo. Anesthesiology 2013;119(3):541–51.

[47] Abouleish E. Postpartum hypertension and convulsion after oxytocic drugs. Anesth Analg 1976;55(6):813–5.

[48] Lavoie A, McCarthy RJ, Wong CA. The ED90 of prophylactic oxytocin infusion after delivery of the placenta during cesarean delivery in laboring compared with nonlaboring women: an up-down sequential allocation dose-response study. Anesth Analg 2015;121(1): 159–64.

[49] George RB, McKeen D, Chaplin AC, et al. Up-down determination of the ED(90) of oxytocin infusions for the prevention of postpartum uterine atony in parturients undergoing Cesarean delivery. Can J Anaesth 2010;57(6):578–82.

[50] Hayashi Y., Ibe To., Kawato H.,et al., Postpartum acute myocardial infarction induced by ergonovine administration, *Intern Med*, 42 (10), 2003, 983–986.

[51] Lin Y.H., Seow K., Hwang J., et al., Myocardial infarction and mortality caused by methylergonovine, *Acta Obstet Gynecol Scand*, 84 (10), 2005, 1022.

[52] Casady GN, Moore DC, Bridenbaugh LD. Postpartum hypertension after use of vasoconstrictor and oxytocic drugs. Etiology, incidence, complications, and treatment. J Am Med Assoc 1960;172:1011–5.

[53] Partridge BL, Key T, Reisner LS. Life-threatening effects of intravascular absorption of PGF2 alpha during therapeutic termination of pregnancy. Anesth Analg 1988;67(11):1111–3.

[54] Hankins GD, Berryman GK, Scott RT, et al. Maternal arterial desaturation with 15-methyl prostaglandin F2 alpha for uterine atony. Obstet Gynecol 1988;72(3 Pt 1):367–70.

[55] Cates W. Jr., Grimes D.A., Haber R.J., et al., Abortion deaths associated with the use of prostaglandin F2alpha, *Am J Obstet Gynecol*, 127 (3), 1977, 219–222.

[56] Cates W Jr, Jordaan HV. Sudden collapse and death of women obtaining abortions induced with prostaglandin F2alpha. Am J Obstet Gynecol 1979;133(4):398–400.

[57] Vaidya VR, Arora S, Patel N, et al. Burden of Arrhythmia in Pregnancy. Circulation 2017;135(6):619–21.

[58] Silversides CK, Harris L, Haberer K, et al. Recurrence rates of arrhythmias during pregnancy in women with previous tachyarrhythmia and impact on fetal and neonatal outcomes. Am J Cardiol 2006;97(8):1206–12.

[59] Practice Advisory for the Perioperative Management of Patients with Cardiac Implantable Electronic Devices: Pacemakers and Implantable Cardioverter-Defibrillators 2020: An Updated Report by the American Society of Anesthesiologists Task Force on Perioperative Management of Patients with Cardiac Implantable Electronic Devices: Erratum. Anesthesiology 2020;132(4):938.

[60] Topf A., Bacher N., Kopp K., et al., Management of Implantable Cardioverter-Defibrillators during Pregnancy-A Systematic Review, *J Clin Med*, 10 (8), 2021, 1675.

[61] Jeejeebhoy FM, Zelop CM, Lipman S, et al. Cardiac Arrest in Pregnancy: A Scientific Statement From the American Heart Association. Circulation 2015;132(18):1747–73.
[62] Peterson AA, Arendt KW, Sharpe EE. Management of Supraventricular Tachycardia in Pregnancy. Pain Med 2020;21(2):426–8.
[63] Mhyre J.M., Tsen L.C., Einav S., et al., Cardiac arrest during hospitalization for delivery in the United States, 1998-2011, Anesthesiology, 120 (4), 2014, 810–818.
[64] Ford N.D., DeSisto C.L., Galang R.R., et al., Cardiac Arrest During Delivery Hospitalization : A Cohort Study, Ann Intern Med, 176 (4), 2023, 472–479.
[65] Lipman S, Cohen S, Einav S, et al. The Society for Obstetric Anesthesia and Perinatology consensus statement on the management of cardiac arrest in pregnancy. Anesth Analg 2014;118(5):1003–16.
[66] Merchant R.M., Topjian A.A., Panchal A.R., et al., Part 1: Executive Summary: 2020 American Heart Association Guidelines for Cardiopulmonary Resuscitation and Emergency Cardiovascular Care, Circulation, 142 (16_suppl_2), 2020, S337–s357.
[67] Rose C.H., Faksh A., Traynor K.D., et al., Challenging the 4- to 5-minute rule: from perimortem cesarean to resuscitative hysterotomy. Am J Obstet Gynecol. 2015;213(5):653-6, 653.e1.
[68] Madden AM, Meng ML. Cardiopulmonary resuscitation in the pregnant patient. BJA Educ 2020;20(8):252–8.

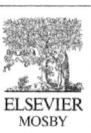

Advances in Anesthesia 41 (2023) 71–85

ADVANCES IN ANESTHESIA

Update and Advances on Post-dural Puncture Headache

Robert Bishop, B Biomed Sci, B Med, FANZCA*,
Amy Chen, MD, William Derois Yates, MD, Julie Fowler, MD,
Stephen Macres, MD, PharmD

Department of Anesthesiology & Pain Medicine, UC Davis Medical Center, 4150 V Street, PSSB
Suite 1200, Sacramento, CA 95817, USA

Keywords
- Dural puncture • Cerebrospinal fluid • Epidual blood patch
- Sphenopalatine nerve block • Occipital nerve block

Key points
- Pathophysiology of post-dural puncture headache (PDPH): PDPH occurs due to dural puncture and subsequent leakage of CSF. The sagging of intracranial structures, meningeal enhancement, and low CSF pressure contribute to the characteristic postural headache. Tearing injury to the dura is preferable for faster healing.
- Risk Factors for PDPH: Female sex, pregnancy, young adulthood, and prior history of headache increase the risk of PDPH. Needle-related factors, such as size, shape, orientation, and multiple attempts also influence the likelihood of PDPH.
- Diagnosis and Treatment of PDPH: Diagnosis is based on characteristic symptoms, occurring within 5 days of dural puncture. Conservative treatment includes oral analgesics, fluid supplementation, and caffeine. Epidural blood patch (EBP) is the gold standard treatment, while alternative injectates (eg, fibrin glue) are considered in specific cases. Regional techniques like sphenopalatine ganglion block and greater occipital nerve block show promise but require further investigation.

A HISTORICAL PERSPECTIVE

The presence of cerebrospinal fluid (CSF) and the encompassing dural membrane has been of interest to all branches of medicine since the time of ancient Egypt. A papyrus scroll estimated to be from 2500 to 3000 BC recorded

*Corresponding author. E-mail address: rbishop@ucdavis.edu

https://doi.org/10.1016/j.aan.2023.05.005
0737-6146/23/Published by Elsevier Inc.

various case reports of traumatic injuries and the resultant anatomic findings. One such case report described an open fracture of the skull, and importantly, the first recorded description of both brain matter and the surrounding liquid. Following this discovery, there were scant references until the Renaissance, when Leonardo DaVinci in 1504 constructed detailed anatomic diagrams that were subsequently improved upon by the anatomist, Niccolò Massa, in 1536 [1]. Following Massa, Mario Valsalva identified spinal fluid during the dissection of the canine spinal cord in 1692, and finally, Francois Magendie in 1842 established CSF as a physiologic component of the central nervous system and gave it the name "liquide cerebrospinal" [2].

Access to the CSF was appealing to physiologists to better understand the function of the central nervous system, as well as to physicians who were interested in the properties of CSF for diagnostic and therapeutic purposes. In 1891, Heinrich Quincke published a series of case reports where he had performed lumbar punctures in order to relieve intracranial pressure. He documented opening and closing pressures as well as analysis of protein concentration [3]. Augustine Bier's seminal paper in 1899 describes the injection of cocaine into the subarachnoid space of both himself and his assistant, with the initial onset of dermatomal anesthesia, and a subsequent positional headache that left Bier bedbound for over a week [4]. The injection of other therapeutic agents to act on the central nervous system was of interest given the ability of intrathecal injection to bypass both the blood-brain barrier and the first-pass metabolism of the liver. In 1900, Romanian surgeon Nicolae Racoviceanu-Pitesti injected morphine into the subarachnoid space [5]. However, nearly 80 years passed before interest piqued in the subject leading to multiple large study publications investigating the role of spinal opioids for the treatment of pain Fig. 1 [6].

Today, accessing the neuraxial space (either epidural or subarachnoid) is routinely indicated for a variety of diagnostic tests and therapeutic interventions. These include: neuraxial anesthesia or analgesia for surgical and obstetric procedures, epidural injection of corticosteroids, implantation of intrathecal catheters or nerve stimulators, drainage of CSF for spinal cord protection during aortic surgery, and diagnostic lumbar puncture for a broad spectrum of neurologic disorders. Of particular interest is the increased utilization of neuraxial anesthesia to reduce or eliminate opioid use in the perioperative period

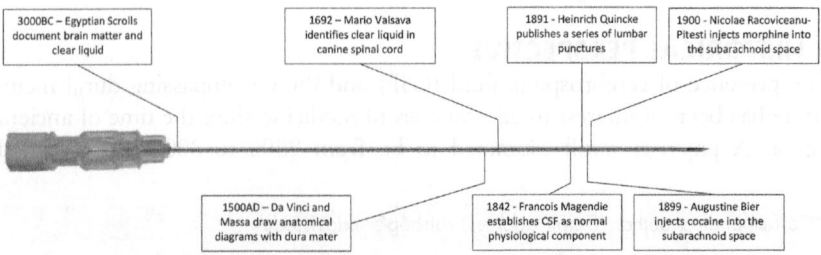

Fig. 1. Investigating the role of spinal opioids for the treatment of pain.

[7], and the implantation of nerve stimulators as alternate means of managing chronic pain. Irrespective of whether the dura is breached intentionally or accidently, there is a risk of post-dural-puncture headache and therefore prompt diagnosis and treatment remain relevant.

Anatomy and physiology

From Massa's original description of *liquide cerebrospinal,* we have progressed to a detailed understanding of the structure and function of CSF. This enhanced understanding of the role of CSF in central nervous system homeostasis has evolved in parallel with advances in imaging technology, as well as the inception and evolution of fields such as molecular biology. CSF plays a critical role in the homeostasis of the interstitial fluid of the brain parenchyma and the regulation of neuronal functioning. The formation and composition of CSF in the choroid plexus is more complex than a plasma ultrafiltrate, and active transport of molecules into the CSF is influenced by cholinergic, adrenergic, serotoninergic, and peptidergic autonomic innervation [8]. Beyond providing a cushion to alleviate the stresses of mechanical force, the CSF gives the brain buoyancy, allowing it to "float" within its compartment and reduce the effective mass to about 50g. The volume of CSF is approximately 150 mL, with approximately 25% of this volume residing in the cerebral ventricles and the remainder distributed in the subarachnoid space and central canal of the spinal cord. The production of CSF is such that the entire volume is replaced 4 times every 24 hours, with flow originating within the choroid plexus and reabsorption via arachnoid villi and granulations into the dural venous sinuses, as well as through cranial and spinal nerve sheaths into the lymphatic outflow system. Flow is unidirectional and pulsatile in nature, influenced by arterial and respiratory pressure oscillations [9].

Cerebrospinal fluid pressure, defined as the intracranial pressure in the prone position, is the result of a dynamic equilibrium between CSF secretion, absorption, and resistance to flow. A normal value in adults is 10 to 15 mm Hg. The Monro-Kellie doctrine states that the sum of volumes of brain, CSF, and intracranial blood is constant. An increase in one should cause a decrease in one or both of the remaining two [10]. CSF overproduction or obstruction to drainage will eventually lead to increased intracranial pressure (ICP) once other compensatory mechanisms are overwhelmed. Conversely, low production of CSF or increased removal will result in low ICP, referred to as intracranial hypotension.

The dura mater arises from the embryonic mesoderm and encases the spinal cord and brain. This continuous membrane differs in the spine compared to the cranium, as the external endosteal layer of the cranial dura mater terminates at the foramen magnum and the descending dura mater of the spine is composed of the innermost cranial meningeal layer. The dura mater terminates at the level of S2, where it forms the coccygeal ligament and anchors the dural sac to the sacrum [11]. The classic description of the microscopic anatomy is that of collagen fibers arranged parallel in a longitudinal (cranial-caudal) direction, however opinions differ whether this structure is consistent throughout all layers of the dura, with some studies demonstrating elastin and collagen fibers arranged without specific orientation [12,13]. The dural sac supports the spinal cord both by forming a protective sheath, as well as suspending the spinal cord via a system of ligaments that attach to the spinal roots. Furthermore, the presence of ligaments and trabeculations in the subdural space are thought to provide additional stability and may be implicated in the phenomenon of an incomplete spinal following what appears to be a successful injection of local anesthetic [11].

Pathophysiology of post-dural puncture headache

The classic pathogenesis of a post-dural puncture headache (PDPH) was first described by Bier as a breach of the dura followed by leakage of CSF, and the development of a postural headache. In patients with a dural defect, Gadolinium-enhanced MRI demonstrates the sagging of the intracranial structures and meningeal enhancement. Periradicular leaks and epidural fluid collections can be seen on CT myelogram or on T2-weighted MRI [14]. The sagging is hypothesized to produce traction on cranial nerves which results in neck and shoulder pain, and the meningeal enhancement seen on MRI is due to the vasodilation of meningeal vessels in an attempt to maintain a constant intracranial volume [15]. The vasodilation and increased blood flow can also be detected with transcranial Doppler [16]. The low-pressure state arises as CSF loss is greater than production, and CSF pressure falls intracranially as the patient moves to an upright position, with pressures falling to 3 mm Hg or less [15].

The dura has been studied in vitro to ascertain the nature of the defect and the effects of various needle designs on the resultant injury [17,18]. Previously, the proposed longitudinal orientation of the fibers dictated the optimal needle approach to minimize the potential for injury. A needle advanced with the bevel parallel to the fibers would cut fewer fibers and thus lead to a smaller injury [19]. However, as this longitudinal arrangement is not consistent throughout the layers of the dura, it is probably not as important as once thought. Instead, it is postulated that a tearing injury is preferable to a cutting injury as the resultant inflammatory response is responsible both for an initial decrease in the size of the defect, and faster healing of the dura [18].

Risk factors for post-dural puncture headache

There are multiple patient factors that increase the risk of PDPH Female sex, pregnancy, young adult age (18–50 years), and a prior history of headache have been identified as common risk factors. Women have been found to be at a two to three times increased risk of PDPH compared to men, and pregnancy may also confer additional risk due to increased cerebral vasodilation [20]. A retrospective study demonstrated in obstetric patients the risk of developing a PDPH following dural puncture is higher with vaginal delivery than the cesarian section. It is thought that bearing down during the second stage of labor increases the pressure gradient for CSF to leak and may also increase the size of the dural defect [21]. Prior history of headaches, including chronic headaches and PDPH, may also increase the risk of PDPH. Obesity, defined as a BMI greater than 30, appears to be protective against PDPH, with increased intra-abdominal and epidural pressure decreasing the pressure gradient for CSF leakage [22].

In addition to patient factors, there are several procedural risk factors that can increase the likelihood of PDPH. Firstly, needle size has been shown in several studies to have an association with PDPH. Unsurprisingly, the risk of PDPH decreases proportionally with decreasing needle diameter. However, there is a limitation, as very small needles (eg 29 gauge) are more prone to bending on insertion, and low CSF flows may contribute to a higher failure rate for spinal anesthesia [15]. As well as size, the shape of the needle tip has evolved from a beveled cutting point with a hollow bore, to pencil point needles with side openings. This style of needle is called "atraumatic," although in vitro studies demonstrate that the resulting dural defect represents a tear rather than a clean cut [18]. It is postulated that the resulting inflammatory response decreases the size of the dural defect and permits faster healing. A meta-analysis of randomized control trials showed that an atraumatic needle reduces the risk of PDPH [23]. For cutting needles such as Quincke or Tuohy, the orientation of bevel insertion is also related to the risk of PDPH. Despite disagreement about the complete orientation of dural fibers throughout the layers, a meta-analysis demonstrated that PDPH incidence is reduced when the cutting bevel is parallel to the longitudinal axis [24]. There is no association with needle orientation and PDPH with pencil point needles given their symmetric cross-section. During multiple attempts, the spinal needle may become deformed due to contact with bone or bending in tissue. This can result in an irregular shape to the needle and produce a greater dural defect for a given size needle. During multiple attempts, or at the completion of the first attempt, there is also an increased risk of PDPH if the stylet is not replaced, and is also seen with needles that do not incorporate a stylet [25]. The summary from Renia and colleagues at the New York School of Regional Anesthesia has a number of high-resolution microscopic images of the dura and the resulting defects from various needles and approaches Fig. 2 [13].

Diagnosis of post-dural puncture headache

The International Headache Society defines a post-dural puncture headache as any headache that develops within 5 days of dural puncture and is not better accounted for by any other cause [26]. The headache is typically characterized as occurring within a minute of standing and is felt throughout the entire head, often in the temporal or occipital regions. It may also cause nausea, sensitivity to light, hearing difficulties, neck stiffness, and can worsen with physical activity, coughing, or straining. PDPH can lead to double vision due to traction on the fourth and sixth cranial nerves. Untreated, it typically resolves in 7 to 14 days; however ,long-term sequelae can include chronic headache and low back pain. In the obstetric population, a recent series of studies have demonstrated that symptoms are may progress well beyond this window and

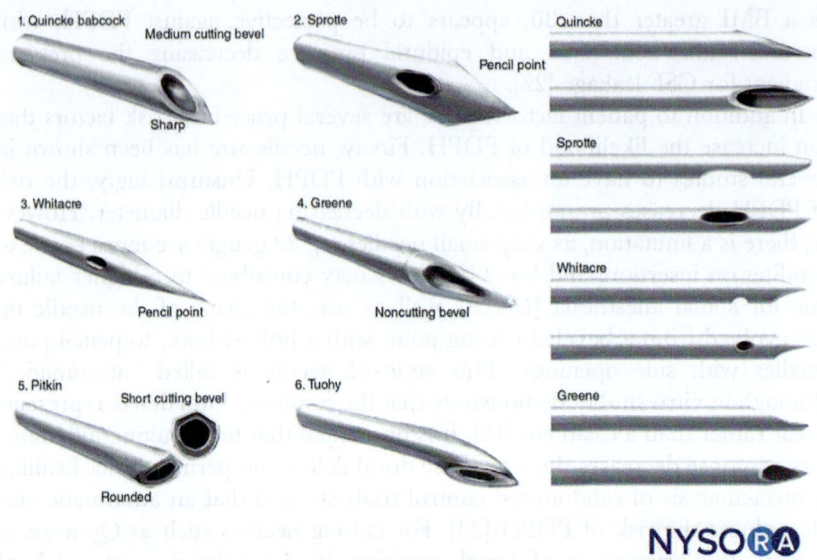

Fig. 2. Regional anesthesia-different types of needles [13].

persisting for up to 24 months [27]. There are also reports of postpartum depression, and bacterial meningitis following PDPH [28].

Following a dural puncture, rare but serious complications include spinal hematoma, abscess, venous sinus thrombosis, and subdural hemorrhage [29]. Thus, a PDPH should be considered early after the presentation of a new-onset headache to expedite treatment, but other causes for headache should be investigated and eliminated. A sudden onset of severe headache, a change in mental status, focal neurologic signs, fever, or a headache that does not respond to treatment should be investigated promptly [30]. The box later in discussion summarizes differential diagnoses Box 1.

Treatment of post-dural puncture headache

Conservative methods
Once the diagnosis of PDPH is established it is important to promptly initiate treatment. Although the headache may be self-limiting,it can impact the patient's quality ofand is is compounded in obstetric patients who typically have a newborn to attend to. The American Society of Anesthesiologists Statement on Post-Dural Puncture Headache Management recommends that treatment is started within 24h and therapy guided by the severity of the symptoms [31].

Conservative treatment traditionally recommended bedrest, supine position, and placement of an abdominal binder. These were considered to decrease the pressure gradient at the level of the dural defect and thus minimize ongoing CSF leakage. However, while the intensity of the headache may decrease, bed-rest does not prevent the onset of a PDPH following a dural puncture, and

Box 1: Differential diagnoses for post-dural puncture headache

Migraine

Non-specific headache

Caffiene or other stimulant withdrawal

Meningitis

Pre-eclampsia

Pituitary infarction

Intracranial hemorrhage

Venous sinus thrombosis

Migraine

Non-specific headache

Caffiene or other stimulant withdrawal

Meningitis

Pre-eclampsia

Pituitary infarction

Intracranial hemorrhage

Venous sinus thrombosis

there is minimal evidence to suggest that bedrest decreases symptoms [32]. Furthermore, prolonged bedrest may increase the risk of venous thromboembolism [33].

Oral and intravenous fluid supplementation has been utilized to alleviate the postural headache. However, aggressive overhydration has not demonstrated any benefit [34] and current recommendations are for normal levels of hydration and to only supplement with intravenous therapy if the oral route cannot be tolerated [33].

Initial drug therapy consists of oral acetaminophen or ibuprofen, a common regimen for analgesia following childbirth. These have provided mild symptomatic relief for PDPH, but efficacy is limited. Opioid analgesics are also prescribed in the post-natal period, but the duration should be limited. Strong evidence for the use of opioids for PDPH is lacking [35]. Intrathecal administration of morphine following accidental dural puncture has not been shown to decrease the incidence or severity of PDPH [36].

Caffeine, by either the oral or intravenous route, has been used to treat moderate PDPH symptoms. The mechanism of action is twofold; it causes cerebral vasoconstriction and increases the production of CSF. It has a long half-life and readily crosses the blood–brain barrier. Intravenous caffeine has been associated with toxicity and seizures, but data is limited to case reports [37]. Even in lower doses it may be poorly tolerated due to restlessness and insomnia. It will also be excreted into breastmilk which should be considered in nursing mothers. Two RCTs comparing caffeine to placebo for the treatment of PDPH demonstrated that caffeine treatment resulted in a significant reduction in the proportion of participants with PDPH persistence and those requiring further intervention [35].

Other medications in use include theophylline and aminophylline which both have a similar mechanism of action to caffeine. DDAVP and ACTH have been utilized in an attempt to increase the circulating blood volume [15]. Gabapentin has demonstrated improvement in headache severity, but one limitation is sedation [38]. Hydrocortisone has also been shown to improve pain scores [39]. With the above drug categories, studies are limited by low patient numbers and the applicability beyond obstetric patients, who make up the bulk of study groups.

Intrathecal catheter
If the dura is inadvertently breached at the time of an epidural catheter placement, one option is to leave the catheter sited in the intrathecal space. The reasoning is that the presence of the catheter will initially allow for the continuation of analgesic therapy, as well as preventing CSF leakage by physically blocking the passage of CSF. Following this, the presence of the catheter would trigger an exaggerated inflammatory response, allowing for faster healing of the defect upon catheter removal. The optimal timing of removal of the catheter has not been determined, with most studies indicating catheter removal between 24 and 36h to allow for a degree of inflammation to occur. Recent studies comparing PDPH incidence and need for further therapy have shown mixed results [40,41]. Per the ASA Position Statement on PHPH, the risk of inadvertent epidural dosing of an intrathecal catheter and the risk of infection should also be considered [42].

Epidural blood patch
The treatment modality that has undergone the most study remains the autologous epidural blood patch (EBP). It is considered the gold standard that other treatment modalities are compared to. The mechanism is that the injection of autologous blood will form a clot to plug the defect and prevent further CFS leakage. A secondary effect is the mass effect of the injectate which can raise CSF pressure back to normal levels and reduce the cerebral vasodilation and traction effect on the nociceptive structures [20]. It is theorized that the second effect is responsible for the immediate relief in symptoms [43].

The technique is well-described in the literature. Previously, a small volume of blood was advocated, however most institutions now recommend an endpoint of 20 to 30 mL of blood, or a subjective feeling of fullness at the site of the injection reported by the patient [15,42,44]. Contraindications for EBP include coagulopathy, fever or infection, and technical difficulty. In the past there has been concern about CNS spread of infections such as COVID-19 [45] or HIV, or seeding of tumor in oncology patients. In these instances, evidence is limited to case studies and consensus remains that it will likely require an individual risk/benefit assessment.

The timing of the EBP has been studied extensively in the obstetric population. Prophylactic EPB can be performed at the time of a recognized dural puncture and has been shown to reduce symptom severity and duration. However, as not all patients with a recognized dural puncture develop a PDPH, there is no consensus on recommending all patients receive a prophylactic EBP [43]. An early EBP should be considered in patients with a severe PDPH, especially if there are associated neurologic symptoms such as visual change, as this can be caused by traction on cranial nerves – a particularly worrisome sign [42]. Previously it was thought that intervention within 24 hours carried a higher failure rate and thus a requirement for a repeat procedure; however, this observation is likely skewed by the fact that early treatment usually corresponds with more severe symptoms and likely a larger dural defect. Most guidelines recommend a graded approach, using conservative measures initially and administering an EBP at about 48h [42,46].

The success rate for EBP is high, with most studies quoting a range from 65% and as high as 98% if a subsequent injection is needed. In the cases of subsequent injection, it is prudent to further investigate the cause of the headache if there was no initial improvement with the first EPB.

Complications following EBP include transient low back pain, and while common it is usually better tolerated than the headache and is short lived. Less common risks include infection, and patients should be counseled to be vigilant if the pain persists or there are other symptoms suggestive of deeper infection. Also, placing the EBP can create a secondary dural tear, especially if the initial attempt was technically difficult. Rarer complications include arachnoiditis or spinal hematoma due to the injection of intrathecal blood [47].

Other epidural injectates
Several alternative products have been investigated to perform the function of autologous blood. Often this is in the setting of repeat failed EBPs and where the diagnosis of ongoing CSF leakage has been determined. Fibrin glue has been utilized with improvement in symptoms, but data is limited to small case series [48]. Dextran has been attempted with similar success, however again the dataset is small [49]. As a last resort, open surgical repair has been reported in patients with persistent symptoms and ongoing CSF leakage [15].

Regional techniques
Sphenopalatine ganglion block (SPGB) has been used for several headache types and chronic or recurrent cranio-facial pain syndromes. It was first described over 100 years ago but has recently gained interest as a treatment for PDPH. Anatomically, the sphenopalatine ganglion (SPG) is a bilateral collection of sympathetic, parasympathetic, and somatosensory nerve cells and is located close to the sphenopalatine foramen posterior to the middle nasal concha. It's appeal lies in the relatively straightforward accessibility via a "blind" technique that enables the practitioner to apply local anesthetic topically to block the ganglion. Given the variety of neurons clustered within the ganglion, the effects of local anesthetic blockade can be widespread, however the proposed mechanism of SPGB is a blockade of parasympathetic nerves which reduces cerebral vasodilation. Typically, patients will have almost immediate

symptom relief following the application of local anesthetic and will remain symptom-free for up to 6 hours. The advantage of the SPGB is the ease of the procedure and the avoidance of accessing the epidural space, however the technique does not address the underlying process driving the headache.

Whilst endoscopic techniques for SPGB have been described, the "blind" technique is simpler. SPGB involves applying local anesthetic to the mucosa of the nasopharynx, via cotton-tipped applicators or specialized, purpose-marketed catheters, in the area over the sphenopalatine ganglion. Subsequent local anesthetic can be added dropwise to flow down the applicator, or a specialized applicator can be constructed as later in discussion Fig. 3.

A suggested technique is.

1. After informed consent, the patient is connected to standard monitors and lays supine.
2. The applicator tip is soaked in the desired local anesthetic.
3. The applicator is advanced into the first nostril.
4. Using a gentle, slow, vertical advancement, the applicator is inserted until it comes to rest on the posterior nasopharynx. The ganglion itself lies superior and lateral to the back of the middle turbinate. A slightly cephalad direction should be taken, between the middle and inferior turbinates, rather than hugging the floor of the nose. The ganglion will lie just lateral to the applicator, so aim to place the tip resting laterally, rather than medially, within the confines of its final location after advancement.
5. Repeat the procedure on the other side.
6. Leave for 10 to 15 mins, checking periodically that the applicators have not come forwards, then add another 0.5 mL to each side. Larger volumes will likely just run down the posterior nasopharynx.
7. Leave for another 10 to 15 mins, then remove the applicators.

The evidence for SPGB remains limited. to case reports or retrospective analysis [50]. One RCT compared SPGB to oral caffeine with improved head-ache scores in the SPGB group, however the study was performed following spinal anesthesia for urologic surgery where one would expect a low PDPH rate and smaller CSF leak [51]. One placebo-controlled RCT demonstrating

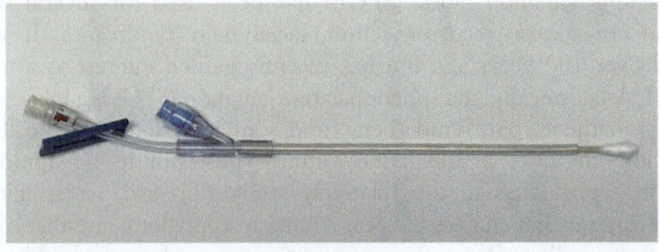

Fig. 3. Image of an SPGB applicator made from a cotton-tip applicator and a J-loop IV extension. The addition of the J-loop allows for additional local anesthetic to be administered to the SPG once the applicator is in place.

improvement in pain and reduced EBP rates but not statistically different to placebo [52].Given the placebo response, some have postulated that the effect may also be attributable to the mechanical stimulation of the SPG and independent of local anesthetic administration [30]. The danger of late complications from a persistent leak, such as subdural hemorrhage or seizure, would not expect to be ameliorated by the SPGB, and one would be cautious in persisting with this as a sole therapeutic technique for persistent PDPH symptoms.

The greater occipital nerve block (GONB) has been frequently used for managing specific types of chronic headache, but it is now being considered for the management of PDPH. It is a superficial block, relatively easy to perform, and accuracy of block placement can be improved with ultrasound guidance [53]. The greater occipital nerve is typically located one-third the distance from the occipital protuberance to the mastoid process. In the landmark technique, the occipital artery can be palpated, and local anesthetic can be injected medial to the artery. Using an ultrasound to perform this block provides direct visualization of the nerve and avoids injury or injection into the occipital artery. As with SPGB, the rate of adverse events following the procedure is very low [54]. The mechanism of the bilateral GONB is to diminish central sensitization by temporarily blocking afferent input to the dorsal horn and trigeminal nucleus neurons [30,55]. The preferred injectate is a long-acting amide local anesthetic (eg, ropivacaine or bupivacaine) combined with dexamethasone to

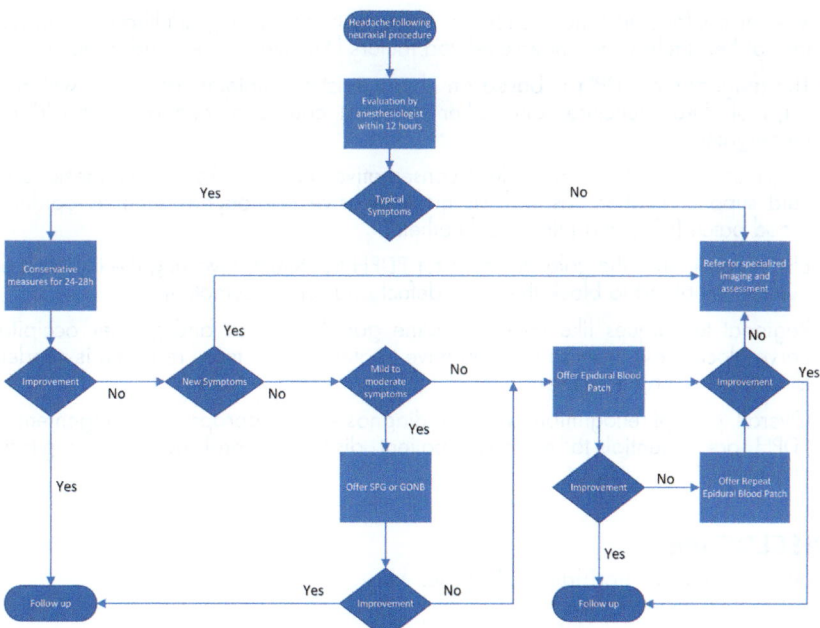

Fig. 4. Suggested decision pathway. GONB, greater occipital nerve block; SPG, sphenopalatine ganglion nerve block.

prolong block duration. Currently, evidence for the procedure is limited to case reports and small prospective trials [56]. Whilst results are encouraging, larger randomized control trials are needed. As with SPGB, the GONB does not treat the underlying process, and an EPB should be considered if the headache does not resolve.

Finally, there is one small case series reporting successful treatment of PDPH with targeted acupuncture. The mechanism of action is via the modulation of neuropeptides and neurotransmitters including substance P and enkephalin. The study is limited to 5 patients who had failed conservative treatment. All subjects had improvement following acupuncture and none required EBP [57]. Given the relative simplicity of the procedure and the high degree of safety, this technique warrants further investigation Fig. 4.

The figure above outlines a proposed algorithm for the management of PDPH. As new evidence emerges, the current gold standard of epidural blood patch may be supplanted by a nerve block, or placement of an alternate injectate into the epidural space. What will remain unchanged is the importance of prompt recognition, consideration of alternate diagnoses, and follow-up to both identify and mitigate potential long-term sequelae.

CLINICS CARE POINTS

- Risk factors for PDPH include female sex, pregnancy, young adulthood, prior history of headaches, and needle-related factors like size, shape, and orientation.
- The diagnosis of PDPH is based on characteristic symptoms, occurring within 5 days of dural puncture, and other potential causes of headache should be investigated.
- Treatment options for PDPH include conservative measures like oral analgesics and fluid supplementation, as well as more invasive approaches such as epidural blood patch (EBP) and intrathecal catheter.
- EBP is considered the gold standard for PDPH treatment, involving the injection of autologous blood to block the dural defect and relieve symptoms.
- Regional techniques like sphenopalatine ganglion block and greater occipital nerve block show promise as alternative treatments, but more research is needed to determine their effectiveness.
- Overall, prompt recognition, accurate diagnosis, and appropriate management of PDPH are essential to minimize patient discomfort and potential long-term sequelae.

DISCLOSURE

The authors have nothing to disclose.

References

[1] Clarke E, O'Malley CD. The human brain and spinal cord; a historical study illustrated by writings from antiquity to the twentieth century. Berkeley (CA): University of California Press; 1968. p. 926, xiii.

[2] Deisenhammer F, Sellebjerg F, Teunissen CE, et al. Cerebrospinal fluid in clinical neurology. Berlin: Springer; 2015. p. 441.

[3] Quincke H. Berliner klinische Wochenschrift: Die Lumbalpunction des Hydrocephalus. Berlin: August Hirschwald; 1891.

[4] Bier A. Experiments on the spinal cord cocainization. Arch Klin Chir Ver Dtsch Z Chir 1899;51:361–8.

[5] Brill S, Gurman GM, Fisher A. A history of neuraxial administration of local analgesics and opioids. Eur J Anaesthesiol. Sep 2003;20(9):682–9.

[6] Kissin I. Clinical studies that initiated the use of spinal opioids for the treatment of pain: A new approach to historical review. Curr Rev Clin Exp Pharmacol 2022;19:61–7.

[7] Wick EC, Grant MC, Wu CL. Postoperative Multimodal Analgesia Pain Management With Nonopioid Analgesics and Techniques: A Review. JAMA Surg 2017;152(7):691–7.

[8] Sakka L, Coll G, Chazal J. Anatomy and physiology of cerebrospinal fluid. European annals of otorhinolaryngology, head and neck diseases 2011;128(6):309–16.

[9] May R, Reddy U. Cerebrospinal fluid and its physiology. Anaesth Intensive Care Med 2020;21(1):60–1.

[10] Mokri B. The Monro–Kellie hypothesis: applications in CSF volume depletion. Neurology 2001;56(12):1746–8.

[11] Nagel SJ, Reddy CG, Frizon LA, et al. Spinal dura mater: biophysical characteristics relevant to medical device development. J Med Eng Technol 2018;42(2):128–39.

[12] Fink BR, Walker S. Orientation of fibers in human dorsal lumbar dura mater in relation to lumbar puncture. Anesth Analg. Dec 1989;69(6):768–72.

[13] Renia MA, Franco CG, Prats-Galino A, Matchés F, López A, de Andrés JA. Ultrastructural Anatomy of the Spinal Meninges and Related Structures. Available at: https://www.nysora.com/topics/anatomy/ultrastructural-anatomy-spinal-meninges-related-structures/. Accessed March 1, 2023.

[14] Wang Y-F, Fuh J-L, Lirng J-F, et al. Cerebrospinal fluid leakage and headache after lumbar puncture: a prospective non-invasive imaging study. Brain 2015;138(6):1492–8.

[15] Turnbull DK, Shepherd DB. Post-dural puncture headache: pathogenesis, prevention and treatment. Br J Anaesth 2003;91(5):718–29.

[16] Mowafy SMS, Abd Ellatif SE. Transcranial Doppler role in prediction of post-dural puncture headache in parturients undergoing elective cesarean section: prospective observational study. J Anesth 2019;33(3):426–34.

[17] Angle PJ, Kronberg JE, Thompson DE, et al. Dural tissue trauma and cerebrospinal fluid leak after epidural needle puncture: effect of needle design, angle, and bevel orientation. Anesthesiology 2003;99(6):1376–82.

[18] Reina MA, de Leon-Casasola OA, Lopez A, et al. An in vitro study of dural lesions produced by 25-gauge Quincke and Whitacre needles evaluated by scanning electron microscopy. Reg Anesth Pain Med 2000;25(4):393–402.

[19] Norris MC, Leighton BL, DeSimone CA. Needle bevel direction and headache after inadvertent dural puncture. Anesthesiology 1989;70(5):729–31.

[20] Patel R, Urits I, Orhurhu V, et al. A comprehensive update on the treatment and management of postdural puncture headache. Curr Pain Headache Rep 2020;24:1–9.

[21] Angle P, Thompson D, Halpern S, et al. Second stage pushing correlates with headache after unintentional dural puncture in parturients. Can J Anesth 1999;46:861–6.

[22] Peralta F, Higgins N, Lange E, et al. The Relationship of Body Mass Index with the Incidence of Postdural Puncture Headache in Parturients. Anesth Analg 2015;121(2):451–6.

[23] Arevalo-Rodriguez I, Muñoz L, Godoy-Casasbuenas N, et al. Needle gauge and tip designs for preventing post-dural puncture headache (PDPH). Cochrane Database Syst Rev 2017;4(4):CD010807.

[24] Richman JM, Joe EM, Cohen SR, et al. Bevel direction and postdural puncture headache: a meta-analysis. Neurol 2006;12(4):224–8.

[25] Strupp M, Brandt T, Müller A. Incidence of post-lumbar puncture syndrome reduced by rein-serting the stylet: a randomized prospective study of 600 patients. J Neurol. Sep 1998;245(9):589–92.

[26] Olesen J. International classification of headache disorders. Lancet Neurol 2018;17(5): 396–7.

[27] Niraj G, Mushambi M, Gauthama P, et al. Persistent headache and low back pain after acci-dental dural puncture in the obstetric population: a prospective, observational, multicentre cohort study. Anaesthesia 2021;76(8):1068–76.

[28] Mims SC, Tan HS, Sun K, et al. Long-term morbidities following unintentional dural puncture in obstetric patients: A systematic review and meta-analysis. J Clin Anesth 2022;79: 110787.

[29] Bos EM, van der Lee K, Haumann J, et al. Intracranial hematoma and abscess after neuraxial analgesia and anesthesia: a review of the literature describing 297 cases. Reg Anesth Pain Med 2021;46(4):337–43.

[30] Li H, Wang Y, Oprea AD, et al. Postdural Puncture Headache-Risks and Current Treatment. Curr Pain Headache Rep 2022;26(6):441–52.

[31] Statement on Post-Dural Puncture Headache Management. American Society of Anesthesi-ologists. Updated October 13, 2021, 2023. Available at: https://www.asahq.org/stan-dards-and-guidelines/statement-on-post-dural-puncture-headache-management. Accessed March 13, 2023.

[32] Arevalo-Rodriguez I, Ciapponi A, Roqué-Figuls M, et al. Posture and fluids for preventing post-dural puncture headache. Cochrane Database Syst Rev 2016;(3); https://doi.org/ 10.1002/14651858.CD009199.pub3:CD009199. Accessed January 21, 2023.

[33] Russell R, Laxton C, Lucas DN, et al. Treatment of obstetric post-dural puncture headache. Part 1: conservative and pharmacological management. Int J Obstet Anesth 2019;38: 93–103.

[34] April MD, Long B. Does Bed Rest or Fluid Supplementation Prevent Post-Dural Puncture Head-ache? Ann Emerg Med 2018;71(5):e55–7.

[35] Basurto Ona X, Uriona Tuma SM, Martínez García L, et al. Drug therapy for preventing post-dural puncture headache. Cochrane Database Syst Rev 2013;2013(2):CD001792.

[36] Peralta FM, Wong CA, Higgins N, et al. Prophylactic Intrathecal Morphine and Prevention of Post-Dural Puncture Headache: A Randomized Double-blind Trial. Anesthesiology 2020;132(5):1045–52.

[37] Bolton VE, Leicht CH, Scanlon TS. Postpartum seizure after epidural blood patch and intra-venous caffeine sodium benzoate. Anesthesiology 1989;70(1):146–9.

[38] Wagner Y, Storr F, Cope S. Gabapentin in the treatment of post-dural puncture headache: a case series. Anaesth Intensive Care 2012;40(4):714–8.

[39] Neves JF, Vieira VL, Saldanha RM, et al. [Hydrocortisone treatment and prevent post-dural puncture headache: case reports]. Rev Bras Anestesiol 2005;55(3):343–9.

[40] Kaddoum R, Motlani F, Kaddoum RN, et al. Accidental dural puncture, postdural puncture headache, intrathecal catheters, and epidural blood patch: revisiting the old nemesis. J Anesth 2014;28(4):628–30.

[41] Jagannathan DK, Arriaga AF, Elterman KG, et al. Effect of neuraxial technique after inadver-tent dural puncture on obstetric outcomes and anesthetic complications. Int J Obstet Anesth 2016;25:23–9.

[42] Statement on Post-Dural Puncture Headache Management. American Society of Anesthesi-ologists. Updated October 13, 2021. Available at: https://www.asahq.org/standards-and-guidelines/statement-on-post-dural-puncture-headache-management. Accessed March 13, 2023.

[43] Zetlaoui PJ, Buchheit T, Benhamou D. Epidural blood patch: A narrative review. Anaesth Crit Care Pain Med 2022;41(5):101138.

[44] Gaiser RR. Postdural Puncture Headache: An Evidence-Based Approach. Anesthesiol Clin 2017;35(1):157–67.

[45] Ibrahim M, Darling R, Oaks N, et al. Epidural blood patch for a post-dural puncture headache in a COVID-19 positive patient following labor epidural analgesia. Int J Obstet Anesth 2021;46:102970.

[46] Treatment of obstetric post-dural puncture headache. Obstetric Anaesthetists' Association. Available at: https://www.oaa-anaes.ac.uk/assets/_managed/cms/files/Guidelines/New%20PDPH%20Guidelines.pdf. Accessed March 1, 2023.

[47] Russell R, Laxton C, Lucas DN, et al. Treatment of obstetric post-dural puncture headache. Part 2: epidural blood patch. Int J Obstet Anesth 2019;38:104–18.

[48] Gandhi J, DiMatteo A, Joshi G, et al. Cerebrospinal fluid leaks secondary to dural tears: a review of etiology, clinical evaluation, and management. Int J Neurosci 2021;131(7): 689–95.

[49] Reynvoet ME, Cosaert PA, Desmet MF, et al. Epidural dextran 40 patch for postdural puncture headache. Anaesthesia 1997;52(9):886–8.

[50] Cohen S, Levin D, Mellender S, et al. Topical Sphenopalatine Ganglion Block Compared With Epidural Blood Patch for Postdural Puncture Headache Management in Postpartum Patients: A Retrospective Review. Reg Anesth Pain Med 2018;43(8):880–4.

[51] Gayathri GA, Karthik K, Saravanan R, et al. A randomized control study to assess the efficacy of the sphenopalatine ganglion block in patients with post dural puncture headache. Saudi J Anaesth 2022;16(4):401–5.

[52] Jespersen MS, Jaeger P, Ægidius KL, et al. Sphenopalatine ganglion block for the treatment of postdural puncture headache: a randomised, blinded, clinical trial. Br J Anaesth 2020;124(6):739–47.

[53] Palamar D, Uluduz D, Saip S, et al. Ultrasound-guided greater occipital nerve block: an efficient technique in chronic refractory migraine without aura? Pain Physician 2015;18(2): 153–62.

[54] Giaccari LG, Aurilio C, Coppolino F, et al. Peripheral Nerve Blocks for Postdural Puncture Headache: A New Solution for an Old Problem? In Vivo 2021;35(6):3019–29.

[55] Matute E, Bonilla S, Girones A, et al. Bilateral greater occipital nerve block for post-dural puncture headache. Anaesthesia 2008;63(5):557–8.

[56] Niraj G, Kelkar A, Girotra V. Greater occipital nerve block for postdural puncture headache (PDPH): a prospective audit of a modified guideline for the management of PDPH and review of the literature. J Clin Anesth 2014;26(7):539–44.

[57] Dietzel J, Witstruck T, Adler S, et al. Acupuncture for treatment of therapy-resistant post-dural puncture headache: a retrospective case series. Br J Anaesth. Nov 2013;111(5):847–9.

Advances in Anesthesia 41 (2023) 87–110

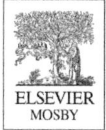

ADVANCES IN ANESTHESIA

ELSEVIER
MOSBY

Reconceptualizing Acute Pain Management in the 21st Century

Stephen Macres, MD[a],*, Robin J. Aldwinckle, BMBS, FRCA[b],
Usha Saldahna, MD[c], Scott G. Pritzlaff, MD[d],
Michael Jung, MD, MBA[e], Josh Santos, MD[f],
Mariya Kotova, PharmD[g],
Robert Bishop, B Biomed Sci, B Med, FANZCA[h]

[a]Department of Anesthesiology and Pain Medicine, University of California, Davis Medical Center, 4150 V. Street, Sacramento, CA 95817, USA; [b]Anesthesiology, Department of Anesthesiology & Pain Medicine, 4150 V. Street, PSSB Suite 1200, Sacramento, CA 95817, USA; [c]Regional Anesthesia Fellowship, Department of Anesthesiology and Pain Medicine, University of California, Davis Medical Center, 4150 V. Street, Sacramento, CA 95817, USA; [d]Division of Pain Medicine, Pain Medicine Fellowship, Department of Anesthesiology and Pain Medicine, University of California, Davis Medical Center, 4860 Y. Street, Suite 3020, Sacramento CA 95817, USA; [e]Pain Fellowship, Department of Anesthesiology and Pain Medicine, UC Davis Medical Center, 4860 Y. Street, Suite 3020, Sacramento CA 95817, USA; [f]Pre-Anesthesia Readiness & Education Program, 4150 V. Street, Sacramento, CA 95817, USA; [g]Department of Pharmacy, UC Davis Medical Center, 1240 47th Avenue, Sacramento, CA 95831, USA; [h]Department of Anesthesiology and Pain Medicine, University of California Davis Medical Center, Sacramento, CA, USA

Keywords

- Acute perioperative pain management • Acute pain team organization
- Peripheral nerve stimulation and acute pain • Cryo-neurolysis and acute pain
- Transitional pain service • Opioid use disorder
- Acute pain management of the opioid-dependent patient • Biased opioid ligand

Key points

- Acute perioperative pain management that uses multimodal opioid-sparing techniques, Enhanced Recovery After Surgery (ERAS) protocols, and a transitional pain service that encourages preoperative assessment of the opioid-dependent patient will improve acute pain management and patient outcomes.

Continued

*Corresponding author. Department of Anesthesiology and Pain Medicine, University of California, Davis Medical Center, 4150 V. Street, PSSB 1200, Sacramento, CA 95817.
E-mail address: smmacres@ucdavis.edu

https://doi.org/10.1016/j.aan.2023.06.006
0737-6146/23/© 2023 Elsevier Inc. All rights reserved.

Continued

- Opioid stewardship encourages a multimodal, multidisciplinary approach to acute perioperative pain management that optimizes analgesia and patient satisfaction while mitigating side effects from opioid analgesics.
- Risk factors for opioid-induced respiratory depression include obesity, advanced age, a diagnosis of obstructive sleep apnea and opioid dependence.
- Peripheral nerve stimulation and cryo-neurolysis are emerging technologies for treating perioperative pain.
- The opioid-dependent patient will benefit from the perioperative administration of subanesthetic doses of the N-methyl-D-aspartate (NMDA) receptor antagonist ketamine.

"Prediction is difficult-particularly when it involves the future."

Mark Twain

INTRODUCTION

Following surgery patients experience acute pain which is a multidimensional phenomenon the etiology of which can be multifactorial. Over 300 million surgeries are carried out annually throughout the world, and many of these surgeries are performed as inpatients. Unfortunately, despite our best efforts acute postoperative pain management continues to be an unresolved worldwide problem [1,2]. Tissue injury associated with surgery can trigger numerous adverse neuroendocrine and sympathoadrenal responses, resulting in detrimental physiologic responses. Adverse consequences of poorly controlled acute pain include the increased risk of adverse cardiovascular and thromboembolic complications, increased hospital length of stay, poor sleep, increased time to first ambulation, increased opioid use, and delirium in the elderly, all of which have the potential of increasing costs for the health care system [3].

Generally speaking, acute pain resolves over about one to 3 months. However, poorly managed acute pain can increase the likelihood of patients developing chronic post-surgical pain (CPSP) (Table 1), which can potentially have negative psychological effects and cause patients to be less satisfied with their surgical experience. It is, therefore, vital that we manage acute pain effectively using multimodal, analgesic techniques.

Table 1
Incidence of chronic postsurgical pain [80,81]

Type of surgery	Incidence of CPSP (%)	Chronic pain at 12 mo
Abdominal surgery	17–21	No data
Amputation	30–85	75% (lower extremity)
Caesarean section	6–55	No data
Hip arthroplasty	7–23	28%
Knee arthroplasty	13–44	18%
Mastectomy	11–57	43%–56% (mastectomy)
Thoracotomy	5–71	41%

Despite the existence of acute pain services and the availability of effective analgesics and non-pharmacological techniques, there is still good evidence that the overall incidence of moderate-to-severe pain in surgical patients remains unacceptably high [4]. Fortunately, a multisociety collective effort was initiated in 2021, which both developed and then promulgated 7 guiding principles for the management of acute perioperative pain [5]. These recommendations include: (1) a thorough preoperative evaluation of the patient prior to surgery that addresses comorbid conditions that can interfere with adequate acute pain control, (2) use of a validated pain assessment tool to monitor treatment, (3) a multimodal approach to acute pain management, (4) education of the patient about treatment options, (5) education of the patient about their treatment plan, (6) adjusting and tailoring the treatment plan to the patient as needed, and (7) access to an acute pain specialist for the high-risk patient when required.

Organizing an acute pain management service

The cost of postoperative pain services in a privatized health system, where postoperative care is only partially reimbursed, is a major barrier to their establishment. Apart from the benefits to patient care, an acute pain service (APS), however, adds value by lowering hospital expenses by enhancing surgical results and promoting patient recovery and early discharge [6]. Depending on the reimbursement model, this added value, of an acute pain service, might balance out the service's initial costs, making it a convincing investment. The APS offers direct patient care, such as managing continuous epidural and regional catheter infusions and other modalities, and can take the lead in patient education as well as the training of other physicians, nurses, and caregivers to ensure their proficiency in accurately identifying, managing, and attending to patients' needs. The surgical patient would ideally receive a continuum of care during the perioperative period by a proactive APS. The main objective is to use "protocol-based systems that optimize resource utilization while improving patient care" [7] to reduce the variability of acute pain management.

For an acute pain service to be successful there must be an institutional commitment to support the establishment of the service. A physician leader with education and experience in acute and chronic pain management must serve as the team's focal point and additional anesthesiologists, with similar training, must also be available to participate in a supervisory role and to maintain continuity of care. Protocolized acute pain management pathways can then be developed, which midlevel providers (registered nurses or nurse practitioners) can follow [3].

The authors' institution offers an ACGME (Accreditation Council for Graduate Medical Education) accredited regional anesthesia and acute pain medicine fellowship that follows this model. The team members include the physician team leader, fellow, registered nurse, anesthesia resident, an intern, a clinical pharmacist, and an anesthesia technician. The APS can take the lead in changing the institutional culture so that alleviating pain and suffering are prioritized [8].

Pre-assessment and perioperative planning

A detailed preoperative assessment is crucial to the management of postoperative pain. The goal of this assessment is to identify risk factors for difficult-to-manage postoperative pain. Ideally, this would take place with enough lead time to allow for optimization of modifiable risk factors and creation of an individually tailored management plan prior to surgery. The assessment commonly occurs as part of a preoperative evaluation in an established pre-anesthesia clinic by a provider with experience in pain management [9]. The advent of a transitional pain service has shown promising results in creating a multidisciplinary, patient-centric approach, with emphasis on individually tailored plans to optimally manage pain throughout the perioperative time continuum [9,10].

Chronic pain conditions, substance abuse, and psychological conditions (mood disorders and high-level catastrophizing behaviors) are known risk factors for severe and/or prolonged postoperative pain [11–13]. A history of chronic pain should prompt further assessment for opioid use, which is linked to higher opioid requirements and pain scores postoperatively [13,14]. If opioid use is present, several strategies can be employed preoperatively to mitigate risk of severe postoperative pain including initiation of non-opioid agents to decrease opioid use preoperatively; cessation of sedative agents which when given concomitantly with opiates increases the risk of adverse events; and patient education to set realistic expectations [9].

Patients with substance use disorder should be counseled on cessation and referred to substance use programs to prevent withdrawal perioperatively. Methadone or buprenorphine initiation is reasonable to prevent untoward effects from substance use disorder, withdrawal, and potentially reduce postoperative pain [15]. A pain management plan that uses non-opioid therapies and regional anesthesia should be considered in response to increased opioid tolerance.

The presence of depression, anxiety, and a high level of catastrophizing also place patients at risk for difficult-to-control postoperative pain. Relaxation therapy focusing on developing coping strategies should be considered preoperatively as this has been shown to reduce pain postoperatively in patients with the previously mentioned psychological conditions [16,17].

Preoperative assessment is also important in screening for comorbidities and medication use that could influence treatment modalities offered to the patient. For example, anticoagulation or antiplatelet agents limit the use of neuraxial and some regional anesthesia techniques unless held with sufficient time prior to the procedure. Furthermore, partial-mu opioid agonists (eg, buprenorphine) used to treat either chronic pain or substance dependence also puts the patient at risk for difficult-to-control postoperative pain. Although a coordinated plan to taper buprenorphine has been suggested [18], current expert opinion recommends against discontinuation of buprenorphine in the perioperative period [19]. A multimodal approach that optimizes the use of regional analgesia is highly recommended. Consultation with an acute pain specialist would be a prudent decision.

The Transitional Pain Service

Since management of acute perioperative pain can be fragmented and unpredictable, we are strong advocates of the development of a Transitional Pain Service (TPS). The TPS is a multidisciplinary organization that employs a multimodal approach to pain management to "bridge the gap between acute and chronic pain" [20] in complex surgical patients who may be opioid dependent, such as patients with "failed back syndrome", opioid use disorder (OUD), or sickle cell disease. There are several staffing models that have been described in the literature [20], which include the "high intensity" model used at the Toronto General Hospital, in Canada, or the "low intensity" model practiced at the Veterans Administration Medical Center (VAMC) in Salt Lake City, Utah. A recent economic analysis of the ratio of savings to cost of the "low intensity" approach has been shown to have a positive economic impact [20]. A TPS can be easily situated within a pre-existing perioperative surgical home and tailored to share resources and cut costs. Examples of interventions that a TPS may offer a patient include opioid weaning, peripheral neuromodulation, relaxation therapies, and cognitive-behavioral therapy [20].

The opioid-dependent chronic pain patient

The opioid-dependent population of patients includes not only patients with substance use disorder but also patients with chronic pain. Although chronic pain has been defined in the past as pain without any apparent biological value that persists for greater than 3 months, it has been further subdivided into chronic primary as well as secondary pain. Chronic primary pain is described as pain in one or more anatomic regions that lasts or returns for more than 3 months that cannot be better explained by another chronic pain condition. Chronic secondary pain on the other hand tends to be linked to other diseases, such as cancer, chronic pain following surgery and trauma, neuropathic pain, visceral pain, and musculoskeletal disorders [3].

The number of patients with chronic pain for whom chronic opioids have been prescribed has dramatically increased since the late 1990s with the thought in mind that opioid therapy would enhance quality of life, function, and pain management. Unfortunately, data indicate that there have been no corresponding declines in the rates of disability or enhancements in health status despite the increased use of opioids for chronic pain [21]. Adverse consequences associated with the long-term use of opioids that complicate the management of this patient population include physical dependence, opioid withdrawal syndrome, tolerance, opioid-induced hyperalgesia (OIH), and respiratory depression.

Tragically, over the past several decades, an opioid crisis of unprecedented proportions has ensured that has exacerbated the problem. It has transpired in 3 waves, with the first wave commencing in the 1990s secondary to the overprescribing of oxycodone due to misleading marketing strategies by the manufacturer of OxyContin. This was followed shortly thereafter by a second wave in 2010, when drug dealers began to market heroin to individuals who were dependent on prescription opioids. The third wave hit in 2014 when fentanyl was illicitly added to sham pharmaceutical pills and peddled to unsuspecting individuals. The COVID-19 pandemic has only served to aggravate the situation.

Since these patients can experience a complicated hospital course, which is compounded by increasing hospital length of stay and high readmission rate, it is mandatory that they receive a comprehensive preoperative evaluation with emphasis on mitigation strategies. The US Food and Drug Administration (FDA) defines the opioid tolerant patient as the patient who consumes more than 60 oral milligram equivalents of morphine daily for 7 days or longer. Because this patient population is particularly vulnerable to respiratory depression (Table 2), it is strongly advised that a multimodal approach toward acute pain management be pursued in this patient population. Consultation with an acute pain specialist would also be practical advice.

Opioid use disorder

Special consideration should be taken when managing acute pain in the patient with OUD who is receiving medication for the treatment of their condition (MOUD). Medications approved by the FDA for the management of OUD include methadone, buprenorphine, and naltrexone. It is not advised to stop taking methadone or buprenorphine before surgery. Patients who are taking maintenance methadone prior to surgery should continue taking it afterward. For better analgesia, instead of administering the drug once daily, it may be divided into 3 doses throughout the day, which may be administered at 8 hour intervals. Serious side effects associated with methadone treatment include QT prolongation, torsades de pointe, and respiratory depression.

Buprenorphine has received FDA approval in the United States to treat chronic pain, OUD, and acute pain. The drug is a nociceptin opioid receptor (ORL-1) agonist, kappa receptor antagonist, and partial mu receptor agonist. Buprenorphine is a potent analgesic with a ceiling effect on respiratory

Table 2
Risk factors for opioid induced respiratory depression [82,83]

Patient characteristics	Perioperative factors
Obesity	Continuous infusion of opioids
Diagnosis of OSA	Multiple prescribers and multiple routes of administration of opioids.
Advanced age > 60 y	Concurrent use of sedative medications
Opioid-dependent patient	Poor nursing assessment
PMH significant for cardiac (CAD, CHF), pulmonary (COPD) and neurologic (CVA) diseases	Increased incidence of post-anesthesia events including hypoventilation, apnea, desaturation, and sedation/ analgesia mismatch.
Lower extremity surgery	

Abbreviations: CAD, coronary artery disease; CHF, congestive heart failure; COPD, chronic obstructive pulmonary disease; CVA, cerebral vascular accident; PMH past medical history.

depression and therefore a potentially safer alternative than methadone for OUD. The drug is available in numerous formulations for administration that include parenteral, transdermal, sublingual, buccal films, subcutaneous, and subdermal implants. Buprenorphine should not be routinely discontinued prior to surgery [19]. It is strongly advised to consult with a specialist in the management of acute pain in this patient population.

Naltrexone is a semi-synthetic opioid antagonist that has been shown to be highly effective in patients dependent on alcohol or opioids who are highly motivated to maintain their abstinence. The drug may be administered orally (50 mg po) once a day or as a depot injection (Vivitrol 380 mg), which is administered monthly. The oral formulation should be discontinued 72 hours prior to surgery in these patients, and surgery should ideally be postponed for at least 4 weeks following the last dose of depot naltrexone. Because naltrexone and chronic opioid antagonism can cause opioid receptor upregulation in these patients, they are more likely to experience opioid-related side effects like respiratory depression. The reader is directed to a few outstanding reviews on the subject [19,22] because a thorough discussion of this subject is outside the purview of this review .

Pharmacologic management of acute pain

Acute pain is caused by a variety of different factors, which include surgery, trauma, burns, and musculoskeletal injuries. Management of acute pain requires the application of multimodal analgesic strategies using enhanced recovery guidelines. The judicious use of opioid medications that optimize analgesia while minimizing opioid related adverse side effects will improve both outcomes and patient satisfaction. Non-opioid analgesics that have proven to be beneficial in opioid-sparing strategies include the para-aminophenol derivatives, non-steroidal anti-inflammatory drugs (NSAIDs), gabapentinoids, N-methyl-D-aspartate (NMDA) receptor antagonists, local anesthetics, magnesium, and alpha-2-agonists. In this section, we will briefly review the efficacy of these drugs, however, a full discussion of this topic is beyond the scope of this article and the reader is referred to other more comprehensive reviews [3,23]. See Tables 3–5) for dosing recommendations of these drugs.

Acetaminophen is a para-aminophenol derivative that inhibits prostaglandin synthesis in the central nervous system and is effective for mild-to-moderate pain. It is available for both oral and intravenous administration. Following major surgery, the addition of acetaminophen to an analgesic protocol can improve pain control, decrease oral morphine equivalents (OMEs), and decrease the incidence of postoperative nausea and vomiting. The drug has a low risk of gastrointestinal (GI), renal and cardiovascular side effects but it should be avoided in patients with severe liver disease [23].

NSAIDs inhibit the cyclooxygenase enzyme (COX) and impair prostaglandin synthesis. Following major surgery, much like acetaminophen, NSAIDs have demonstrated a reduction in the 24 hour morphine requirement as well as a reduction in postoperative nausea and vomiting. NSAIDs have also

Table 3
Guidelines for preoperative analgesia (single dose) in adults [3,4,22,23]

Drug	Dosing guidelines
Acetaminophen intravenous dosing	Weight>50 kg: 650 mg q4h or 1000 mg q6h Weight<50 kg: 12.5 mg/kg q4h or 15 mg/kg q6h Avoid in patients with severe liver failure. Maximum dose: <50 kg: 3.75g/d >50 kg: 4 g/d
Celecoxib	400 mg po, age < 65 y 200 mg po, age > 65 y Avoid in patients with renal failure
Gabapentin	300 mg po, age < 65 y 100–300 mg po age > 65 y Adjust dose in renal failure

Table 4
Guidelines for intraoperative multimodal analgesia [3,4,22,23,84]

Drug	Adult Intravenous Dosing guidelines
Lidocaine	Dosing is based on ideal body weight. Bolus: 0.5–1.5 mg/kg Infusion: 1–1.5 mg/kg/h The infusion may be continued postoperatively on a monitored floor per institution protocol. Decrease the dose in patients with liver disease.
Ketamine	Bolus: 0.1–0.35 mg/kg Infusion: 0.1–1 mg/kg/h May consider postoperative infusion in a monitored setting per institution protocol. Consider the addition of a benzodiazepine or alpha-2-agonist to moderate adverse side effects such as agitation or hypertension.
Magnesium	Bolus: 1–3 g (30–50 mg/kg) Infusion: 0.5–1 g/h
Dexmedetomidine	Bolus: 0.5 MCG/kg over 10–15 min if hemodynamically stable Infusion: 0.3–1 MCG/kg/h
Esmolol	Bolus: 500 MCG/kg Infusion: 5–50 MCG/kg/min
Dexamethasone	1–10 mg (usual dosing range is 0.1–0.2 mg/kg) once at the beginning of the case. Higher doses may provide better analgesia.
Methadone	0.1–0.3 mg/kg (do not exceed 30 mg) once at the beginning of the case [22]. Plasma T1/2 can be > 24 h. Monitor closely for postop opioid related side effects, particularly respiratory depression. Do not combine the drug with other opioids.

Abbreviations: MCG, microgram; mg, milligram.

Table 5
Guidelines for postoperative inpatient analgesia [3,4,22,23,84]

Drug	Adult Dosing guidelines
Acetaminophen (APAP)	650 mg po q4h while awake or, 975 mg po q6h.
Celecoxib	100–200 mg po q12–24h
Meloxicam	15 mg po qd
Ibuprofen	400 mg po TID or q6h with meals
Ketorolac	15–30 mg IV q6–8h (weight ≥ 50 kg, or age < 65 y) 15 mg IV q6–8h not to exceed 60 mg/24 h (weight < 50 kg or age >65 y) The drug is recommended for short term use only, not to exceed 5 days. Avoid ketorolac in patients with moderate to severe renal impairment.
Gabapentin	100 mg po TID or 100 mg po at breakfast and lunch then 300 mg po at hs.
Pregabalin	25–50 mg po BID
Oxycodone	Opioid naïve patient: 5 mg po q4h PRN moderate to severe pain.
Hydrocodone	Same dosing as with oxycodone
Ketamine	Bolus dose: 0.1–0.35 mg/kg or 5–10 mg IV push once or q2h PRN for refractory pain. Consult acute pain service for specific guidelines.

been shown to be synergistic with acetaminophen so they can be combined for enhanced analgesia [23]. NSAID-related side effects include GI side effects such as nausea and vomiting, bleeding risk secondary to platelet dysfunction, acute kidney injury, cardiac events, and bone healing impairment [24]. GI side effects appear to be dose-dependent with a lower risk at ibuprofen doses of 1200 mg/ d or less [25]. Likewise, meloxicam may be a safer alternative at lower doses since it is a selective COX-2 inhibitor at 7.5 mg/d but non-selective at 15 mg/d [26]. Ketorolac is available for intravenous administration and is recommended for short-term use not to exceed 5 days. The dose should be adjusted for renal failure and is contraindicated in patients with severe kidney disease. See table for dosing recommendations. When there is no contraindication, begin the NSAID at the lowest dose for the shortest duration possible.

The gabapentinoids, gabapentin and pregabalin, are anticonvulsants that display antinociceptive properties that can be ascribed to attenuation of dorsal horn sensitivity primarily through modulation of calcium-mediated neurotransmitter release at the α-2-δ calcium channel subunit. Gabapentinoids can increase the risk of postoperative sedation and in combination with opioids may also increase the risk of postoperative respiratory depression [3]. Before initiation of the gabapentinoid, consider patient-specific factors such as advanced age, renal function, concomitant CNS depressants, and side effect profile such as drowsiness and dizziness [27].

Ketamine is an NMDA receptor antagonist that has been shown to be particularly efficacious in the opioid tolerant patient [3]. The perioperative administration of intravenous ketamine can reduce 24 and 48 hour postoperative morphine requirements and patient-reported pain intensity. Surgical procedures that produce the most severe postoperative pain, such as upper abdominal, thoracic, lower abdominal, intra-abdominal, and orthopedic procedures all benefit the most from the perioperative use of subanesthetic ketamine [28].

Although Enhanced Recovery after Surgery (ERAS) guidelines [29] have recommended the use of intravenous (IV) lidocaine for perioperative pain management its efficacy is unclear. A recent 2018 Cochrane review [30] could not state with certainty whether intravenous lidocaine-reduced opioid requirements or improved 4 hour postoperative pain scores and a 2020 meta-analysis [31] could not demonstrate a significant reduction in pain scores. Additional trials are needed to identify if there is any perioperative benefit to IV lidocaine.

The perioperative administration of intravenous magnesium for abdominal and orthopedic surgery and hysterectomy can reduce 24 hour postoperative OME requirements and pain scores. Ongoing trials continue to investigate the pain benefit and opioid reduction profile of perioperative IV magnesium.

The alpha-2-agonists, clonidine and dexmedetomidine, can reduce the 24 hour morphine requirements and pain intensity and are anxiolytic. Adverse effects include sedation, bradycardia, and hypotension.

Opioids are a mainstay in managing acute postoperative pain. Judicious use of opioid medication is encouraged using a multimodal strategy that optimizes the use of the non-opioid analgesics combined with regional analgesia techniques and procedures. We strongly recommend that you perform a thorough preoperative opioid use assessment and risk stratification analysis as described by Edwards and colleagues [32] prior to surgery when evaluating your patient (Table 6). A full discussion of opioid analgesic pharmacology and dosing guidelines is beyond the scope of this chapter. Prudence dictates consultation with an acute pain specialist when managing the opioid-dependent patient.

The *biased opioid ligand* TRV-130 (oliceridine) is a unique addition to our analgesic armamentarium that was recently approved for the management of acute pain [3]. The drug selectively activates the G-protein pathway versus the beta-arrestin pathway of the mu receptor, and it is the biased nature of this binding that allows for targeted and efficient pain relief, and potentially fewer opioid-related side effects [33]. These advantages make TRV-130 an attractive alternative for the treatment of moderate to severe pain, especially in cases where traditional opioids are ineffective or pose a high risk of adverse effects. Although oliceridine displays a lower risk of GI and respiratory side effects, vis-a-vis morphine, a dose-dependent increase in respiratory depression has been described. Careful monitoring of the patient for respiratory depression is therefore still indicated. The drug has a rapid onset of action, achieving peak pain relief within 15 minutes of administration. The recommended dose of the drug is 1 to 2 mg IV q 1 to 3 hours not to exceed 27 mg in any 24 hour

Table 6
ONET (opioid naive, exposed, tolerant) Classification System[32]

Preop opioid use assessment (oral morphine equivalent: OME)	
Opioid naïve	No opioid exposure in the previous 90 d
Opioid exposed	Any amount of opioid 60 mg OME per day in previous 90 d
Opioid tolerant	≥60 mg OME per day in the 7 d prior to surgery.

Risk modifiers
1. History of substance use disorder (eg, alcohol or opioid)
2. Surgery associated with moderate to severe postoperative pain and chronic postoperative pain such as thoracotomy or spinal fusion.

period [34]. Further studies are needed to fully evaluate the long-term safety and efficacy of the *biased opioid ligand* TRV-130 in the clinical setting.

Precision medicine and *pharmacogenetics* are emerging fields of medicine that aim to provide personalized treatment options for patients based on their genetic makeup. Two of the key genes involved in pharmacogenetics include CYP2D6 and CYP2D9 that code for the cytochrome P450 enzymes responsible for the metabolism of both the opioid and NSAID analgesics, respectively [35,36]. Individual variations in the CYP2D6 and CYP2C9 gene can impact the efficacy and toxicity of the medications metabolized by these enzymes. Pharmacogenetic testing can identify individuals who are poor metabolizers or ultra-rapid metabolizers that may require dosage adjustments of specific drugs to achieve therapeutic effects and minimize toxicity. These emerging technologies will enable health care providers to tailor treatment to individual patients based on their genetic make-up leading to improved efficacy and reduced adverse events.

Regional anesthesia

Regional anesthesia is an important and often defining feature of an acute pain service [4,22,37]. Regional anesthesia (commonly referred to as "nerve blocks") generally involves placement of local anesthetic (eg, ropivacaine) and other injectable medications near neural structures such as peripheral nerves to induce analgesia and anesthesia [38,39]. These injections may include "single shot" injections or indwelling catheters, often placed with image guidance such as with ultrasound imaging [40–42]. Classically, a block involved injecting perineurally around a large, combined motor-sensory nerve such as the femoral nerve; however, other blocks such as interfascial "plane blocks" (eg, transversus abdominis plane [TAP] block) have become more common [43–45]. A broader definition of regional anesthesia procedures can include the placement of neuraxial blocks such as spinal and epidural anesthesia; however, such techniques may also be considered a distinct modality.

Regional anesthesia is a versatile pain management modality and often considered a cornerstone of multimodal or ERAS pathways due to their high effectiveness in providing analgesia and opioid-sparing benefits [46–48]. The blocks are specific to "regions" of the body (as shown in Table 7) and may reduce the need for systemic medications such as intravenous pain medications. An overview of the technique and specific indications for every block is beyond the scope of this overview; however, many dedicated resources exist [38,39]. Additional desired effects of regional anesthesia may include improved blood flow (desirable in surgeries such as arteriovenous fistula creation), sympathectomy (eg, stellate ganglion block [SGB] for refractory ventricular tachycardia), and avoidance of general anesthesia (eg, in cesarean section thus allowing immediate mother–baby bonding among other benefits). See Table 7 for specific recommendations.

Regional anesthesia can have risks, including periprocedural pain, bleeding, infection, and injury to surrounding structures such as blood vessels and nerves. Guidelines regarding specific safety considerations such as anticoagulation are available [49]. Local anesthetic systemic toxicity may occur with high volumes and concentrations of local anesthetic and have defined management [50]. Clinicians performing blocks should be well trained in regional anesthesia, and fellowship training is often a valuable educational experience for practitioners.

Interventional approaches
Peripheral Nerve Stimulation
Peripheral nerve stimulation (PNS) is an established technique that involves applying electrical stimulation to peripheral nerves or nerve roots to relieve pain. PNS involves placing specialized leads that are placed percutaneously, usually with high-resolution ultrasound or even fluoroscopy. Permanent and temporary systems are available, but the evidence surrounding acute pain mainly focuses on temporary systems. Because of the small design (300 μm diameter), leads can be kept in place for up to 60 days. The benefits of PNS over peripheral nerve catheters include no motor blockade, low infection risk, and compact device profile (Fig. 1).

The mechanism of PNS for acute pain is thought to involve the modulation of pain signals as they travel from the peripheral nerves to the central nervous system. Classically, it was thought that gate control theory was a prominent mechanism by stimulating Aβ afferent fibers, pain transmission via Aδ, and c fibers can be reduced. Additional mechanisms of action include peripheral effects like decreasing the release of inflammatory mediators and even modulation of central or spinal pathways [51]. Furthermore, the electrical stimulation from PNS can activate inhibitory pathways in the spinal cord, reducing the transmission of

Table 7
Peripheral nerve blockade recommendations [3]

Anatomic location	Preferred block	Comments
Upper extremity		
Total shoulder arthroplasty	Interscalene block	The superior trunk block can potentially spare the phrenic nerve.
Rotator cuff tear	Superior trunk block	The ICBN provides cutaneous sensation to the lateral chest, medial aspect of the upper arm, and the axilla.
AVF creation: Supraclavicular block (SCB) is very useful. Combine with intercostobrachial nerve (ICBN) block.	SCB	Continuous catheter: consider infraclavicular approach.
	Infraclavicular approach	
Elbow	Axillary approach	
Wrist surgery		
Lower extremity		
Total hip arthroplasty	Pericapsular nerve group (PENG) block	An epidural may be useful if bilateral limbs are involved, and anticoagulation status does not preclude placement.
Hip fracture	Fascia Iliaca block	Consider addition of an adductor canal block to cover the medial aspect of the limb.
Total knee arthroplasty	Quadratus lumborum block	
Patella fracture or torn tendon	Adductor canal block and iPACK (infiltration between popliteal artery and capsule of the knee) block	
Below the knee amputation	Femoral nerve block	
Above the knee amputation	Popliteal block or subgluteal sciatic nerve block	
Ankle surgery		
Abdomen	Bilateral rectus sheath blocks for mid-line incision	If there is no contraindication, a thoracic epidural placed congruent to the surgical incision is an option.
Exploratory laparotomy	Lateral TAP block for kidney transplant. Bilateral blocks if the incision crosses the midline	**External oblique intercostal blocks** for upper midline and lateral abdominal incisions.
Kidney transplant		
Cesarean section		

(continued on next page)

Table 7
(continued)

Anatomic location	Preferred block	Comments
Chest wall		If there is no contraindication, a thoracic epidural placed congruent to the surgical incision is an excellent option.
Mastectomy	Pectoralis (PECS) block	
Thoracotomy	Paravertebral blocks	
Rib fractures	Anterior serratus block	
	Erector spinae plane block (ESPB)	
Other		
Ophthalmic surgery	Peribulbar/retrobulbar block	
Carotid endarterectomy	Cervical plexus block (deep and superficial)	
Lumbar spine surgery	Erector spinae plane block	
Refractory ventricular tachycardia	Stellate ganglion block	
Intractable hiccups	Phrenic nerve blockade	

Abbreviation: AVF, arteriovenous fistula.

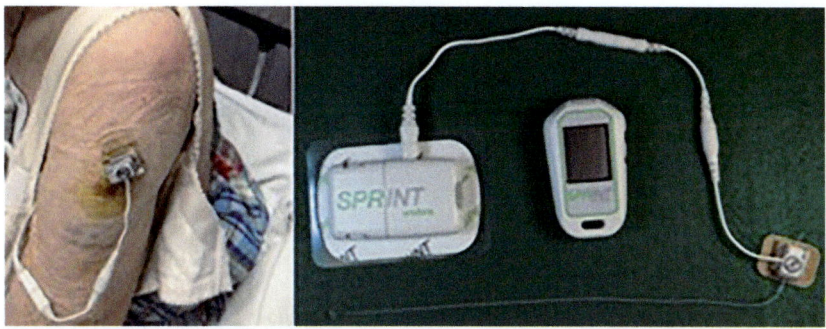

Fig. 1. PNS lead placed at the axillary nerve as it emerges from the quadrangular space for a patient with subacute shoulder pain after hemiarthroplasty (left). A temporary, percutaneous PNS system with externalized microlead, pulse generator, and patient controller (right). (*Courtesy of* S Pritzlaff, MD, Sacramento, CA.)

pain signals to the brain. These central mechanisms can explain why PNS can be helpful in conditions like post-amputation and hemiplegic shoulder pain [52,53].

Several types of acute pain have been shown to respond to PNS, including postoperative pain, cancer pain, and acute pain due to traumatic injury. In postoperative pain, PNS is an effective alternative to traditional pain management techniques, such as opioid analgesics. Increasing evidence indicates that PNS can be helpful in the acute pain setting [54,55]. For example, a recent randomized controlled trial demonstrated significant reductions in pain and opioid consumption at 7 days postop in patients undergoing rotator cuff repair or foot/ankle surgery. Leads were placed at the brachial plexus and sciatic nerve, respectively [55].

Despite the promising results, there are some limitations to using PNS for acute pain. One of the significant limitations is the need for patient compliance and cooperation. Lead migration is also possible, particularly if the site of the implanted lead is near a large joint or mobile area of the body. Additionally, PNS is not always effective in all patients, and some may experience increased pain or discomfort during the stimulation. Furthermore, current PNS systems are MRI conditional at best or even MRI incompatible. This can limit postsurgical imaging, and the system may need to be explanted if an MRI needs to be completed. Finally, the long-term effects of PNS are not well understood, and further research is required to fully understand its efficacy for treating acute pain.

Cryoneurolysis

Cryoneurolysis is a medical procedure that uses extreme cold to temporarily or permanently block nerve signals and relieve pain. This procedure was performed as an open procedure by surgeons intraoperative, but the availability of percutaneous cannulae has allowed anesthesiologists and pain physicians to perform cryoneurolysis percutaneously with ultrasound. Several

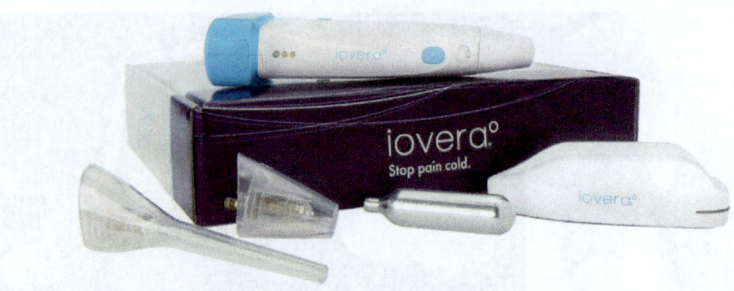

Fig. 2. Photo of commercially available handheld, percutaneous cryoneurolysis device with single and multitoned tips. (©Pacira Pharmaceuticals, Inc. All Rights Reserved. Used Under License.)

commercially available systems use pressurized nitrous oxide or carbon dioxide to cool the cryoprobe tip, which freezes the target nerve(s). An "ice ball" forms around the probe's tip with temperatures between $-20°C$ and $-100°C$ (Fig. 2). After exposure to these temperatures, nerves undergo Wallerian degeneration, but the connective tissues surrounding the axon (epineurium, perineurium, and endoneurium) remain intact. As a result, the scaffolding architecture of the nerve remains intact, and the nerve can regenerate over weeks to months. Although not permanent, cryoneurolysis will cause numbness and weakness if a mixed motor/sensory nerve is treated.

Several studies have shown that cryoneurolysis is effective in managing acute pain [56–58]. In addition, cryoneurolysis has been shown to be effective in reducing pain and opioid consumption in patients with acute pain following total knee arthroplasty. Nerves targeted for knee pain include the infrapatellar branch of the saphenous nerve and the genicular nerves [59]. Other applications for cryoneurolysis include targeting intercostal nerves for thoracotomy pain, but data are limited [58].

The evidence suggests that cryoneurolysis is an effective technique for managing acute and postsurgical pain. However, more research is needed to fully understand its long-term effects and compare it to other pain management techniques.

NON-SURGICAL CONSULTS FOR THE ACUTE PAIN TEAM
Intractable hiccups
There have been several case reports of the successful use of phrenic nerve block for intractable hiccups not responding to conservative and pharmacologic treatment [60–63]. A single injection ultrasound-guided right phrenic nerve block was successful in the immediate resolution of hiccups that had prolonged a hospital stay after minor spine surgery for 7 days [61]. A patient with an esophageal stent for esophageal cancer had relief of hiccups and mediastinal

pain after a left, and, subsequently, a right phrenic nerve block. Hiccups were still relieved at follow up at 2 and 4 weeks after the procedure. A single injection phrenic nerve block performed intraoperatively relieved hiccups within a few minutes during abdominal surgery under low-dose epidural anesthesia. Renes [62] reported a case where a phrenic nerve catheter was successful in resolving hiccups not responsive to conservative measures. Pre-injection scanning of the diaphragm revealed abnormal movement of the right side, so a right phrenic nerve catheter was placed to prevent involvement of the normal functioning side. The hiccups resolved after the initial injection and infusion but recurred when the initial infusion was stopped. The catheter allowed recommencement of the infusion and complete resolution after a further 24 hours of infusion. It is well reported that phrenic nerve block causes a decrease in ratio of the forced expiratory volume (FEV1)/forced vital capacity of the lungs (FVC) of approximately 25% [64], and imaging of the diaphragm should be considered prior to placement of a phrenic nerve block [62], and should be avoided in patients with significant respiratory impairment.

Refractory ventricular tachycardia

Stellate ganglion block (SGB) has shown to be an effective treatment for ventricular arrhythmias (VAs), and its ability to be performed at bedside using ultrasound is a significant advantage over fluoroscopy. Studies have shown that the autonomic nervous system has an important role in the triggering and maintenance of VA, especially in electrical storm (ES). Two meta-analyses (35 cases, 22 studies, and 38 cases, 23 studies) showed that SGB for drug refractory ES was associated with a reduced burden of VA episodes and defibrillation events [65,66]. The stellate ganglia do not appear to have equivalent sympathetic effects on the myocardium, with the left side appearing to have greater influence in both a canine model and after coronary occlusion [67]. Hence, most human studies use a left SGB for treatment of VA. However, it should be noted that myocardial damage may lead to remodeling of both the left and right stellate ganglia, which supports the use of bilateral SGB for the treatment of VA [68].

Unilateral or bilateral SGB can reduce arrhythmia burden and defibrillation events for 24 to 72 hours in refractory VT. The efficacy of SGB appears to be consistent despite the type (monomorphic vs polymorphic) or etiology (ischemic vs non-ischemic cardiomyopathy) of the VA [67] and may allow time for use of other therapies like catheter ablation, surgical sympathectomy, or heart transplantation. Consideration should be given to the timing of the block, if possible, in relation to anticoagulant dosing, but given the urgency of the procedure and the risk of holding anticoagulant medication in this group of patients this is not always possible or prudent. Bilateral blocks should be reserved for intubated patients given the potential effect on the recurrent laryngeal and phrenic nerves. Overall, ultrasound-guided SGB is a relatively safe procedure with a low risk for complications, even when performed on the anticoagulated patient.

Rib fractures management

Rib fractures are a common thoracic injury encountered in more than 20% of patients [69] with blunt thoracic trauma, and represent a substantial health burden. There is no universally agreed upon risk stratification score, but the Rib Score and Chest Trauma Score (CTS) are commonly used. Significant risk factors for mortality include age and number of rib fractures, along with pre-existing lung disease, use of anticoagulants prior to injury, and oxygen saturation at presentation. Prompt pain management may decrease the incidence of pulmonary complications such as atelectasis, pneumonia, ICU admission, and mechanical ventilation as it improves the altered respiratory mechanics that usually peak 48 to 72 hours after the injury. Analgesia follows a stepwise fashion, from simple analgesics, through opioids (including PCA), and regional analgesia, depending on patient risk stratification and patient assessment. The Eastern Association for the Surgery of Trauma (EAST) recommends the use of epidural analgesia for rib fractures as the preferred analgesic technique [70]. However, epidural analgesia is an invasive procedure and polytrauma patients often have multiple contraindications, including hemodynamic instability, cervical or thoracic spine injuries, coagulation abnormalities, and are technically harder to perform in the intubated critically ill patient. Fascial plane blocks are easier to perform and are less limited by patient positioning or anticoagulation compared to epidurals. In addition, they have a more favorable risk/benefit profile, and appear to have non-inferior analgesia [71,72], although the current evidence base for their use is limited. There is some evidence for improved spirometry after erector spinae block (ESB) [71] and serratus anterior plane block (SPB) [73]. Fascial plane blocks for rib fractures include SPB for anterolateral rib fractures, and ESB for posterior fractures. Paravertebral block or epidural is usually reserved for poor response to the other fascial plane blocks. Bilateral fascial plane blocks or an appropriately positioned epidural may be used for bilateral rib fractures.

Acute burn injury

Burn injury can be severe and debilitating and presents as one of the most painful injuries sustained by an individual. Inflammatory responses are initiated within minutes of injury and can last for days leading to sensitization of nociceptors at the area of injury. The primary hyperalgesia that results from the intrinsic burn pain itself can progress to sensitization of the area surrounding the tissue injury. This is mediated by repeated stimulation of nociceptive-afferent fibers, and further exacerbated by painful procedures including debridement of the wound, daily wound care, surgery, and physical therapy, leading to secondary hyperalgesia. The complex nature of burn pain requires a multifaceted approach [74]. Opioids are the mainstay of treatment in the acute phase of burn pain and often the most efficacious perioperatively. The increased risk of side effects compounded by significant opioid dose escalation can require burn patients to extend hospital length of stay and impact the cost of hospitalization. Prolonged opioid use can also escalate to opioid tolerance as well as the intensification of pain in the context of opioid use known as opioid induced hyperalgesia (OIH). OIH can occur regardless of the duration of opioid exposure or dose and leads to increased pain from both painful and non-painful stimuli [75]. Regional anesthesia is a promising modality to mitigate the boomerang effect of poorly controlled acute pain which can result in the unrelenting propagation to chronic pain [76]. Peripheral nerve blocks have a useful role after split thickness skin grafting, a reconstructive procedure used in the treatment of deep burn injuries. Skin is typically harvested from the anterolateral thigh and is reported as a dominant site of pain due to localized activation of nociceptors in the epidermal layer of the skin and the potential for continued aggravation. Continuous nerve block catheters and their utility in burn donor site pain is poorly studied. The fascia iliaca compartment block provides blockade of both the lateral femoral cutaneous nerve and the femoral nerve and is a useful technique to manage burn donor pain [77]. Fascia iliaca catheter placement can facilitate extension of analgesia beyond the grafting procedure itself when daily dressing changes may be necessary for several days after surgery [78]. Ultrasound-guided percutaneous cryoneurolysis is an FDA-cleared technique that offers the potential for a prolonged sensory block of the lateral femoral cutaneous nerve that can last several weeks to months [79]. This is an alternative to a peripheral nerve block, especially in those patients with less than 5% burns where management occurs on an outpatient basis. Overall, regional anesthesia is a key player in the multimodal approach to the often-underappreciated burn donor site pain.

CONCLUDING REMARKS

Enhanced recovery protocols should include standardized acute perioperative pain management techniques that optimize patient care through the prudent use of evidence-based opioid stewardship strategies [5]. Likewise, incorporation of procedure-specific regional anesthesia techniques that can reduce the risk of opioid-related adverse drug events must be included in perioperative acute pain management. Communication and cooperation between health care professionals will be crucial for the success of this endeavor. It presents the opportunity for physicians to develop a patient-focused perspective that offers the patient a positive perioperative experience and improved postoperative recovery. Finally, the addition of systems within hospitals such as a transitional pain service and addiction specialist consultation has the potential to improve patient outcomes.

CLINICS CARE POINTS

- Enhanced recovery pathways, that emphasize perioperative pain strategies, lead to shorter hospital stays, faster recovery, lower complication rates, improved patient satisfaction, and cost savings in healthcare.
- Ultrasound-guided peripheral nerve blocks improve accuracy, safety, and effectiveness in anesthesia and pain management, enabling targeted pain relief and minimizing complications during procedures and recovery.

- A transitional pain service offers specialized pain management, smoother postoperative recovery, reduced opioid use, improved patient education, and enhanced long-term pain outcomes.

DISCLOSURE

S. Macres, R.J. Aldwinckle, U. Saldahna, M Jung, J. Santos, R. Bishop; No Disclosures or Commercial Interests. S.G. Pritzlaff; Consultant-SPR Therapeutics, Nalu Medical, BT Medical, Bioventus. Educational Grants: Nevro, United States, Abbott, Medtronic. Royalties: Wolters Kluwer (UpToDate), Oxford University Publishing (book). M. Kotova, ; No Disclosures.

References

[1] Buvanendran A, Fiala J, Patel KA, et al. The Incidence and Severity of Postoperative Pain following Inpatient Surgery. Pain Med 2015;16(12):2277–83.

[2] Gan TJ, Habib AS, Miller TE, et al. Incidence, patient satisfaction, and perceptions of post-surgical pain: results from a US national survey. Curr Med Res Opin 2014;30(1):149–60.

[3] Macres S.M., Saldana U., Zhou J., et al., Chapter 55: Acute Pain Management. In: Cullen, Stock, Ortega, et al., eds. Clinical anesthesia. 9th edition: Wolters Kluwer; 2023 In Press.

[4] Small C, Laycock H. Acute postoperative pain management. Br J Surg 2020;107(2): e70–80.

[5] Mariano ER, Dickerson DM, Szokol JW, et al. A multisociety organizational consensus process to define guiding principles for acute perioperative pain management. Reg Anesth Pain Med 2022;47(2):118–27.

[6] Stadler M, Schlander M, Braeckman M, et al. A cost-utility and cost-effectiveness analysis of an acute pain service. J Clin Anesth 2004;16(3):159–67.

[7] Zaccagnino MP, Bader AM, Sang CN, et al. The Perioperative Surgical Home: A New Role for the Acute Pain Service. Anesth Analg 2017;125(4):1394–402.

[8] Berry PH, Dahl JL. The new JCAHO pain standards: implications for pain management nurses. Pain Manag Nurs 2000;1(1):3–12.

[9] Walters T, Mariano ER, Clark JD. Perioperative Surgical Home and the Integral Role of Pain Medicine. Pain Med 2015;16(9):1666–72.

[10] Buys MJ, Bayless K, Romesser J, et al. Multidisciplinary Transitional Pain Service for the Veteran Population. Fed Pract 2020;37(10):472–8.

[11] Chou R, Gordon DB, de Leon-Casasola OA, et al. Management of Postoperative Pain: A Clinical Practice Guideline From the American Pain Society, the American Society of Regional Anesthesia and Pain Medicine, and the American Society of Anesthesiologists' Committee on Regional Anesthesia, Executive Committee, and Administrative Council. J Pain 2016;17(2):131–57.

[12] Doan LV, Blitz J. Preoperative Assessment and Management of Patients with Pain and Anxiety Disorders. Curr Anesthesiol Rep 2020;10(1):28–34.

[13] Patanwala AE, Jarzyna DL, Miller MD, et al. Comparison of opioid requirements and analgesic response in opioid-tolerant versus opioid-naive patients after total knee arthroplasty. Pharmacotherapy 2008;28(12):1453–60.

[14] Rapp SE, Ready BL, Nessly ML. Acute pain management in patients with prior opioid consumption: a case-controlled retrospective review. Pain 1995;61(2):195–201.

[15] Ward EN, Quaye AN, Wilens TE. Opioid Use Disorders: Perioperative Management of a Special Population. Anesth Analg 2018;127(2):539–47.

[16] Lin PC. An evaluation of the effectiveness of relaxation therapy for patients receiving joint replacement surgery. J Clin Nurs 2012;21(5–6):601–8.

[17] Powell R, Scott NW, Manyande A, et al. Psychological preparation and postoperative outcomes for adults undergoing surgery under general anaesthesia. Cochrane Database Syst Rev 2016;2016(5):CD008646.

[18] Quaye AN, Zhang Y. Perioperative Management of Buprenorphine: Solving the Conundrum. Pain Med 2019;20(7):1395–408.

[19] Kohan L, Potru S, Barreveld AM, et al. Buprenorphine management in the perioperative period: educational review and recommendations from a multisociety expert panel. Reg Anesth Pain Med 2021;46(10):840–59.

[20] Sun EC, Mariano ER, Narouze S, et al. Making a business plan for starting a transitional pain service within the US healthcare system. Reg Anesth Pain Med 2021;46(8):727–31.

[21] Sites BD, Beach ML, Davis MA. Increases in the use of prescription opioid analgesics and the lack of improvement in disability metrics among users. Reg Anesth Pain Med 2014;39(1):6–12.

[22] Hyland SJ, Brockhaus KK, Vincent WR, et al. Perioperative Pain Management and Opioid Stewardship: A Practical Guide. Healthcare (Basel) 2021;9(3):333.

[23] Mariano E.R., Approach to the management of acute pain in adults, In: UpToDate, Section ed. Robert Maniker, Deputy ed. Marianna Crowley, 2023, Available at: www.uptodate.com. Accessed February 12, 2023.

[24] Chang RW, Tompkins DM, Cohn SM. Are NSAIDs Safe? Assessing the Risk-Benefit Profile of Nonsteroidal Anti-inflammatory Drug Use in Postoperative Pain Management. Am Surg 2021;87(6):872–9.

[25] Varrassi G, Pergolizzi JV, Dowling P, et al. Ibuprofen Safety at the Golden Anniversary: Are all NSAIDs the Same? A Narrative Review. Adv Ther 2020;37(1):61–82.

[26] Haffar A., Fillingham Y.A., Breckenridge L., et al., Meloxicam versus Celecoxib for Postoperative Analgesia after Total Knee Arthroplasty: Safety, Efficacy and Cost, J Am Acad Orthop Surg Glob Res Rev, 6(4), 2022, e22.00032. doi: 10.5435/JAAOSGlobal-D-22-00032.

[27] Peng PW, Wijeysundera DN, Li CC. Use of gabapentin for perioperative pain control – a meta-analysis. Pain Res Manag 2007;12(2):85–92.

[28] Schwenk ES, Viscusi ER, Buvanendran A, et al. Consensus Guidelines on the Use of Intravenous Ketamine Infusions for Acute Pain Management From the American Society of Regional Anesthesia and Pain Medicine, the American Academy of Pain Medicine, and the American Society of Anesthesiologists. Reg Anesth Pain Med 2018;43(5):456–66.

[29] Gustafsson UO, Scott MJ, Hubner M, et al. Guidelines for Perioperative Care in Elective Colorectal Surgery: Enhanced Recovery After Surgery (ERAS((R))) Society Recommendations: 2018. World J Surg 2019;43(3):659–95.

[30] Weibel S, Jelting Y, Pace NL, et al. Continuous intravenous perioperative lidocaine infusion for postoperative pain and recovery in adults. Cochrane Database Syst Rev 2018;6(6):CD009642.

[31] Rollins KE, Javanmard-Emamghissi H, Scott MJ, et al. The impact of peri-operative intravenous lidocaine on postoperative outcome after elective colorectal surgery: A meta-analysis of randomised controlled trials. Eur J Anaesthesiol 2020;37(8):659–70.

[32] Edwards DA, Hedrick TL, Jayaram J, et al. American Society for Enhanced Recovery and Perioperative Quality Initiative Joint Consensus Statement on Perioperative Management of Patients on Preoperative Opioid Therapy. Anesth Analg 2019;129(2):553–66.

[33] Viscusi ER, Skobieranda F, Soergel DG, et al. APOLLO-1: a randomized placebo and active-controlled phase III study investigating oliceridine (TRV130), a G protein-biased ligand at the micro-opioid receptor, for management of moderate-to-severe acute pain following bunionectomy. J Pain Res 2019;12:927–43.

[34] Oliceridine (Olinvyk™) (package insert). Chesterbrook, PA, 19087 USA: Trevena Inc.; 2020.

[35] Chadwick A, Frazier A, Khan TW, et al. Understanding the Psychological, Physiological, and Genetic Factors Affecting Precision Pain Medicine: A Narrative Review. J Pain Res 2021;14:3145–61.

[36] Smith DM, Stevenson JM, Ho TT, et al. Pharmacogenetics: A Precision Medicine Approach to Combatting the Opioid Epidemic. J Am Coll Clin Pharm 2022;5(2):239–50.

[37] Albrecht E, Chin KJ. Advances in regional anaesthesia and acute pain management: a narrative review. Anaesthesia 2020;75(Suppl 1):e101–10.

[38] Neal JM, Gerancher JC, Hebl JR, et al. Upper extremity regional anesthesia: essentials of our current understanding, 2008. Reg Anesth Pain Med 2009;34(2):134–70.

[39] Tran DQ, Salinas FV, Benzon HT, et al. Lower extremity regional anesthesia: essentials of our current understanding, Reg Anesth Pain. Med 2019;44:143–80.

[40] Ilfeld BM. Continuous Peripheral Nerve Blocks: An Update of the Published Evidence and Comparison With Novel, Alternative Analgesic Modalities. Anesth Analg 2017;124(1):308–35.

[41] Levene JL, Weinstein EJ, Cohen MS, et al. Local anesthetics and regional anesthesia versus conventional analgesia for preventing persistent postoperative pain in adults and children: A Cochrane systematic review and meta-analysis update. J Clin Anesth 2019;55:116–27.

[42] Suksompong S, von Bormann S, von Bormann B. Regional Catheters for Postoperative Pain Control: Review and Observational Data. Anesth Pain Med 2020;10(1):e99745.

[43] Chan EY, Fransen M, Parker DA, et al. Femoral nerve blocks for acute postoperative pain after knee replacement surgery. Cochrane Database Syst Rev 2014;2014(5):CD009941.

[44] Elsharkawy H, Pawa A, Mariano ER. Interfascial Plane Blocks: Back to Basics. Reg Anesth Pain Med 2018;43(4):341–6.

[45] Sanderson BJ, Doane MA. Transversus Abdominis Plane Catheters for Analgesia Following Abdominal Surgery in Adults. Reg Anesth Pain Med 2018;43(1):5–13.

[46] Grant MC, Sommer PM, He C, et al. Preserved Analgesia With Reduction in Opioids Through the Use of an Acute Pain Protocol in Enhanced Recovery After Surgery for Open Hepatectomy. Reg Anesth Pain Med 2017;42(4):451–7.

[47] Mancel L, Van Loon K, Lopez AM. Role of regional anesthesia in Enhanced Recovery After Surgery (ERAS) protocols. Curr Opin Anaesthesiol 2021;34(5):616–25.

[48] Tan M, Law LS, Gan TJ. Optimizing pain management to facilitate Enhanced Recovery After Surgery pathways. Can J Anaesth 2015;62(2):203–18.

[49] Horlocker TT, Vandermeulen E, Kopp SL, et al. Regional Anesthesia in the Patient Receiving Antithrombotic or Thrombolytic Therapy: American Society of Regional Anesthesia and Pain Medicine Evidence-Based Guidelines (Fourth Edition). Reg Anesth Pain Med 2018;43(3):263–309.

[50] Neal JM, Barrington MJ, Fettiplace MR, et al. The Third American Society of Regional Anesthesia and Pain Medicine Practice Advisory on Local Anesthetic Systemic Toxicity: Executive Summary 2017. Reg Anesth Pain Med 2018;43(2):113–23.

[51] Deer TR, Naidu R, Strand N, et al. A review of the bioelectronic implications of stimulation of the peripheral nervous system for chronic pain conditions. Bioelectron Med 2020;6:9.

[52] Gilmore C, Ilfeld B, Rosenow J, et al. Percutaneous peripheral nerve stimulation for the treatment of chronic neuropathic postamputation pain: a multicenter, randomized, placebo-controlled trial. Reg Anesth Pain Med 2019;44(6):637–45.

[53] Wilson RD, Bennett ME, Nguyen VQC, et al. Fully Implantable Peripheral Nerve Stimulation for Hemiplegic Shoulder Pain: A Multi-Site Case Series With Two-Year Follow-Up. Neuromodulation 2018;21(3):290–5.

[54] Ilfeld BM, Ball ST, Gabriel RA, et al. A Feasibility Study of Percutaneous Peripheral Nerve Stimulation for the Treatment of Postoperative Pain Following Total Knee Arthroplasty. Neuromodulation 2019;22(5):653–60.

[55] Ilfeld BM, Plunkett A, Vijjeswarapu AM, et al. Percutaneous Peripheral Nerve Stimulation (Neuromodulation) for Postoperative Pain: A Randomized, Sham-controlled Pilot Study. Anesthesiology 2021;135(1):95–110.

[56] Finneran Iv JJ, Ilfeld BM. Percutaneous cryoneurolysis for acute pain management: current status and future prospects. Expert Rev Med Devices 2021;18(6):533–43.

[57] Gabriel RA, Ilfeld BM. Extending Perioperative Analgesia with Ultrasound-Guided, Percutaneous Cryoneurolysis, and Peripheral Nerve Stimulation (Neuromodulation). Anesthesiol Clin 2022;40(3):469–79.

[58] Park R, Coomber M, Gilron I, et al. Cryoanalgesia for postsurgical pain relief in adults: A systematic review and meta-analysis. Ann Med Surg (Lond). 2021;69:102689.

[59] Mihalko WM, Kerkhof AL, Ford MC, et al. Cryoneurolysis before Total Knee Arthroplasty in Patients With Severe Osteoarthritis for Reduction of Postoperative Pain and Opioid Use in a Single-Center Randomized Controlled Trial. J Arthroplasty 2021;36(5):1590–8.

[60] Arsanious D, Khoury S, Martinez E, et al. Ultrasound-Guided Phrenic Nerve Block for Intractable Hiccups following Placement of Esophageal Stent for Esophageal Squamous Cell Carcinoma. Pain Physician 2016;19(4):E653–6.

[61] Kuusniemi K, Pyylampi V. Phrenic nerve block with ultrasound-guidance for treatment of hiccups: a case report. J Med Case Rep 2011;5:493.

[62] Renes SH, van Geffen GJ, Rettig HC, et al. Ultrasound-guided continuous phrenic nerve block for persistent hiccups. Reg Anesth Pain Med 2010;35(5):455–7.

[63] Zhang Y, Duan F, Ma W. Ultrasound-guided phrenic nerve block for intraoperative persistent hiccups: a case report. BMC Anesthesiol 2018;18(1):123.

[64] Urmey WF, McDonald M. Hemidiaphragmatic paresis during interscalene brachial plexus block: effects on pulmonary function and chest wall mechanics. Anesth Analg 1992;74(3):352–7.

[65] Fudim M, Boortz-Marx R, Ganesh A, et al. Stellate ganglion blockade for the treatment of refractory ventricular arrhythmias: A systematic review and meta-analysis. J Cardiovasc Electrophysiol 2017;28(12):1460–7.

[66] Meng L, Tseng CH, Shivkumar K, et al. Efficacy of Stellate Ganglion Blockade in Managing Electrical Storm: A Systematic Review. JACC Clin Electrophysiol 2017;3(9):942–9.

[67] Ganesh A, Qadri YJ, Boortz-Marx RL, et al. Stellate Ganglion Blockade: an Intervention for the Management of Ventricular Arrhythmias. Curr Hypertens Rep 2020;22(12):100.

[68] Saddic LA, Howard-Quijano K, Kipke J, et al. Progression of myocardial ischemia leads to unique changes in immediate-early gene expression in the spinal cord dorsal horn. Am J Physiol Heart Circ Physiol 2018;315(6):H1592–601.

[69] de Moya M, Nirula R, Biffl W. Rib fixation: Who, What, When? Trauma Surg Acute Care Open 2017;2(1):e000059.

[70] Bulger EM, Edwards T, Klotz P, et al. Epidural analgesia improves outcome after multiple rib fractures. Surgery 2004;136(2):426–30.

[71] Adhikary SD, Liu WM, Fuller E, et al. The effect of erector spinae plane block on respiratory and analgesic outcomes in multiple rib fractures: a retrospective cohort study. Anaesthesia 2019;74(5):585–93.

[72] Bhalla PI, Solomon S, Zhang R, et al. Comparison of serratus anterior plane block with epidural and paravertebral block in critically ill trauma patients with multiple rib fractures. Trauma Surg Acute Care Open 2021;6(1):e000621.

[73] Hernandez N, de Haan J, Clendeninn D, et al. Impact of serratus plane block on pain scores and incentive spirometry volumes after chest trauma. Local Reg Anesth 2019;12:59–66.

[74] James DL, Jowza M. Principles of Burn Pain Management. Clin Plast Surg 2017;44(4):737–47.

[75] Holtman JR Jr, Jellish WS. Opioid-induced hyperalgesia and burn pain. J Burn Care Res 2012;33(6):692–701.

[76] Grunzweig KA, Son J, Kumar AR. Regional Anesthetic Blocks for Donor Site Pain in Burn Patients: A Meta-Analysis on Efficacy, Outcomes, and Cost. Plast Surg (Oakv). 2020;28(4):222–31.

[77] Town CJ, Strand H, Johnson J, et al. Ultrasound-Guided Fascia Iliaca Plane Block for the Treatment of Donor Site Pain in the Burn-Injured Patient: A Randomized Control Trial. J Burn Care Res 2021;42(5):981–5.

[78] Cuignet O, Pirson J, Boughrouph J, et al. The efficacy of continuous fascia iliaca compartment block for pain management in burn patients undergoing skin grafting procedures. Anesth Analg 2004;98(4):1077–81.

[79] Finneran JJ, Swisher MW, Gabriel RA, et al. Ultrasound-Guided Lateral Femoral Cutaneous Nerve Cryoneurolysis for Analgesia in Patients With Burns. J Burn Care Res 2020;41(1): 224–7.

[80] Glare P, Aubrey KR, Myles PS. Transition from acute to chronic pain after surgery. Lancet 2019;393(10180):1537–46.

[81] Rosenberger DC, Pogatzki-Zahn EM. Chronic post-surgical pain - update on incidence, risk factors and preventive treatment options. BJA Educ 2022;22(5):190–6.

[82] Gupta K, Prasad A, Nagappa M, et al. Risk factors for opioid-induced respiratory depression and failure to rescue: a review. Curr Opin Anaesthesiol 2018;31(1):110–9.

[83] Lee LA, Caplan RA, Stephens LS, et al. Postoperative opioid-induced respiratory depression: a closed claims analysis. Anesthesiology 2015;122(3):659–65.

[84] Schwenk E.S., Non-opioid pharmacotherapy for acute pain in adults, In: UpToDate, Section ed. Robert Maniker, Deputy ed. Marianna Crowley, 2023, Available at: www.uptodate.com. Accesed February 12, 2023.

Advances in Anesthesia 41 (2023) 111–125

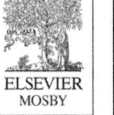

ELSEVIER
MOSBY

ADVANCES IN ANESTHESIA

Expert Advice for the Expert Witness

Richard P. Dutton, MD, MBA

US Anesthesia Partners, Dallas, TX, USA

Keywords

- Malpractice • Litigation • Expert witness • Forensic medicine • Plaintiff
- Defendant

Key points

- The US malpractice system has many flaws, but failure to engage will lead to determination of the anesthesia standard of care by nonanesthesiologists, to the detriment of our profession.
- Anesthesiologist expert witnesses should understand the flow of typical malpractice cases and their role in the process.
- Anesthesiologist expert witnesses, whether engaged by the plaintiff or the defendant, should be truthful in representing the profession's standards of practice and should educate the court regarding possible causes of adverse events.
- Both the American Medical Association and the American Society of Anesthesiologists (ASA) offer Guidelines for physician expert witnesses. The ASA maintains a process for review of inappropriate expert testimony.

INTRODUCTION

My goal in writing this article is to provide practical advice for the anesthesiologist engaged as an expert witness in a medical malpractice case. I review the structure and function of the medical jurisprudence system in the United States, the timeline of a malpractice case, professional society guidelines for expert witnesses, and the specific perspectives of the plaintiff and defense experts. The literature offers few resources specifically for anesthesiologists, but I have

Note: The author prepared the article, figures, and tables, and approved the final manuscript.

Funding source: None.

The opinions expressed in this work are the author's alone and do not reflect the opinions of the American Society of Anesthesiologists or US Anesthesia Partners.

E-mail address: richard.dutton@usap.com

https://doi.org/10.1016/j.aan.2023.06.001
0737-6146/23/© 2023 Elsevier Inc. All rights reserved.

synthesized guidance from work regarding physician experts in general and have included the published guidelines of the American Medical Association (AMA) and the American Society of Anesthesiologists (ASA).

This presentation is guided by my own experience as an expert witness, on both the plaintiff and the defense side, and from participation as an anesthesiology expert in a federal class action lawsuit, as a consultant to a self-insurance trust, as a researcher into aggregated closed claims data, and even as a pro bono expert in a death penalty case. Where facts are available, I have referenced them; the opinions in between are mine alone and do not represent the official views of the AMA, the ASA, or US Anesthesia Partners.

MEDICAL MALPRACTICE IN THE UNITED STATES

The US malpractice system was estimated to cost 55 billion dollars in 2008, or about 2.4% of all health care expenditures [1,2]. Extrapolating to the 3 trillion dollar US health care budget in 2023, this means an annual cost of about 72 billion dollars today. Few experts believe this expenditure brings value to patient care [1,3–5].

Every clinician must understand the malpractice system or risk becoming its victim. Most of us will be sued at some point in our career [6], and many of us will be drawn into a malpractice case as a fact witness or requested as an expert. Some anesthesiologists passively protest against malpractice litigation by refusing to engage as expert witnesses, or by restricting participation only to defense cases. However, failure to participate risks damaging the standing of all anesthesiologists by allowing lay opinions or uninformed experts to determine the standard of care. As a profession, anesthesiologists must self-regulate; if we fail to do so, we will be regulated by others.

In accordance with this principle, the stated policy of the AMA is that:

1. The giving of medicolegal testimony by a physician expert witness is considered the practice of medicine, and
2. All medicolegal expert witness testimony given by a physician is subject to peer review [7].

Medical malpractice is a component of the tort system of civil law, designed to deliver remedies to those harmed by the negligence of others. This is in contrast to criminal law, which is based on injuries arising from deliberate acts of malevolence. Criminal cases must be proven "beyond a reasonable doubt," whereas civil cases are decided only by "more likely than not." Although the term "forensic medicine" is sometimes conflated with the work of expert witnesses in medical malpractice cases, it is important to note the difference between the two. Forensic medicine is defined as the application of medical knowledge to investigation of a crime [8], and indeed the specialty of Psychiatry has a board-certified subspecialty of Forensic Medicine focused on determining the competence of accused criminals to stand trial in criminal cases [9]. Anesthesiologists have been found guilty of deliberately harming patients, but such cases are vanishingly rare, and the resulting criminal prosecution is not controversial. Malpractice litigation, on the other hand, is a common civil law event and reflects the uncertainties of practicing medicine. A recent publication noted that 75% of physicians in low-risk specialties will be named in a malpractice lawsuit over the course of their career, rising to 99% in high-risk specialties, such as obstetrics, orthopedic surgery, or neurology [6,10].

For anesthesia clinicians, being named in a malpractice suit is a life-changing event on par with marriage, divorce, or death of a loved one. Much like being diagnosed with a serious illness, the clinician can anticipate years of unrewarding busy-work, professional criticism by strangers, career uncertainty, and the possibility of a significant financial penalty. Some recent evidence has linked malpractice claims against clinicians to deterioration in personal wellness, and even to a decrease in the quality of care for future patients [11–14]. This condition has a diagnosis of its own: Medical Malpractice Stress Syndrome [15]. Any clinician who has been sued, even frivolously, will agree that the implied criticism of one's worth is a significant and life-changing psychological challenge.

Malpractice claims against clinicians are based on 4 legal requirements.

- That the defendant (clinician) owed the patient a duty of care
- That this duty was breached by a violation of the standard of care
- That the plaintiff (patient) suffered an injury
- Proof that the breach of the duty was the cause of the injury (proximate cause)

Anesthesia clinicians have a duty of care when they are assigned a specific case or patient, whether through elective scheduling or when stepping into an emergency case. Clinicians in this circumstance are expected to provide unsolicited and unbiased advice to their patients, to obtain informed consent for treatment whenever possible, and to maintain confidentiality of personal information. Although a lay person providing medical care in an emergency may be sheltered from legal consequences by a state's Good Samaritan laws, a licensed clinician is expected to provide the technical elements of anesthesia care in accordance with known best practices and is subject to civil litigation if they fail to do so.

Standard of care is the slipperiest component of malpractice litigation, and the area where expert witnesses most commonly battle. Historically, the standard of care is based on what a reasonable practitioner in the clinician's local community would do in a similar situation. Although this local standard is still relevant in rural and underserved areas, for most malpractice claims in the Information Age, the standard is now a national one. The proliferation of published Guidelines and Protocols from national organizations has contributed to this shift; for major malpractice claims against anesthesia clinicians, it is common for expert witnesses to be drawn from any part of the country. Because clinical medicine, even in anesthesiology, still involves as much art as science, reasonable people may disagree on what represents "standard" care. Hence the need for expert witnesses.

Patient injury is usually obvious, in the form of death or lasting disability of the patient. Increasingly, though, "injury" may include psychiatric issues, such as posttraumatic stress disorder, social issues such as loss of consortium, or emotional distress, all of which are more subjective. More contentious is the degree to which the injury is caused by a specific action or inaction of the clinician. At one extreme, a medication administration error leading to cardiac arrest illustrates an obvious link between action and injury. At the other extreme, a postoperative nerve injury diagnosed weeks after surgery may have been caused by a mispositioned regional block needle, by chronic inflammation, by a positioning injury, or by surgical manipulation, with no easy way to determine which was the real cause. In addition to debates over the standard of care, discussion of the cause of injury—and which clinician was responsible to what degree—occupies much of the attention of expert witnesses. In cases whereby the hospital, surgeon, and anesthesiologist are in different corporations—each with their own legal representation—it is easy for the plaintiff's attorney to play one off against the other. It is not unusual for one or more of these entities to "settle out" early in the defense, often leading the defendant with the most insurance or greatest institutional resources to manage the defense alone.

Fig. 1 illustrates the normal course of a medical malpractice claim, showing both the flow of legal actions and the role of the expert witness. Variation may arise from different state or federal procedural regulations, such as the requirement in some states for mediation efforts before proceeding to trial. About one-third of cases are settled with a payment to the patient; most of the remainder are dismissed before trial. Only about 5% of cases proceed as far as a jury

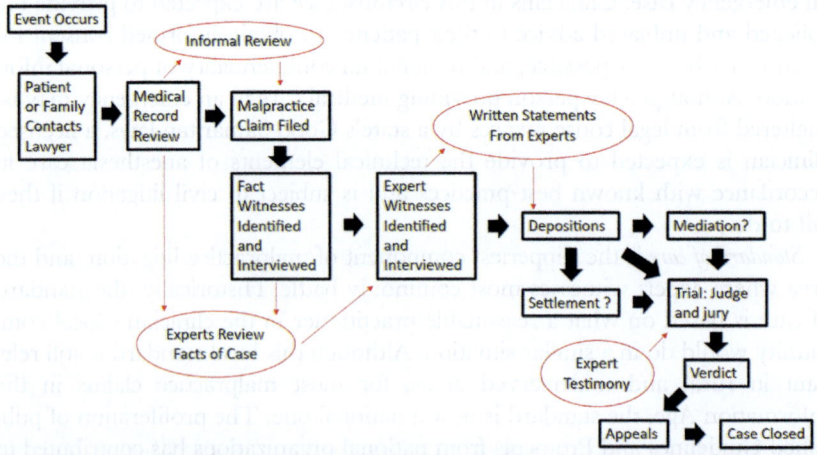

Fig. 1. A generic timeline for a medical malpractice claim, showing the key legal steps in black and the role of expert witnesses in red. Some cases require written statements from experts before depositions; some states require mediation efforts before proceeding to trial. Cases can be settled at any point in the process, but the most common time is after facts and expert opinions are collected.

verdict [15]. Cases that go to trial are idiosyncratic and involve battles of expert opinions, decided by a lay jury: this leads to variability in outcome and uncertainty about the standard of care. Juries often feel sympathy for the patient, regardless of the quality of care provided, and seek to compensate them from the faceless "deep pockets" of the hospital or practice group. In cases that go to trial, the defendant wins approximately 80%, but the occasional well-publicized jackpot award encourages plaintiff's attorneys to file marginal and frivolous cases. One of the key functions of expert witnesses, on both sides of the claim, is to help the legal system establish causality and determine fair compensation for a given injury.

Financial penalties awarded at trial are divided into several categories: payment of direct medical expenses incurred, payment of predicted future medical expenses (established by actuarial experts), and a penalty payment for the patient's pain and suffering. This last category, known as "noneconomic damages," is the most subjective and the most variable. In the 1980s, out-of-control escalation in noneconomic payments led to a crisis in access to health care in many parts of the United States. Physicians in high-risk specialties could no longer afford malpractice insurance and were moving to other states, refusing high-risk patients and procedures, or retiring from practice. To date, 19 states have imposed maximum limits on noneconomic damages; 5 states have capped total damages, and 2 states have done both [3]. These efforts have contributed to greater stability of malpractice payments in recent decades, with moderation or even a decrease in malpractice insurance rates. However, the patchwork nature of these laws has led to greater variability in outcomes, and malpractice risk, from state to state. Some experts have opined that tort reform limiting punitive damages improves the quality of care by reducing the need for excess spending on defensive medicine that does not improve population health outcomes [3,4]. Confidentiality agreements as part of some settlements hinder public transparency regarding the overall costs of malpractice and make it hard to determine the benefits of tort reform. As Studdert and Hall [3] noted: "For the most part ... such reform hasn't happened, and the system in place for more than 150 years grinds on, largely disconnected from wider efforts to improve the quality and safety of patient care."

Forty states have now adopted "apology laws," more formally known as Communication and Resolution Programs, that shield clinician and hospital efforts to acknowledge errors and compensate patients for unintended harm. Under these rules, an apology from the hospital or clinicians cannot be taken as an admission of liability [15]. Although these programs are well-intentioned mechanisms for providing closure to patients and families without attorney involvement, they have been cynically manipulated by plaintiffs' attorneys as a means of gathering presuit information.

On the other hand, every state has a law requiring any settlement made on behalf of a clinician, any adverse change to their license or hospital credentials, and any trial judgment against them to be reported to the National Practitioner Data Bank (NPDB) [15]. The NPDB is a clearinghouse for malpractice claim information nationwide. The NPDB is routinely queried by state medical boards as part of the licensure process, and by practices, hospitals, and systems when credentialing clinicians. Whereas decades ago, hospital-employed clinicians could be shielded from NPDB reporting (by the hospital assuming full liability for a given event), this loophole has largely been closed by subsequent state laws. Physicians who have been named once in a malpractice suit are more likely to be named multiple times (Fig. 2).

The number of malpractice claims against physicians leading to a payment to the patient has decreased by 75% in the past 20 years, although the median payment has remained roughly constant [3]. One-third of all paid claims involve a missed or delayed diagnosis. In anesthesia, examples of this category include failure to recognize unexpected hemorrhage, delay in managing airway obstruction, and reluctance to escalate care when the patient is in distress.

Although it would be lovely to imagine that health care will someday be so safe and consistent that malpractice claims are eliminated, in reality this is unlikely. For one thing, we have decades of recent history in which every gain in medical society has been reinvested in performing more complicated surgeries

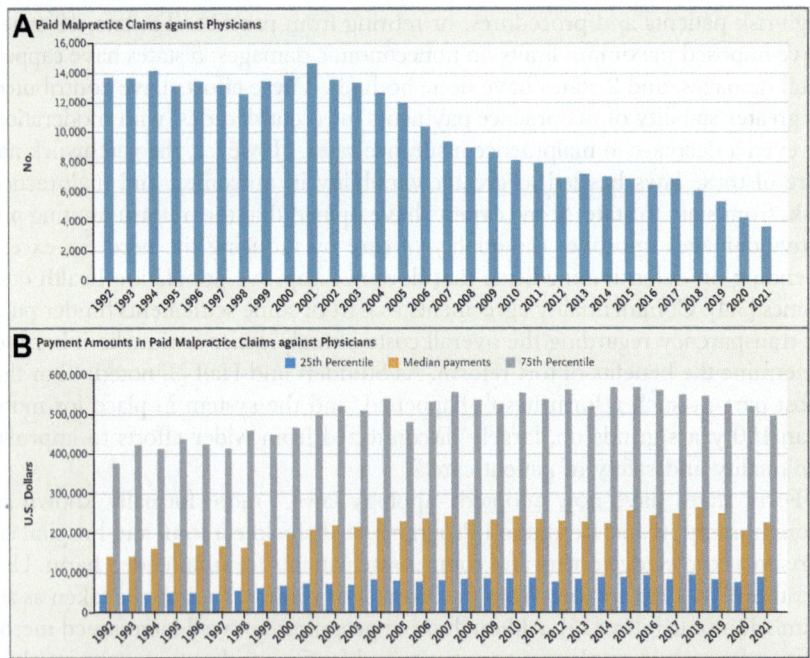

Fig. 2. Paid malpractice claims against physicians over time. Physicians include medical doctors and doctors of osteopathy. Payments have been adjusted to 2021 dollars using the consumer price index for all urban consumers (https://data.bls.gov/PDQWeb/cu). (Bernard Black, David A. Hyman, Joshua Y. Lerner, Physicians with multiple paid medical malpractice claims: Are they outliers or just unlucky?, International Review of Law and Economics, 58, 2019, 146-157 https://doi.org/10.1016/j.irle.2019.03.006.)

on higher-risk patients. In their landmark paper of 1952, Beecher and Todd [16] documented a 4% in-hospital mortality for patients admitted for an elective surgical procedure. A major procedure of the day was open cholecystectomy, and a major cause of mortality was anesthesiologist inexperience with use of curare. Fifty years later, mortality for surgical inpatients continues to hover between 2% and 4% [17], although most occur outside of the operating room (OR) and most involve desperately ill patients having procedures not dreamed of in 1950. Humans are likely to require complex anesthesia care for the foreseeable future.

A second variable is the inevitability of error in any process dependent on human decisions. Although humans are enormously creative at solving problems, they are also creative at producing errors. Humans are not built by nature for consistent performance of repetitive tasks [18]. The quality movement in health care, and anesthesiology in particular, has done exceptional work at mitigating the consequences of human error through design of safer systems—putting more safety filters between the event and the patient—but it is certain that errors will continue to occur. One way or another there will be an enduring need to compensate patients experiencing iatrogenic injury.

DUTIES OF THE EXPERT WITNESS

As was noted above, the AMA considers provision of expert testimony to be part of the practice of medicine. Both AMA and ASA have published on the topic of expert witnesses; Box 1 shows qualifications and guidelines for expert witnesses from the ASA Web site [19]. Most noteworthy is that the expert should be engaged in active clinical practice, with relevant, contemporary knowledge. Our specialty, and others, has been plagued by "professional experts": anesthesiologists who devote most of their time to testifying in malpractice cases. These individuals are appealing to the legal profession (and especially plaintiffs' attorneys) because they are a known quantity, they already understand the legal process, and they are willing to make definitive statements regarding violations of the standard of care. To that extent, the opinions are honest, and supported by the scientific literature, there is nothing illegal about this activity, although it is unseemly. When the bias of the "hired gun" to find deviations from the standard of care to favor their client violates known science or does not reflect real practice in the community, a greater problem arises [20]. At the local level, the impartiality of the judicial process is threatened, whereas at the national level this kind of internal cannibalism damages the professional standing of anesthesiology and the public reputation of anesthesiologists.

The first recommendation for any anesthesiologist expert witness is thus "Be Honest." This includes honesty about your training, credentials, and current practice, honesty about the clinical facts of the case in question, and honesty about community standards of practice. The last of these points can be controversial, and the prospective expert is advised to keep an open mind about how peers might practice, especially in the absence of objective data. An intellectual hazard of our specialty is projecting our personal belief about best practice onto

Box 1: Expert witness qualifications and guidelines

Qualifications:

1. The physician (expert witness) should have a current, valid, and unrestricted license to practice medicine.
2. The physician should be board certified in anesthesiology or hold an equivalent specialist qualification.
3. The physician should have been actively involved in the clinical practice of anesthesiology at the time of the event and should have relevant clinical experience and knowledge in the clinical practice areas that are the subject of the proceeding.

Guidelines:

1. The physician's review of the medical facts should be truthful, thorough, and impartial. The physician should not exclude any relevant information to create a view favoring either the plaintiff or the defendant.
2. The physician's testimony should reflect scientific evidence and accepted practice standards prevalent at the time of the event in question.
3. The physician should make a clear distinction between medical malpractice and adverse outcomes not necessarily related to negligent practice.
4. The physician should make every effort to assess whether the alleged substandard practice was causally related to the adverse outcome.
5. The physician's fee for expert testimony should relate to the time spent and in no circumstances should be contingent upon outcome of the claim.
6. The physician should be willing to submit such testimony for review.

Qualifications:

4. The physician (expert witness) should have a current, valid, and unrestricted license to practice medicine.
5. The physician should be board certified in anesthesiology or hold an equivalent specialist qualification.
6. 5wThe physician should have been actively involved in the clinical practice of anesthesiology at the time of the event and should have relevant clinical experience and knowledge in the clinical practice areas that are the subject of the proceeding.

Guidelines:

7. The physician's review of the medical facts should be truthful, thorough, and impartial. The physician should not exclude any relevant information to create a view favoring either the plaintiff or the defendant.
8. The physician's testimony should reflect scientific evidence and accepted practice standards prevalent at the time of the event in question.
9. The physician should make a clear distinction between medical malpractice and adverse outcomes not necessarily related to negligent practice.
10. The physician should make every effort to assess whether the alleged substandard practice was causally related to the adverse outcome.
11. The physician's fee for expert testimony should relate to the time spent and in no circumstances should be contingent upon outcome of the claim.
12. The physician should be willing to submit such testimony for review.

From https://www.asahq.org/standards-and-guidelines/guidelines-for-expert-witness-qualifications-and-testimony.

our colleagues, abetted by a clinical environment in which we rarely see exactly what a colleague is doing, even if it is just one OR away. There are many ways to skin a cat–or provide a safe anesthetic–and often no definitive evidence to indicate which might produce the best outcome.

The observation that medicine is as much art as science, although true, defies the legal system's desire for black and white outcomes. Most malpractice attorneys recognize this fact internally, but do not reflect it in the questions they ask of experts, especially when on the record in a deposition or at trial. Because medicine is complex and nuanced and takes years to learn, malpractice cases are notoriously complex even within the legal system and lead to longer trials with substantial effort devoted to education of the jury. This puts a premium on simple and clear-cut answers to simple and clear questions. However, as H.L. Mencken famously noted, "For every complex problem there is an answer that is clear, simple, and wrong." An important tip for prospective experts is to resist oversimplification of nuanced issues, despite almost certain pressure to do so from the attorneys on both sides of the case.

The work of the expert witness begins with outreach from an attorney, asking the anesthesiologist to look at a case. Both plaintiffs' and defendants' attorneys have networks of specialists on tap, developed over years of interaction with the health care system. Anesthesiologist experts are found through individual referral or outreach. If you wish to become involved, the best approach is to ask your peers to keep you in mind when lawyers reach out. It is common for senior anesthesiologists who are contacted often to hand-off "opportunities" to junior colleagues [21].

From the attorney's perspective, the ideal expert is one with subject matter expertise, the ability to express themselves clearly, a good "bedside manner," and enough experience with the legal system to know the normal rules and protocols [21]. Professional experts are appealing in some ways–as described above–but concerning in others, because their limited clinical practice can easily be portrayed as a negative.

Initial outreach typically includes a quick presentation of the case, and solicitation of an off-the-cuff opinion about its merits. In most cases the appropriate response is "I'll be happy to take a look at it in detail and give my opinion." This should happen when there is a legitimate question of malpractice: a patient injury, practice outside the standard of care, and evidence of causation by the anesthesia clinician. If the case is clearly frivolous, the expert should say so. The attorney will likely seek another opinion or two, but if the expert consensus agrees the case has no merit, they will typically drop it. Cutting off inappropriate suits at this early stage is a valuable contribution of plaintiff's experts to the overall system.

If the expert agrees to look at the case, there will follow a brief discussion of rates and expenses, which the anesthesiologist should be prepared for. For the first-time expert, this can be a delicate moment, because there is little public information about an appropriate hourly rate for chart review, or day rate for depositions and trial testimony. My recommendation is consultation with peers (ideally in advance of the first conversation with an attorney) about the current rates and charges in the local community. The expert's fee schedule should include 3 components: an hourly consultation rate for review of documents and discussions with the attorney, an hourly or flat fee for in-person deposition or trial testimony, and payment of all business expenses for travel and in-person participation. The legitimate basis for these charges is typically the opportunity cost of a lost day in the OR. There is little transparency in the medical community about these rates, but in my experience, hourly rates range from $200 to $600 per hour and day rates for testimony range from $2000 to $5000.

Expert witnesses on either side of an issue can expect to answer certain common questions, regardless of the facts of the suit. These are listed in Box 2. As an expert, you will answer these questions informally for the lawyer who brought you into the case, in a series of calls or meetings over the weeks to months that you are reviewing medical records and deposition testimony. You will have the chance to answer them again, in a more confrontational way, during your deposition under oath by the opposing legal team. Deposition is the opportunity for the opposing side to learn everything about you, your credentials as an expert, and your theory of the case. During the deposition, the attorneys (on both sides) will be assessing your suitability as a witness at trial: your presentability, your professional demeanor, your calm under fire,

---

Box 2: Common deposition questions for the expert witness

- Your name, title, and current professional responsibilities
- Your training and work experience, from college onward and including an explanation of any gaps in time
- A description of your active practice of anesthesiology
- Your personal history with malpractice: "have you ever been sued?" If the answer is yes, expect to be asked about details and expect the attorneys to dig into the key themes and outcomes of the case
- A record of any previous work as an expert witness, including trial testimony, depositions, or record review, and especially in any case similar to the present one. Depending on jurisdiction, your prior malpractice testimony may be discoverable in future cases
- Your relevant academic publications or presentations. Again, anything in public can be reviewed by the opposing legal team and presented for discussion at deposition
- A description of how you got involved with the case and your relationship—if any—with any of the involved patients, clinicians, or lawyers
- A description of your fee structure for reviewing medical records and testifying in malpractice cases
- Your theory of the case. How did the injury occur? What were the causes?
- And the bottom line: your opinion on whether the standard of anesthesia care was met

and your ability to simplify and explain complex medical issues. Importantly, standard rules of evidence do not apply during depositions and virtually any question may be asked. The attorneys on your side will challenge and object to inappropriate questions, but you will normally have to answer them anyway.

Given this purpose, you can expect to experience a variety of conversational tactics during the deposition, ranging from comfortable down-home banter designed to put you at ease, to feigned ignorance, to hyperbolic twisting of your words, to straight-up efforts to make you angry. As an expert you should:

- Dress and present yourself professionally; many depositions today are videotaped, and excerpts may be shown in court.
- Be punctual and accommodating.
- Speak slowly and carefully. Do not be afraid to pause to organize your thoughts and do not hesitate to ask for a break if you need one.
- Do your homework, but do not expect to remember every detail of the case. It is OK to ask to look at case records or deposition testimony to refresh your memory.
- Answer the questions being asked, no more and no less. Avoid the temptation to lecture or editorialize.
- Above all, keep your cool and maintain perspective! I used to tell myself (silently) that what I do every day in the OR is far more dangerous (and important) than the events of a deposition.

Malpractice cases are often settled following collection and review of all expert depositions. At this point, the attorneys on both sides will have a good understanding of the facts, the opinions (and performance) of the experts, and the medical expenses of the patient. This will permit both sides to estimate the likelihood of a favorable verdict at trial and the potential costs of a win or a loss. A negotiated settlement saves time, effort, reputation, money, and uncertainty for all concerned, and in some cases, gets the patient the support they need in a timely fashion.

In the next 2 sections I provide some specific observations from the perspective of first the plaintiff's expert and then the expert for the defense.

PERSPECTIVE OF THE PLAINTIFF'S EXPERT

As noted above, many anesthesiologists will refuse to review cases or serve as a plaintiff's expert, based on believing the system as a whole is a predatory violation of our profession. This approach may be unwise, as it leaves an important component of self-regulation in the hands of those with less knowledge and expertise. In fact, engagement of anesthesiologist experts with plaintiff's attorneys can be beneficial in cutting off frivolous cases and enabling rapid settlement of those with merit, to the benefit of the injured patient and their family.

To meet this lofty ideal, the plaintiff's expert must be scrupulously honest, especially when citing published guidelines. The expert must meet the criteria spelled out in Box 1, and especially in the area of active clinical practice in a setting similar to the defendant. "Hired gun" professional experts are more common on the plaintiff's side. The most significant objection to this activity is the distortion or misinterpretation of the standard of care by someone who is not in day-to-day clinical practice [20]. The plaintiff's expert may legitimately point out controversial areas and differing approaches to anesthesia care but when making a statement, such as "this is how I always manage this kind of patient," it must be supported in real life.

A good plaintiff's expert will remember their obligation to the court (and oath) to provide an unbiased view of the medical facts of the case, taking into consideration the inevitable "fog of war" that confuses any rapidly evolving clinical situation. Although it may be clear in retrospect what happened and what should have been done, an honest plaintiff's expert will view the case from the eyes of the defendant and present to the attorneys— and ultimately the judge and jury—a dispassionate view of events, with appropriate acknowledgment of normal clinical uncertainty.

ASA members who feel the opinions of a plaintiff's expert are inappropriately biased may request a review by the Committee on Expert Witness Testimony Review (see https://www.asahq.org/about-asa/office-of-general-counsel/expert-witness-testimony-review).

This is a standing committee of ASA, composed of senior anesthesiologists. The Committee will undertake a confidential review of the case or cases in question and is empowered by the Society to recommend action if they feel the complaint has merit. Past actions have included public or private censure of the expert; suspension or revocation of the expert's membership in ASA; and filing of official objections to the expert's testimony with the relevant court or courts. Actions of the ASA and individual complainants have led to discreditation of experts who testify frequently and unfairly, or who go on record with egregious misinterpretations of the standard of care. Courts, in turn, have refused to accept testimony in future cases from anesthesiologists censored in this way.

PERSPECTIVE OF THE DEFENSE EXPERT

Service as an expert witness for the defense is less controversial and stigmatizing than service as a plaintiff's expert but is more difficult from a clinical perspective. The Latin principal res ipse loquitor—"the thing speaks for itself"—makes the point that patient injuries in the course of health care are usually obvious; this, plus a natural human sympathy for others, makes the task easier for the plaintiff's expert. Also, there is the inevitable triumph of anecdote over data. The plaintiff's expert is explaining something that did happen, whereas the defense expert is frequently tasked with describing how unlikely it was. It can be hard for the defense expert to explain the rarity of adverse outcomes in the overall course of care when the court can see such an outcome in front of them—or to quote a line we all heard as interns: "Rare diseases are common in patients who have them."

Practicing clinicians know that few things in medicine are 100% certain or predictable, whereas the legal system is built on a desire for black and white verdicts. The defense expert must often explain nuance and controversy in the standard of care that the courts—and the public—would prefer to think of as an arbitrary and definable thing. Statistics are inherently less exciting than stories. To draw from my own experience: when a diabetic patient experiences a deep tissue infection after knee replacement surgery, it is easy to create a plausible story about bacteria wafted into the surgical wound by the forced hot air system, despite consistent scientific evidence that keeping the patient warm is orders of magnitude more important in preventing infection than concern over air flow.

For anesthesia cases, in particular, the "fog of war" concept mentioned above is often in play but can be difficult to explain. Consider the case of a patient who suffers life-threatening hemorrhage as the result of an unrecognized iliac vein injury during an orthopedic procedure. In retrospect, it is obvious what the problem was, and correspondingly easy to criticize the anesthesiologist for being slow to recognize ongoing hemorrhage. In reality though—and we have all been there—it can be difficult to arrive at the correct diagnosis for a hypotensive patient in the heat of the moment and in the face of confounders ranging from anesthetic overdose to cardiac dysfunction to methylmethacrylate anaphylaxis.

As with the plaintiff's expert, the first duty of the defense expert is the honest presentation of the relevant standard of care. Citation of Guidelines from professional societies can be helpful, as can presentation of alternative mechanisms by which the patient's injury could have occurred absent a violation of the standard of care. An example of this kind of "alternative theory of causation" might be the patient who experiences an unexpected cardiac arrest during a surgical procedure. The plaintiff might make the case that this was caused by an overdose of anesthesia, whereas the defense expert could point out that an intercurrent pulmonary embolus would have the same presentation.

Cases with competing theories of causation are often the hardest fought, as each side becomes entrenched in their opinion and aggrieved by the attitude of the opposition. Adverse outcomes in which the anesthesia team were innocent bystanders to the clinical event—in the wrong OR at the wrong time (eg, when the pulmonary embolus occurred)—are among the hardest to review and defend. These cases may hinge on the collateral evidence that either side can bring to bear in support of their theory, ranging from autopsy findings to minutiae of documentation to postmorbid genetic testing. Good defense experts have the creativity to identify diagnostic alternatives that may have contributed to unusual events or delay in diagnosis.

Defense experts must be patient when educating the court regarding the nuance and uncertainty of clinical practice and must resist the temptation—often encouraged by the plaintiff's attorney—to become dogmatic in defiance of clinical reality. The credible defense expert must be sympathetic to both the injured patient and the accused clinicians and must maintain an open mind regarding causation: able and willing to discuss alternative theories while remaining honest and realistic about the most common possibilities.

SUMMARY

I hope this brief overview will be of use to anesthesiologists engaged as expert witnesses, because I feel strongly that participation in the system—as flawed as it may be—is an important aspect of professionalism. If we do not regulate ourselves, we have little grounds for complaint when others do it for us, and less well.

CLINICS CARE POINTS

- Anesthesiologists are not frequently named in malpractice suits.
- Malpractice suits against anesthesiologists may involve large settlements.
- There is a need for anesthesiologists willing to participate as expert witnesses for the legal system.

CONFLICTS-OF-INTEREST DISCLOSURE

The author has no conflicts of interest related to this topic.

References

[1] Mello MM, Frakes MD, Blumenkranz E, et al. Malpractice liability and health care quality: a review. JAMA 2020;323(4):352–66.
[2] Mello MM, Chandra A, Gawande AA, et al. National costs of the medical liability system. Health Aff 2010;9:1569–77.
[3] Studdert DM, Hall MA. Medical malpractice law – doctrine and dynamics. N Engl J Med 2022;387(17):1533–7.
[4] Bilimoria KY, Sohn MW, Chung JW, et al. Association Between State Medical Malpractice Environment and Surgical Quality and Cost in the United States. Ann Surg 2016;263(6):1126–32.
[5] Frakes M, Jena AB. Does medical malpractice law improve health care quality? J Public Econ 2016;143:142–58.
[6] Jena AB, Seabury S, Lakdawalla D, et al. Malpractice risk according to physician specialty. N Engl J Med 2011;365:629–36.
[7] https://policysearch.ama-assn.org/policyfinder/detail/expert%20witness?uri=%2FA-MADoc%2FHOD.xml-0-1842.xml, accessed April 11, 2023.
[8] https://en.wikipedia.org/wiki/Forensic_medicine, accessed April 11, 2023.
[9] https://abfp.com/accessed April 11, 2023.
[10] Guardado JR. Medical Liability Claim Frequency Among U.S. Physicians. Policy Research Perspectives. 2017. Accessed April 29, 2022. https://www.ama-assn.org/sites/ama-assn.org/files/corp/media-browser/public/government/advocacy/policy-research-perspective-medical-liability-claimfrequency.
[11] Austin EE, Do V, Nullwala R, et al. Systematic review of the factors and the key indicators that identify doctors at risk of complaints, malpractice claims or impaired performance. BMJ Open 2021;11(8):e050377.
[12] Maroon JC. Catastrophic cardiovascular complications from medical malpractice stress syndrome. J Neurosurg 2019;130:2081–5.
[13] Paterick ZR, Patel N, Chandrasekaran K, et al. Medical malpractice stress syndrome: a "forme fruste" of posttraumatic stress disorder. J Med Pract Manag 2017;32:283–7.
[14] Vizcaíno-Rakosnik M, Martin-Fumadó C, Arimany-Manso J, et al. The impact of malpractice claims on physicians' well-being and practice. J Patient Saf 2022;18:46–51.

[15] Liang BA, Maroulis J, Mackey TK. Understanding medical malpractice lawsuits. Stroke 2023;54(3):e95–9.

[16] Beecher HK, Todd DP. A study of the deaths associated with anesthesia and surgery: based on a study of 599, 548 anesthesias in ten institutions 1948-1952, inclusive. Ann Surg 1954;140(1):2–35.

[17] Pearse RM, Moreno RP, Bauer P, et al. European Surgical Outcomes Study (EuSOS) group for the Trials groups of the European Society of Intensive Care Medicine and the European Society of Anaesthesiology. Mortality after surgery in Europe: a 7 day cohort study. Lancet 2012;380(9847):1059–65.

[18] Daniel K. Thinking, fast and slow. New York: Farrar, Straus and Giroux; 2011.

[19] https://www.asahq.org/standards-and-guidelines/guidelines-for-expert-witness-qualifications-and-testimony Accessed April 11, 2023.

[20] Radvansky BM, Farver WT, Svider PF, et al. A comparison of plaintiff and defense expert witness qualifications in malpractice litigation in anesthesiology. Anesth Analg 2015;120(6):1369–74.

[21] Benumof Jonathan LMD. Lawyers choose specific experts for many different reasons. Anesth Analg 2016;122(1):293.

Advances in Anesthesia 41 (2023) 127–142

ADVANCES IN ANESTHESIA

Pediatric Anesthesia in the Community

Richard P. Dutton, MD, MBA[a],*, Robert B. Bryskin, MD[b],
Marion 'Red' Starks, MD, MBA[c],
Aesha S. Shukla, MHA, MBA, CPHQ[d], Olivia Lounsbury, MS[e]

[a]Department of Anesthesiology, Texas A&M College of Medicine, Baylor University Medical Center, Dallas, TX, USA; [b]USAP Florida, Orlando, FL, USA; [c]USAP North Texas, Dallas, TX, USA; [d]Quality, Analytics & Patient Experience, US Anesthesia Partners; [e]Quality and Safety Department, Johns Hopkins Children's Center

Keywords
- Pediatric anesthesia • Specialization • Demographics • Outcomes
- Patient experience

Key points
- Pediatric anesthesia is performed at a wide range of surgical and dental facilities.
- Pediatric anesthesia is performed by Board-certified pediatric anesthesiologists, fellowship-trained but noncertified anesthesiologists, and generalists.
- Pediatric anesthesia, regardless of location or clinician, is generally very safe, with high patient and family satisfaction and rare adverse events.

INTRODUCTION

Patients aged younger than 18 years account for 15% to 20% of anesthesia case volume in the United States [1]. The number of pediatric surgical cases in the main operating room has increased slightly in recent decades, although many traditional hospital cases are now done in ambulatory surgery facilities. This has been accompanied by a rapid increase in nonoperating room pediatric anesthetics (nonoperating room anesthesia [NORA]), including both diagnostic procedures such as MRI, cardiac catheterization, endoscopy, and an increasing number of minimally invasive therapeutic procedures [2].

*Corresponding author. US Anesthesia Partners, 12222 Merit Drive, Suite 700, Dallas, TX 75251. E-mail address: richard.dutton@usap.com

https://doi.org/10.1016/j.aan.2023.06.002
0737-6146/23/

Despite the rapid advancements in anesthesia care, the distribution of pediatric patients is not straightforward and not well described in current literature. Dedicated Children's Hospitals perform most high risk, high complexity cases—as they should—but more routine cases are performed in a variety of other environments including children's hospitals within adult hospitals, mixed adult and pediatric ambulatory surgical centers, pediatric ambulatory surgical centers, and dental offices. Similarly, the anesthesia clinicians caring for these patients range from Fellowship-trained and Pediatric Anesthesia Board-certified anesthesiologists to generalists seeing pediatric patients as less than 10% of their practice [3].

A recent effort by the American College of Surgeons, in consultation with the Society for Pediatric Anesthesia (SPA), created the Children's Surgery Verification (CSV) program [4]. The CSV is a quality improvement effort to establish standards for Level 1, Level 2, and Level 3 pediatric surgical facilities. Publication of these guidelines was applauded by the network of children's hospitals but caused consternation in the broader group of community hospitals providing pediatric surgeries. The guidelines, in specifically recommending fellowship-trained and Board-certified pediatric anesthesiologists, have called into question the capabilities of nonspecialized anesthesiologists, many of whom have been providing care for pediatric patients over many years. On the one hand, more training and a rigorous certification policy are likely to promote better outcomes; however, on the other hand, there are not enough qualified subspecialists to meet the national demand for pediatric anesthesia care, and there is little objective evidence of a difference in outcomes based on the credentials of the clinician, especially with regard to routine cases.

More data are required to understand the needs of the population, including both community access to anesthesia and the demand for higher risk procedures, and to define the difference in outcome between highly specialized care in children's hospitals versus pediatric cases performed by generalist anesthesiologists in community facilities.

Our purpose in producing this review is to pragmatically describe the landscape of pediatric anesthesiology in the United States, using the resources of US Anesthesia Partners (USAP), a nationwide private practice serving a broad swath of facilities (academic hospitals, community hospitals, specialty centers, and ambulatory surgery centers) across the country. USAP includes both pediatric anesthesiology specialists and general practitioners, who collectively completed more than 165,000 anesthetics in 2023 in patients aged younger than 18 years. These cases included a range of patient ages, comorbidities, and surgical case types. While a retrospective review cannot provide definitive data on risk versus outcome in pediatric anesthesia, and while our data is only a convenience sample of US anesthesia practice, we trust that the demographic data provided will guide researchers, policy makers and educators to an understanding of the current landscape of care.

METHODS

The primary source of data for the descriptions below is the USAP Clinical Data Warehouse. USAP is a national anesthesia private practice with local groups in Seattle, Las Vegas, Denver, Dallas/Fort Worth, Austin, San Antonio, Houston, Ft. Wayne, Nashville, Ft. Myers, Orlando, Jacksonville, Baltimore, and Washington D.C. Clinical decision-making in USAP, including hospital partnerships, hiring, and daily assignment of personnel to cases, resides with physician leadership in each local "platform," whereas the national practice management infrastructure makes investments in common resources for revenue cycle management, quality improvement (QI), clinician benefits, legal support, and operational efficiency. USAP invests in national-scale data and analytics [5]. Every case is documented in the data warehouse, and used to generate performance scorecards at the group, facility, and individual level [6]. Aggregate data in the Warehouse is used for QI and research projects at multiple levels of the practice.

Captured in the data warehouse are more than 50 demographic, operational, clinical, and quality datapoints for every case, supported by inclusion of the preanesthetic assessment, intraoperative record, and postanesthesia note. USAP conducts routine audits of this information, focused on the correlation between clinician attestation and the medical records and maintains an extremely high rate of compliance with accurate and complete documentation. Case information is further supplemented by inclusion—when available—of patient satisfaction data. Within 10 days of every case USAP solicits the patient (or family) by text and/or email to complete the Anesthesia Patient Satisfaction Questionnaire, Version 2 (APSQ2), a nationally validated instrument used to report Medicare quality measure AQI-48 Patient-Reported Overall Anesthesia Experience. The current USAP survey response rate is 28% to 32% of all patients with demographic data, adding a wealth of unique, and highly actionable, data on patient satisfaction to the Clinical Data Warehouse [7].

For purposes of this review, we abstracted data from every patient aged younger than 18 years cared for by a USAP clinician for a nonobstetric case in calendar years 2016 to 2022. For every case in this dataset, we noted the site of service, the clinicians involved in the patient's care, the date and time of the surgery, the specific case and anesthesia types, and patient demographics including age, sex, and ASA physical status. When the patient or family returned a satisfaction survey, we included the results. This dataset was linked to the USAP Credentials file, providing the training and Board Certification status of each clinician, and to data describing each of the facilities where pediatric anesthesia was performed, including the type, size, and specialization of the facility.

Clinicians were characterized both by their training and by the percentage of their cases, which were pediatric anesthetics, yielding 2 separate dimensions of expertise. Similarly, facilities were sorted based on the percentage of their cases, which were pediatric.

For each of the demographic metrics, we present both the current state (2022) and, if applicable, changes noted during the 7 years of data collected. USAP Tennessee and Indiana are recent platforms who joined USAP in September of 2022; therefore, this dataset does not represent their full scope of pediatric practice for the year.

RESULTS

Location of procedures

From 2016 to 2022, the number of pediatric anesthetics performed by USAP clinicians increased from 83,000 to more than 165,000 annually (Fig. 1). Cases were performed in 505 sites representing roughly 2.6% of the 6 million pediatric anesthetics performed each year in the United States [8]. Year-on-year growth in pediatric case volume was due to both growth of USAP (expansion into new sites) and to increased volume on a same-facility basis. The trend line on Fig. 1 shows the number of pediatric cases as a percentage of all USAP cases in each year, increasing to the current value of 6.70% of total practice volume. In aggregate, the 7 years of data represent more than 800,000 pediatric anesthetics.

USAP clinicians perform pediatric anesthesia across 10 states (Fig. 2). More than 50% of USAP pediatric anesthetics were performed in the state of Texas at 261 sites of service. In Florida, 32,100 pediatric anesthetics were performed in 52 sites of service, while in Colorado and Nevada roughly 20,000 anesthetics occurred in 83 sites. The number of USAP-served stand-alone and attached-but-dedicated children's hospitals (hospital in a hospital) in each state is represented by a number above each state's bar graph, with 7 facilities in Texas, and one each in Colorado, Florida, Nevada, and Oklahoma. The "hospital in a hospital" model is common in community pediatric care, allowing for concentration of resources and expertise in a building dedicated to pediatric care but attached to a larger adult hospital.

Concordant with the pattern of place of service distribution within each state was the distribution of anesthetizing locations. The majority of all pediatric cases were performed on an outpatient basis, either in hospitals, outpatient facilities attached to the hospital, ambulatory surgical centers, or dental offices. In

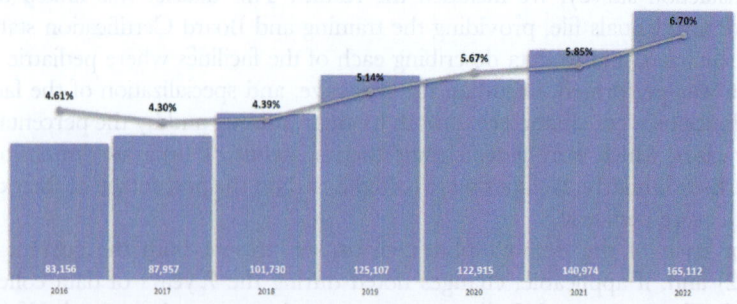

Fig. 1. Total pediatric cases: year over year. Excludes obstetric cases. The trend line shows the percentage of all USAP anesthetics involving pediatric patients.

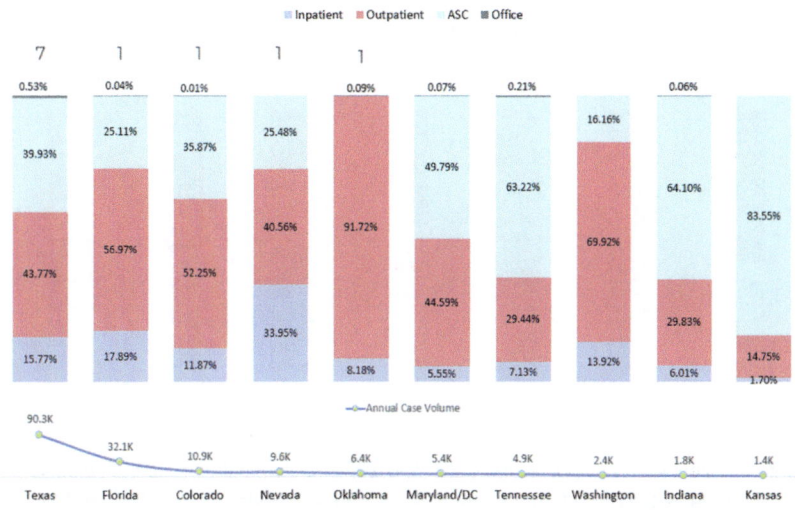

Fig. 2. Pediatric volume by state and place of service. The number above each bar is the count of children's hospitals in each state. The states are sorted by pediatric case volume. The trendline shows volume by state. ASC, Ambulatory Surgery Center.

Indiana, Kansas, Maryland/Washington DC, and Tennessee, the majority of pediatric anesthetics were performed in Ambulatory Surgery Centers (ASCs). In Colorado, Florida, Oklahoma, and Washington, most pediatric anesthetic procedures were performed on an outpatient basis in hospital settings or in surgical centers attached to a hospital. Inpatient hospitals included dedicated, freestanding children's hospitals, children's hospitals attached to a larger general or academic hospital, and community hospitals with pediatric cases mixed with adults. Outpatient hospitals were defined as on-campus outpatient operating rooms caring for both children and adults. ASCs included ambulatory surgery centers caring for both children and adults, and ambulatory surgery centers specializing in pediatric procedures. Office-based anesthesia consisted for the most part of pediatric dental procedures.

From 2016 to 2022, the distribution of place of service across all USAP sites has undergone subtle changes because procedures shifted from inpatient to an outpatient setting (Fig. 3). The proportion of cases occurring in the ASC and Outpatient setting outnumbers the number of inpatient cases. Moreover, the 25% to 30% increase in the proportion of pediatric anesthetics performed at ASCs during the 7 years is consistent with the 40% increase in ASC's utilization trend previously observed during a 10 year period (from 1996 to 2006) by the US National Center for Healthcare Statistics [9]. Outpatient cases performed at a hospital were 49.76% in 2016, growing to 56.97% in 2018 before declining steadily to 47.47% in 2022. During the same period, inpatient cases declined marginally from 17.76% to 16.74%. The volatility of the COVID-19 pandemic likely impedes interpretation of this trend.

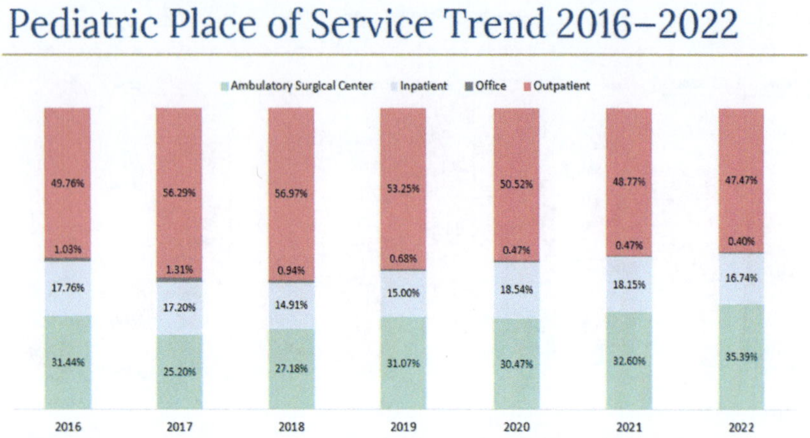

Pediatric Place of Service Trend 2016–2022

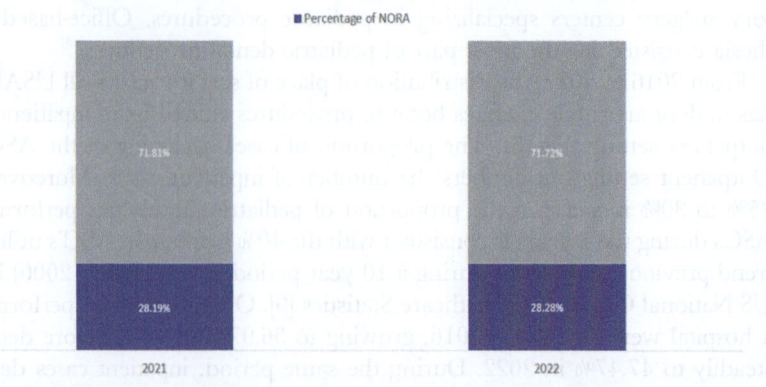

■ Ambulatory Surgical Center   ■ Inpatient   ■ Office   ■ Outpatient

	2016	2017	2018	2019	2020	2021	2022
Outpatient	49.76%	56.29%	56.97%	53.25%	50.52%	48.77%	47.47%
Office	1.03%	1.31%	0.94%	0.68%	0.47%	0.47%	0.40%
Inpatient	17.76%	17.20%	14.91%	15.00%	18.54%	18.15%	16.74%
Ambulatory Surgical Center	31.44%	25.20%	27.18%	31.07%	30.47%	32.60%	35.39%

Fig. 3. Inpatient versus outpatient trend 2016 to 2022. Outpatients include both ambulatory patients having surgery in a hospital and those having procedures in an ambulatory surgery center or office.

Across 7 years, between 14% and 19% of USAP pediatric cases were performed on an inpatient basis, with one children's hospital and 4 dedicated pediatric units (hospital-in-a-hospital) accounting for more than 40% of all inpatient cases.

The need for NORA service in pediatrics has expanded dramatically during the past decade. Previous reports suggested that NORA represents 10% to 24% of the pediatric cases [10]. Our data (Fig. 4) demonstrated a higher percentage of pediatric NORA cases (28.24% avg during the past 2 years) with an upward

Percentage of NORA Pediatric Cases

■ Percentage of NORA

	2021	2022
	71.81%	71.72%
	28.19%	28.28%

Fig. 4. Proportion of remote-site anesthetic procedures.

trajectory from 2021 to 2022 at 28.19% and 28.28%, respectively. This may represent an ongoing evolution in the scope and number of diagnostic and nonsurgical procedures performed at NORA locations.

Patient demographics

Fig. 5 illustrates the number of USAP pediatric cases by age as of 2022. Consistent with national data, about 25% of pediatric anesthetics were in neonates or infants, and more than half occurred in patients aged 6 years or younger [8]. Anesthetics for school-age children were relatively less common until the teen years. There were 1683 neonates cared for across the USAP platforms in 2022, with a gradual increase from 779 in 2016 to 1683 in 2022. Although neonatal anesthetics make up only 1% to 2% of all pediatric cases, they are disproportionately complex and are a notable percentage of all neonatal anesthetics each year in the United States.

Fig. 6 shows the trend from 2018 to 2022 of patient complexity in pediatric patients. USAP has seen a reduction in ASA 1 and 2 patients and an increase in ASA 3, ASA 4, and ASA 5/6 patients. Patients with life-threatening comorbidities, ASA greater than 3, represented 14.68% of pediatric cases in 2022 (24,238 patients).

Procedures

Using groupings based on the Agency for Healthcare Research and Quality's Clinical Classification Software, Fig. 7 shows the most common case types for each age of patient [11]. Beginning in infancy, Ear, Nose and Throat (ENT) cases predominate. Orthopedic surgery is common in older children, while cardiac surgery is almost exclusively confined to neonates and infants.

Figs. 8 and 9 show counts of fellow-level index cases by age and service line, as defined by the Accreditation Council for Graduate Medical Education (ACGME) for the purpose of reviewing and accrediting Pediatric Anesthesia

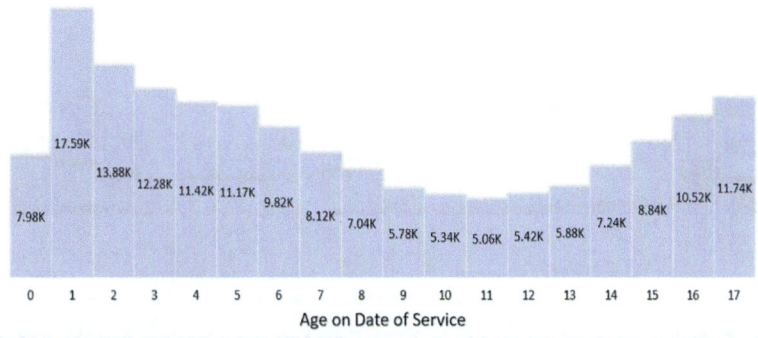

Fig. 5. USAP pediatric cases by age in 2022.

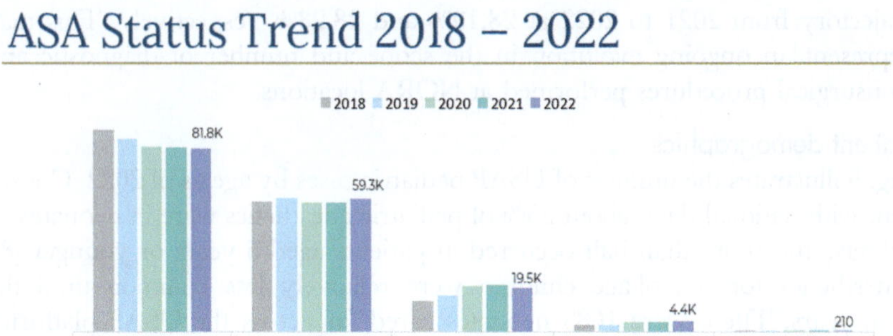

ASA Status Trend 2018 – 2022

■ 2018 ■ 2019 ■ 2020 ■ 2021 ■ 2022

	P1	P2	P3	P4	P5/P6
■ 2018	54.74%	35.16%	8.28%	1.74%	0.08%
■ 2019	52.19%	36.15%	9.65%	1.92%	0.09%
■ 2020	49.95%	34.93%	12.44%	2.56%	0.11%
■ 2021	49.76%	34.93%	12.55%	2.66%	0.11%
■ 2022	49.45%	35.86%	11.84%	2.71%	0.13%

Fig. 6. Pediatric cases by ASA physical status trend from 2018 to 2022.

Fellowship programs [12]. Ensuring sufficient availability of these complex cases for Fellows and Anesthesiology Residents is a requirement for specialty training. The number of fellow-level pediatric index cases performed by USAP clinicians supports the necessity of having an expanded case-log requirement in graduating pediatric anesthesia fellows to adequately prepare them for independent clinical practice [13].

The 1194 congenital heart surgeries performed by USAP clinicians further demonstrate complexity in community pediatric anesthesia practice. This number represents 3.5% of the 33,610 pediatric cardiac cases recorded in the STS database for 2021 [14].

PROCEDURE MIX BY AGE DISTRIBUTION

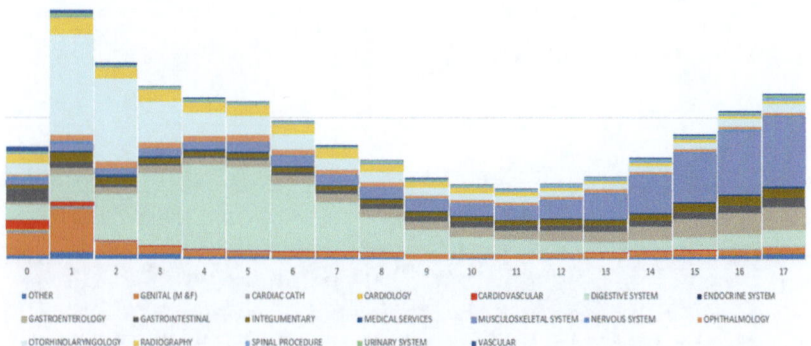

Fig. 7. Pediatric procedures by age in 2022. Case-type groupings are from the Agency for Healthcare Research and Quality Clinical Classification Software.

Pediatric: Complex Cases

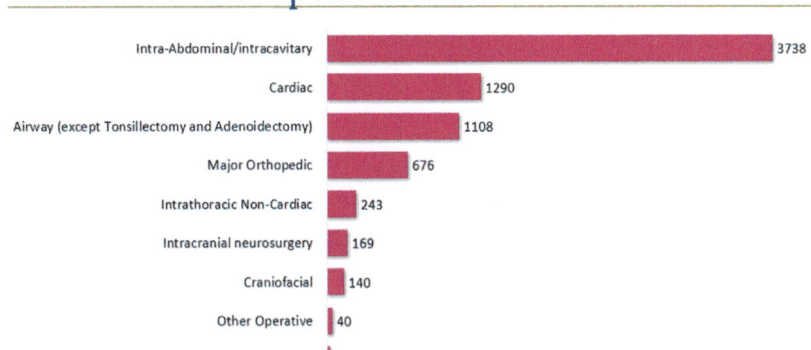

Fig. 8. Complex cases performed by USAP clinicians in 2022.

Clinicians

Fig. 10 describes the population of 4410 USAP clinicians who delivered pediatric anesthesia in 2022 (approximately 90% of all USAP clinicians), their credentials, and the percentage of overall practice dedicated to pediatric anesthesia cases. This total included 2123 anesthesiologists and 2287 Certified Registered Nurse Anesthetists (CRNAs) and Certified Anesthesiologist Assistants (CAAs). For the anesthesiologists involved, we categorized as follows.

- Experts—Anesthesiologists with Pediatric Anesthesia Subspecialty Boards, or Board Certified in Pediatrics in addition to Anesthesiology

Complex Case Category by Age

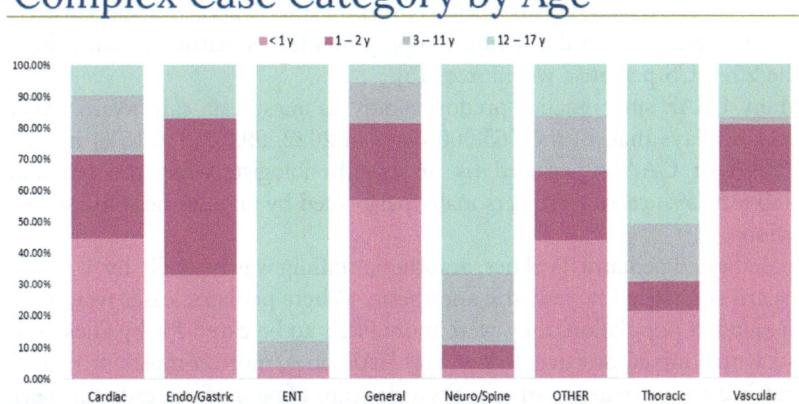

Fig. 9. Complex procedures performed by USAP physicians in 2022 across various pediatric age groups.

Anesthesiologist Categorization

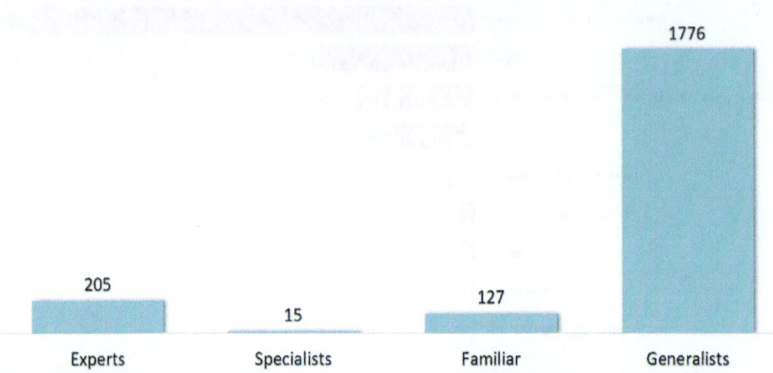

Fig. 10. Number of Unique Anesthesiologists Performing Pediatric Cases by Certification and Percent Volume of Pediatric Patients in Total Volume in 2022. "Experts" are defined as anesthesiologists with Pediatric Anesthesia Subspecialty Boards, or Board Certified in Pediatrics in addition to Anesthesiology. "Specialists" are defined as anesthesiologists with greater than 50% of their cases in patients aged 0 to 17 years. "Familiar" are defined as anesthesiologists with greater than 10% and less than 50% of their cases in patients aged 0 to 17 years. "Generalists" are defined as anesthesiologists with less than 10% of their cases in patients aged 0 to 17 years.

- Specialists—Anesthesiologists with greater than 50% of their cases in patients aged 0 to 17 years but without formal subspecialty training or certification
- Familiar—Anesthesiologists with greater than 10% and less than 50% of their cases in patients aged 0 to 17 years
- Generalists—Anesthesiologists with less than 10% of their cases in patients aged 0 to 17 years

The 220 USAP anesthesiologists comprising the expert and specialist categories, represent 5% of the national supply of 4377 pediatric anesthesiologists in the 2020 US pediatric workforce [15].

Many USAP sites practice predominantly as anesthesia care teams (ACT). Fig. 11 displays that, of the 165,000 cases in 2022, 99,323 (60.15%) involved a CRNA or CAA supervised by an anesthesiologist, while the remaining 65,789 (39.85%) cases were personally performed by an anesthesiologist working alone.

In dedicated pediatric facilities, anesthesia staffing was typically by a group of clinicians specialized in pediatric anesthesia. Where pediatric cases were mixed with an adult population, they were more likely to be cared for by anesthesiologists with a mixed practice. In several USAP cities, more complex or high-risk pediatric cases were assigned to a citywide team of pediatric anesthesia specialists who travel between hospitals to provide this service. This model is effective in community practice because it mirrors activities of the pediatric surgeons. In Las Vegas, for example, pediatric cardiac surgery may be performed in several

Cases Performed: Anesthesiologist vs Anesthesia Care Team

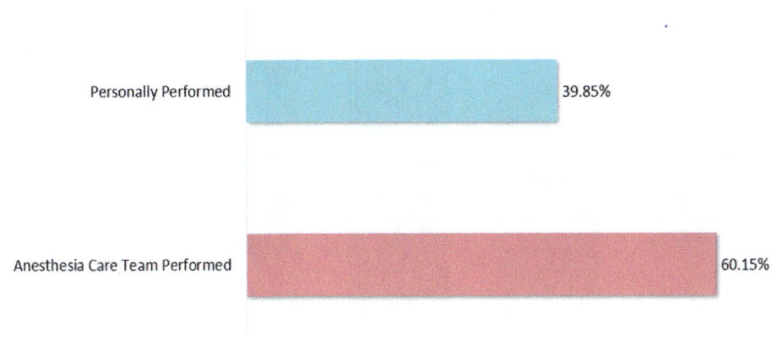

Personally Performed — 39.85%

Anesthesia Care Team Performed — 60.15%

Fig. 11. Percentages of cases performed by only anesthesiologist versus anesthesia care team.

hospitals but always by the same team of surgeons, thus enabling a "follow the surgeon" anesthesia model. While moving between hospitals is less time-efficient for the anesthesiologists involved, this ensures consistent surgeon-anesthesiologist dyads for these cases.

Fig. 12 shows the distribution of ASA III, IV, and V patients and the ACT used, whether an ACT or personally performed by only the anesthesiologist. In ASA physical status groups 1 to 4, ACTs cared for most patients.

Fig. 13 illustrates the ASA distribution by category of pediatric clinician in 2022. The graphic demonstrates that 82.4% of ASA 3 to 5 patients were cared for by "Expert" anesthesiologists, per the categories above. However, 3.3% of

Cases by Anesthesia Model & ASA Status

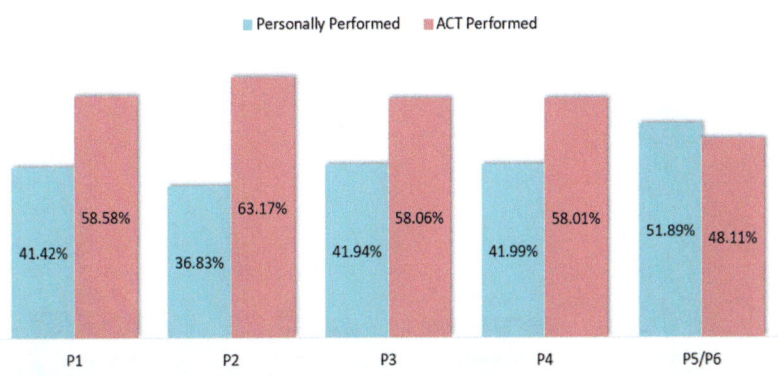

■ Personally Performed   ■ ACT Performed

	P1	P2	P3	P4	P5/P6
Personally Performed	41.42%	36.83%	41.94%	41.99%	51.89%
ACT Performed	58.58%	63.17%	58.06%	58.01%	48.11%

Fig. 12. ASA distribution by anesthesia model in 2022.

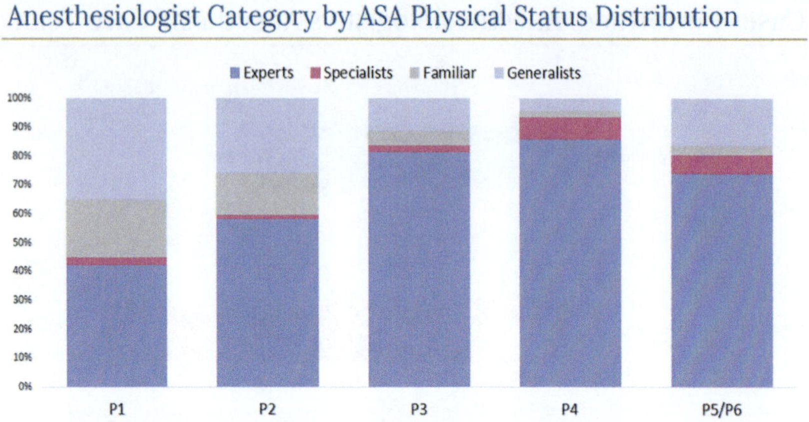

Anesthesiologist Category by ASA Physical Status Distribution

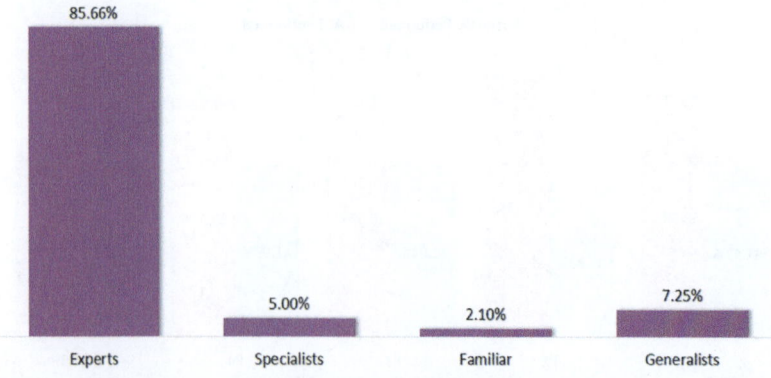

Fig. 13. Pediatric Clinician Category by ASA Distribution in 2022. Categories defined above.

ASA 3 to 5 patients were cared for by "Specialist" anesthesiologists and 4.6% by "Familiar" anesthesiologists. The figure also demonstrates that as patient acuity increases, the percent of cases covered by "Generalists" and "Familiar" anesthesiologists decreases.

The distribution of index cases by category of anesthesiologists, as defined above, is represented in Fig. 14. The figure demonstrates that "Experts" and "Specialist" anesthesiologists perform the majority of anesthetics for sicker patients. However, a fraction of these cases is still performed by "generalists" and "familiar." This reflects the reality of community anesthesia practice that pediatric emergencies can arise at any time or site of service and emphasizes the importance of training and experience in pediatric care for any anesthesia clinician.

Index Cases by Anesthesiologist Categorization

Fig. 14. Distribution of index cases by category of anesthesiologist.

Index cases were more likely to have been performed at a facility that identified itself as a pediatric facility than one that did not (Fig. 15). With the exception of ASA 1 and 2, no index cases were performed at an ASC.

The percentage of index cases performed by each pediatric board-certified anesthesiologist (Expert) is listed in Fig. 16. Pediatric Anesthesiology Board-Certified physicians were 85% more likely to be responsible for the care of an index case. Pediatric board-certified anesthesiologist index cases were performed by single-posted physicians 40% of the time, and by care team 60% of the time.

Safety and outcomes

The USAP Quality program records patient safety outcomes for all anesthesia cases, which are reviewed by the local USAP Risk and Quality Directors and Clinical Quality Committees. In addition, for pediatric cases, the USAP Patient Safety Organization shares demographics and narratives with the Wake Up Safe Patient Safety Organization of the SPA [16]. The most common events reported in pediatric patients were laryngospasm/bronchospasm, intraoperative hypothermia, and transient desaturation. A serious adverse event occurred in less than 1% of all pediatric cases, consistent with national experience and the overall safety of anesthesia in ASA 1 and 2 patients of any age.

Patient satisfaction

Patient experience data has been collected through a robust system for more than 7 years. The adaptive survey, APSQ2, asks questions specific to anesthesia in communication, comfort, easing anxiety, time spent with anesthesiologists/anesthesia care team before and after anesthesia, nausea and vomiting, clinician satisfaction, and overall anesthesia experience. USAP values this feedback; USAP meticulously analyzes that data to provide aggregated feedback to providers and uses the data to further improve patient interactions and experience. Patient and family satisfaction with pediatric anesthesia is generally high,

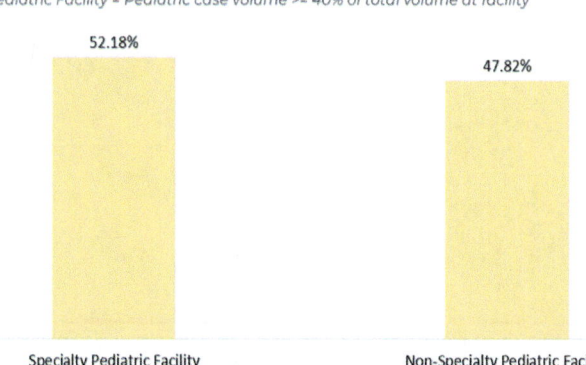

Index Cases by Facility Type

Specialty Pediatric Facility = Pediatric case volume >= 40% of total volume at facility

52.18% — Specialty Pediatric Facility

47.82% — Non-Specialty Pediatric Facility

Fig. 15. Distribution of index cases performed by facility.

Index Cases Personally Performed vs ACT

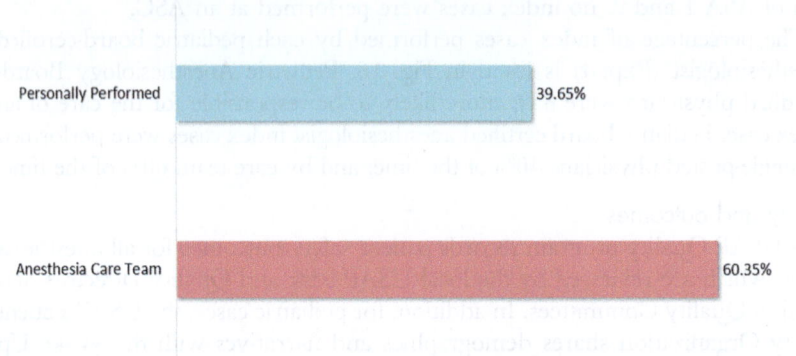

Fig. 16. Distribution of index cases performed by single pediatric board-certified anesthesiologists versus by an ACT.

with greater than 96.94% of returned surveys rating overall anesthesia care as 4 "good" or 5 "great" out of 5 on a Likert scale (Fig. 17). Positive comments outnumber negative comments by a wide margin.

STRENGTHS AND LIMITATIONS

The data presented here are a convenience sample from a nationwide anesthesia private practice and may not reflect the demographics of pediatric anesthesia in other locations. Urban and suburban sites in Texas, Colorado, and Florida are overrepresented. Although USAP practice sites range from freestanding children's hospitals to individual dentist offices, we do not know if

Overall Anesthesia Care Experience

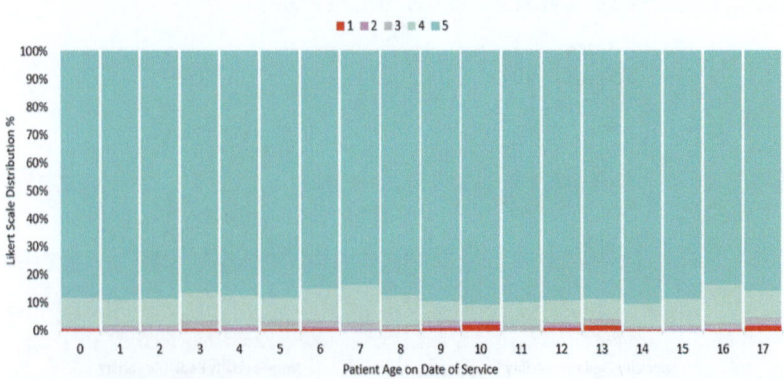

Fig. 17. Overall anesthesia care experience by patient age.

the relative volumes across sites are representative of national practice. These data will be most useful as an illustration of what pediatric anesthesia looks like in nonacademic practice, and as an example of the range of cases, patients, and clinicians involved.

SUMMARY

The practice of pediatric anesthesiology continues to evolve in step with requirements of pediatric surgical societies, regulatory oversight, voluntary hospital verification programs, and credentialing changes. Previous research in this area relied on surveys, membership databases, and enrollment in pediatric anesthesia board certification process to glean geographic distribution, workforce quality, and daily responsibilities of pediatric anesthesiologists [3]. Notable has been the lack of perspective from nonacademic pediatric anesthesiologists. The collective experience of USAP allows a detailed view of pediatric anesthesiologists taking care of children across a wide variation of geographies and facilities, and across the continuum from office-based care, ASCs, community hospitals to dedicated children's facilities. In USAP's experience, a higher percentage of pediatric cases are done in ASCs than for adult anesthesia.

The literature contains relatively little information about the private practice of pediatric anesthesiology. Our report may be valuable for stakeholders, including pediatric anesthesiology fellowship directors, residency program directors, policy makers and, perhaps most importantly, to resident anesthesiologists interested in pursuing a career in pediatric anesthesiology. This last group will benefit from an understanding of opportunities for practice outside of dedicated children's hospitals. As the USAP data illustrate, there is an abundance of cases available in the community, and many nonacademic centers performing substantial volumes of high-acuity work.

One commonly heard description is that private practice pediatric anesthesiology consists of mostly simple cases in healthy patients for whom subspecialized training is not needed. Our experience confirms that, in general, most pediatric patients are healthy, ASA 1 or 2. However, USAP pediatric anesthesia specialists exceed the required number of ACGME Verification Index number of cases used to define a Pediatric Anesthesiologist, each year, while caring for thousands of ASA 3 to 6 patients. Moreover, ACTs are highly involved in the care of our patients, indicating an ongoing need for pediatric-focused CRNAs and CAAs as well as anesthesiologists.

CLINICS CARE POINTS

- Every anesthesiologist must be prepared to care for pediatric patients.
- Most pediatric patients are ASA status 1 or 2, having short and simple procedures.
- Private practice pediatric anesthesia includes the full range of cases and patient acuity.

DISCLOSURE

All authors contributed to preparation of the article, figures, and tables, and approved the final article.

FUNDING SOURCE

None.

CONFLICTS OF INTEREST

The authors have no conflicts of interest related to this topic.

References

[1] Rabbitts JA, Groenewald CB. Epidemiology of Pediatric Surgery in the United States. Paediatr Anaesth 2020;30(10):1083–90.

[2] Nagrebetsky A, Gabriel RA, Dutton RP, et al. Growth of Nonoperating Room Anesthesia Care in the United States: A Contemporary Trends Analysis. Anesth Analg 2017;124(4):1261–7.

[3] Muffly M, Singleton M, Agarwall R. etc., The Pediatric Anesthesiology Workforce: Projecting Supply and Trends 2015-2035. Anesth Analg 2018;126(2):568–78.

[4] Wang KS, Cummings J, Stark A, et al. Section on surgery, committee on fetus and newborn, section on anesthesiology and pain medicine. Optimizing Resources in Children's Surgical Care: An Update on the American College of Surgeons' Verification Program. Pediatrics 2020;145(5); https://doi.org/10.1542/peds.2020-0708.

[5] Dutton RP, Swygert TH, Maloney M, et al. Scaling up quality in anesthesia practice. Int J Qual Health Care 2023;35(1):mzad011.

[6] Dutton RP, Davidson S, Shukla AS. Setting up a quality program: defining the value proposition for anesthesiology. Int Anesthesiol Clin 2021;59(4):1–11.

[7] Pozdnyakova A, Tung A, Dutton R, et al. Factors Affecting Patient Satisfaction With Their Anesthesiologist: An Analysis of 51,676 Surveys From a Large Multihospital Practice. Anesth Analg 2019;129(4):951–9.

[8] Sun LS, Li G, DiMaggio CJ, et al. Feasibility and pilot study of the Pediatric Anesthesia Neurodevelopment Assessment (PANDA) project. J Neurosurg Anesthesiol 2012;24(4):382–8.

[9] Rabbitts J, Groenewald C, Moriarty J, et al. Epidemiology of Ambulatory Anesthesia for Children in the United States: 2006 and 1996. Anesth Analg 2010;111(4):1011–5.

[10] Campbell K, Torres L, Stayer S. Anesthesia and sedation outside the operating room. Anesthesiol Clin 2014;32(1):25–43.

[11] Agency for Healthcare Research and Quality. Clinical Classifications Software Refined (CCSR) for ICU-10-CM Diagnoses. 2022. Available at https://hcup-us.ahrq.gov/toolssoftware/ccsr/dxccsr.jsp. Accessed May 13, 2023.

[12] American College of Graduate Medical Education. Pediatric Anesthesiology Fellowship Minimum Case Numbers. Available at https://www.acgme.org/globalassets/PFAssets/ProgramResources/042_Peds_AN_Minimums.pdf. Accessed May 13, 2023.

[13] Ambardekar A, Furukawa L, Eriksen W, et al. A consensus-driven revision of the accreditation council for graduate medical education case log system: Pediatric anesthesiology fellowship education. Anesth Analg 2023;136(3):446–54.

[14] Kumar S, Gaynor J, Jones L, et al. The Society of Thoracic Surgeons Congenital Heart Surgery Database: 2022 Update on Outcomes and Research. Ann Thorac Surg 2023;115(4):807–19.

[15] Muffly M, Scheinker D, Muffly T, et al. Practice Characteristics of Board-certified Pediatric Anesthesiologists in the US: A Nationwide Survey. Cureus 2019;11(9):e5745.

[16] Buck DW, Claure R, Tjia IM, et al. How the Wake Up Safe pediatric anesthesia collaborative increased quality improvement capability and collaboration. Paediatr Anaesth 2022;32(11):1246–51.

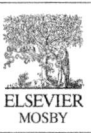

Advances in Anesthesia 41 (2023) 143–162

ADVANCES IN ANESTHESIA

Trauma Anesthesiology Perioperative Management Update

Ryan Perlman, MSc, MD, FRCPC[a],*, Kevin Tsai, MD[b], Jessie Lo, MD[c]

[a]Trauma Anesthesia, Department of Anaesthesia, Cedars-Sinai Medical Center, 8700 Beverly Boulevard, North Tower, Suite 8211, Los Angeles, CA 90048, USA; [b]Department of Anaesthesia, Cedars-Sinai Medical Center, 8700 Beverly Boulevard, North Tower, Suite 8211, Los Angeles, CA 90048, USA; [c]Trauma Education Program, Department of Anaesthesia, Cedars-Sinai Medical Center, 8700 Beverly Boulevard, North Tower, Suite 8211, Los Angeles, CA 90048, USA

Keywords

• Trauma anesthesia • POCUS • TCA • REBOA • Hypothermia • RSI • TBI

Key points

• In cases of traumatic cardiac arrest, volume resuscitation and relieving an obstructive cause of shock may take priority over chest compressions.

• The role of epinephrine in traumatic cardiac arrest is not conclusive; its benefits and potential risks should be considered based on individual cases.

• Cerebral perfusion pressure-based medical management for rising intracranial pressure should be considered based on each case, comorbidities, and the likelihood of impending herniation.

• A restrictive transfusion strategy with a target Hg of 7 to 9 g/dL is generally appropriate for patients with traumatic brain injury.

INTRODUCTION

Several studies have shown that among those younger than 44 years old, trauma is still the leading cause of death [1]. Recent progress in trauma anesthesia has resulted in the creation of innovative resuscitative procedures and treatment strategies that attempt to improve patient outcomes for this

*Corresponding author. Department of Anaesthesia, Cedars-Sinai Medical Center, 8700 Beverly Boulevard, North Tower, Suite 8211, Los Angeles, CA 90048. E-mail address: ryan.perlman@cshs.org

https://doi.org/10.1016/j.aan.2023.06.003
0737-6146/23/Crown Copyright © 2023 Published by Elsevier Inc. All rights reserved.

vulnerable demographic. The effective resuscitation of traumatic cardiac arrest (TCA), the timing of chest compressions, the use of epinephrine, and the specific indications for thoracotomy and endovascular control of bleeding remain controversial despite the advanced implementation of balanced transfusion practice and a greater understanding of the significance of whole blood in our massive transfusion protocols.

Traumatic brain injury (TBI) occurs when the brain parenchyma sustains a physical injury as a consequence of an external application of energy; this causes secondary inflammation to persist for an extended period of time, including an increase in cerebral edema and breakdown of the blood–brain barrier, metabolic dysfunctions, and oxidative stress [2,3]. Restrictive transfusion targets in TBI, appropriate hyperosmolar drugs, preventive and therapeutic hypothermia, and the need for decompressive craniectomy (DC) are controversial in the therapy of patients with TBI.

This article reviews these current controversies in trauma anesthesia, with presentation of the most recent evidence for and against each approach.

PREHOSPITAL AIRWAY MANAGEMENT
Paramedic airway management
The approach to managing airway compromise in the setting of traumatic injury, which may contribute to cardiac and respiratory arrest, is discussed across a number of specialties. Outside of the hospital setting, management of the airway generally falls on external providers or bystanders without the aid of advanced monitoring, rescue airway devices, or specialized training. In recent decades, initiatives by organizations such as the American Red Cross and the American Heart Association have provided resources and certifications in early resuscitative measures or basic life support (BLS) targeting nonhospital staff and potential providers in the general public [4,5]. Among these early measures, airway assessment and management are emphasized, focusing on ventilation assistance and maneuvers to promote oxygenation and protect against aspiration. The use of advanced airway techniques including endotracheal intubation (ETI), the province of prehospital anesthesiologists in some countries, is performed by emergency medical services (EMS) personnel and emergency medicine specialists in the United States.

The value of prehospital airway management has undergone significant review, in large part by EMS system leaders and trauma hospital logistical transport developers, with the aim to match airway management techniques with patient needs following trauma, cardiac arrest, or other medical emergencies while recognizing the limitations of out-of-hospital resources [6]. This subject remains controversial. A multicenter randomized controlled trial (RCT) in 2018, comparing favorable neurologic function after the use of bag-mask ventilation (BMV) versus ETI in prehospital airway management proved inconclusive with neither noninferiority nor inferiority demonstrated between the 2 treatment groups [7]. A systematic review coordinated by the Agency for Healthcare Research and Quality comparing the use of BMV and more invasive techniques involving the supraglottic airway (SGA) and ETI showed low to moderate strength of evidence of no additional benefit in prehospital airway management incorporating invasive approaches (SGA, ETI) in terms of mortality, neurologic function, or return of spontaneous circulation (ROSC) [6]. The *Journal of Paramedic Practice* similarly published a review of data among BVM, SGA, and ETI in cardiac arrest and trauma patients, identifying greater success in securing the airway on the first attempt with the use of SGA, but no evidence of difference among these approaches for ROSC, neurologic outcomes, or survival [8].

Preoxygenation or denitrogenation is a critical component of airway management because of its ability to increase oxygen reserve and delay hypoxemia during apneic periods. The approach to preoxygenation can be patient-driven (continuous positive airway pressure [CPAP] in spontaneously breathing obese patients), passive (nasal cannula or face mask), provider-driven as in apneic oxygenation by mask ventilation, or a combination of these practices [9]. Nasal cannula should be avoided in cases of basal skull fracture or any sign of a cerebrospinal fluid leak [3]. The decision on which method of preoxygenation to use is made case by case, and the effectiveness in prolonging apnea without desaturation varies based on several factors, including patient physiology (increased metabolic requirements) and cooperation. The use of a nasal cannula at 5 to 10 L per minute may provide apneic oxygen and important extra seconds during traumatic intubation to reduce the relative risks of hypoxemia and secondary injury, especially if airway management is not expected to be difficult [9].

Barriers to coordinating comprehensive analyses of prehospital airway management include the challenge of performing RCTs in the prehospital setting. As a result, out-of-hospital studies are generally observational, as such there remain many issues with obtaining consent or identifying patients who fulfill certain inclusion criteria. Though the prehospital approach is still up for debate, it is clear that when the goal is to protect the patient from aspiration and maintain adequate oxygenation, advanced interventions are indicated. Patients may benefit from basic airway maneuvers and supplemental oxygen for transport to a clinical facility where induction and intubation can be performed in a more controlled setting. The focus remains on early transport to a designated trauma center [10].

Paralytic agents

A critical part of RSI is the use of paralytic agents to create optimal conditions for securing the airway. Succinylcholine 1 to 2 mg/kg is traditionally used, based on its fast onset, short half-life, and short duration of action. Rocuronium has been increasingly used as an alternative, especially with the advent of sugammadex, a rapid nondepolarizing neuromuscular blocker reversal agent, in the early 2000s. Advantages of achieving paralysis with rocuronium include avoidance of potentially catastrophic side effects of succinylcholine including hyperkalemia, bradycardia, and increased intracranial pressure (ICP).

Furthermore, sugammadex allows for reliable prompt reversal of paralysis in "cannot intubate, cannot ventilate" scenarios following administration of rocuronium (duration of action of succinylcholine and rocuronium are 10–15 minutes and 30–90 minutes, respectively). This provides an appealing alternative in RSI scenarios involving major trauma, burns, and other common trauma presentations [11].

A database review of intubating conditions in RSI and modified RSI comparing the use of succinylcholine (minimum dose 1 mg/kg) and rocuronium (minimum dose 0.6 mg/kg) up until 2007 was published and expanded to include RCTs and clinical control trials through 2015 [12]. These reviews concluded that while succinylcholine was superior in facilitating clinically acceptable intubating conditions at the described doses, there was no statistical difference in intubation conditions comparing succinylcholine with a higher initial dose of rocuronium (1.2 mg/kg), noting that the former was clinically superior due to its shorter duration of action [12]. Historically, succinylcholine was the preferred agent in trauma due to its rapid onset and short duration of action. When used correctly, rocuronium can also provide neuromuscular blockade as quickly and effectively as succinylcholine. Rocuronium was previously avoided due to its prolonged duration of action, which precluded early neurologic examination. With sugammadex now being widely available, the patient can be adequately reversed and assessed in a timely manner [13].

In trauma resuscitation, major accidents may involve intracranial injuries. For patients with TBI, RSI is the standard of care because of the association between hypoxemia and adverse neurologic outcomes. Fasciculations due to succinylcholine may contribute to increased ICP, which may negatively affect neurologic outcomes in patients with closed head trauma or those with associated ocular globe injuries [14]. A literature review yielded poor evidence of clinically significant changes in ICP; however, increased electroencephalogram (EEG) arousal, elevated cerebral blood flow, and subsequently increased ICP have been demonstrated in animal models and associated with increased mortality as compared to rocuronium paralysis [15–18]. Clinically significant increases in ICP or brain herniation are not reported in the human literature and it is still unknown if preventing fasciculations with a nondepolarizing neuromuscular blocker prior to administration of succinylcholine will improve neurologic outcomes for patients with intracranial injuries.

Cricoid pressure

The greatest point of controversy in the RSI protocol involves the use of anterior cricoid pressure, with proponents for this maneuver often citing compression of the esophagus as a theoretic precaution against regurgitation of abdominal contents [19]. Compression of the esophagus to prevent gastric distention during mask ventilation was first observed by Sellick in a cadaver model, and then subsequently reproduced in 26 anesthetized, paralyzed patients deemed high risk for aspiration. Notably, in 3 of these patients, regurgitation of gastric contents occurred following intubation and release of cricoid pressure. Studies that followed included both pediatric and adult populations, and cricoid pressure was soon thereafter introduced into the standard RSI protocol [20,21].

A number of studies, however, show no evidence to support the use of cricoid pressure. In the largest randomized double-blinded trial, which included 3472 patients undergoing RSI with either cricoid pressure or a sham procedure, the incidence of pulmonary aspiration was the same in both groups. It was also found that the grade of view was worse and the time to intubation was longer when cricoid pressure was used [22]. Nevertheless, the British Difficult Airway Society (DAS) has affirmed its recommendation to perform cricoid pressure during RSI to prevent gastric distention during mask ventilation [23]. Proof of mask ventilation following induction is not routinely obtained during RSI, and many providers agree that the additional application of cricoid pressure, especially when performed by a provider other than the one performing intubation or by someone who is unfamiliar with the technique (a minimum of 30N of pressure), in fact, skews the view of the laryngeal opening and makes the passage of an endotracheal tube, placement of an SGA, and even BMV more challenging. Current data analysis, therefore, suggests there is not enough evidence for the application of cricoid pressure as a guideline-imposed measure against preventing aspiration during intubation [24].

The use of cricoid pressure as a necessary part of RSI is declining. If used, immediate release is recommended if vision deteriorates during difficult laryngoscopy. If cricoid pressure is attempted, the British DAS guidelines similarly recommend early relief of cricoid pressure in cases of difficult laryngoscopy. However, the European Resuscitation Council, Scandinavian Clinical Practice Guidelines, and German Airway Management Guidelines do not routinely support the use of cricoid pressure in emergency and trauma intubations [25,26]. More recently, a trauma simulation study evaluated the use of new airway tools for traumatic airways, including channeled and nonchanneled video laryngoscopes, which allow for intubation without removal of the cervical collar. When performing RSI using cricoid pressure with the cervical collar in place, the video laryngoscope was faster and encouraged a shared mental model approach to resuscitation during simulation when compared to other techniques [27].

TRAUMATIC CARDIAC ARREST
Deferral of resuscitation
It is still up for discussion how long resuscitation should proceed in the case of an unobserved TCA. After observing 3 baboons with tamponade, bleeding, and traumatic-induced cardiac arrest in 1989, Luna and colleagues were the first to propose deferring chest compressions following prolonged traumatic arrest [28]. Improvements in blood pressure with chest compressions in normovolemic cardiac arrest were not replicated in hypovolemic cardiac arrest and diastolic blood pressure decreased even further, likely severely affecting coronary perfusion pressure [28]. The authors suggested that extended cardiopulmonary

resuscitation (CPR) is futile for thoracotomy patients in TCA who cannot be transported to a trauma hospital within a short timeframe. Advanced Trauma Life Support (ATLS) does not recommend initiation of CPR for patients in asystole in most cases. [3]. According to the American College of Surgeons Committee on Trauma, resuscitation should be deferred if there are no indications of life after a prolonged cardiac arrest with absence of organized electrical activity [29].

Survival from TCA with asystole has historically been dismal. Fewer than 2% of trauma patients are expected to survive a cardiac arrest during transit to the hospital. Studies looking back at the outcomes of patients with pulseless electrical activity (PEA) have shown very poor outcomes, particularly when the heart rate is less than 40 beats per minute [30]. Recent research suggests that resuscitation is unsuccessful in 80% of cases when an unwitnessed arrest is combined with advanced age (> 80 years) and PEA [30]. In a UK research study, a shockable initial rhythm and air ambulance availability were helpful, whereas advanced age, longer prehospital response time, and the use of epinephrine were associated with poor outcomes [31] (Box 1).

Treatment for TCA deviates from that for an acute coronary ischemic event because of the greater importance placed on the patient population, hemorrhage control, and obstructive shock prevention [3,32]. Despite their importance in a medical emergency, chest compressions can interfere with urgent therapeutic interventions in TCA including needle decompression, rapid transfusion, thoracotomy for cardiac tamponade, etc. Point-of-care ultrasonography (POCUS) has been widely adopted to assess cardiac contractility in TCA when patients arrive with PEA or pseudo-PEA but still exhibit some signs of life [33]. Early use of POCUS in TCA for its prognostic ability to determine those individuals where withdrawal of resuscitation might be considered has been shown to have a 100% sensitivity in some trials [33].

Until intravascular blood resuscitation has been initiated, it may be advisable to delay performing chest compressions in TCA depending on the severity of bleeding and the specific cause of TCA. Even though animal studies have shown that external chest compressions can produce 30% of cardiac output, this may not be the case in tamponade or severe hypovolemic conditions. It is more important to restore normal intravascular blood volume and remove any barrier to heart filling (eg, tamponade, tension pneumothorax) before beginning chest compressions. Animal studies on injured pigs have shown

---

Box 1: Favorable prognostic factors following traumatic arrest

1. Penetrating mechanism of injury, particularly thoracic
2. Vital signs at any time since first medical contact
3. Signs of life at any time since first medical contact for example, spontaneous movement, respiratory efforts, organized electrical activity, reactive pupils
4. The short duration of cardiac arrest (<10 minutes)
5. Cardiac contractility on point-of-care ultrasonography

that closed cardiac compressions lead to higher mortality rates than primary whole-blood resuscitation [34]. It has been shown that open cardiac massage has no additional benefits over closed cardiac chest compression in TCA; therefore, performing specific interventions targeting treatable causes of TCA may be advisable prior to initiation of chest compressions depending on the injuries [35].

However, in another study, patients who received prehospital external chest compressions after TCA had a 6% higher survival rate, according to the ROC Epistry-Trauma and PROPHET registries. Nonetheless, the distance to a level one trauma center remains the most significant risk factor affecting mortality, with times less than 15 minutes associated with improved outcome [36]. Predictive evidence at the bedside (signs of life and POCUS), delaying chest compressions when indicated, lung-protective breathing, relief of tamponade or obstructing pneumothorax, hemorrhage control, and balanced massive transfusion regimens are the cornerstones of TCA treatment. Further studies are necessary to evaluate the role and timing of chest compressors in TCA in the prehospital environment.

Role of epinephrine

Epinephrine, a directly acting sympathomimetic amine, is used in CPR to improve coronary and cerebral perfusion through alpha-mediated peripheral vasoconstriction, thereby potentially increasing blood supply and improving the chance of survival. There is controversy over whether or not epinephrine should be used in prehospital resuscitation. One meta-analysis, from 2014, found that patients who received epinephrine prior to hospital arrival had a 3-fold greater chance of achieving prehospital restoration of spontaneous circulation, but this had no appreciable effect on discharge survival [37,38]. It is, nevertheless, recommended by the ATLS curriculum to continue the use of epinephrine on patients who have suffered trauma or cardiac arrest (TCA). There has been no recorded rise in prehospital ROSC rates (OR: 4.67, 95% confidence interval [CI]: 0.50–32.50) when the patient has been found down for greater than 20 minutes [38].

TCA patients accounted for 1.5% of sampled patients in a large randomized study but the use of epinephrine was not associated with a greater 30-day survival rate [39]. Furthermore, Chiang and colleagues found that epinephrine delivery in the prehospital setting boosted short-term survival, particularly for patients with longer prehospital times, but was unrelated to 1-month survival [40]. Because of the lack of improvement in prehospital ROSC and the possible risks posed by vasoactive agents in hypovolemic TCA, the usage and benefit of epinephrine in this context should be evaluated in accordance with particular life-threatening conditions.

In 2017, it was established that vasopressors should be used when fluids and blood products are insufficient to maintain blood pressure [3,41]. In prehospital settings, the administration of epinephrine was related to an increased chance of ROSC but did not enhance short or long-term survival in instances of

TCA, according to the findings of another systematic review [41]. Therefore, it is recommended that epinephrine be used cautiously in cases of TCA and that the decision to administer the medication should be based on a comprehensive evaluation of the patient's condition and the cause of the cardiac arrest, as well as a consideration of the potential benefits and risks of epinephrine administration.

Resuscitative thoracotomy versus resuscitative endovascular balloon occlusion of the aorta

As a hemodynamic bridge to definitive hemorrhage control, aortic closure by clamp or balloon increases proximal cardiac and cerebral perfusion. Uncontrolled hemorrhagic shock from pelvic fractures and abdominal bleeding typically calls for resuscitative endovascular balloon occlusion of the aorta (REBOA), while resuscitative thoracotomy (RT) is performed on patients with TCA after approximately 10 minutes of prehospital CPR (Fig. 1) [42]. Although thoracotomy improves outcomes for penetrating trauma relative to blunt injury, the survival advantages of REBOA relative to RT in imminent cardiac arrest due to bleeding have not been well described. The recommended time frame for contemplating a thoracotomy rises from 10 minutes for blunt trauma to 15 minutes for penetrating injuries, as stated by the Western Trauma Association [43].

The inclusion of open cardiac massage following RT has not resulted in significant changes in end-tidal CO_2 or recovery of spontaneous circulation. With the development of REBOA, a thoracotomy is no longer required to perform cardiac massage since open cardiac massage may not offer extra benefits. The choice to perform REBOA or RT in cases of bleeding or cardiac arrest depends on the severity and suspected location of the injury. Chest trauma may be

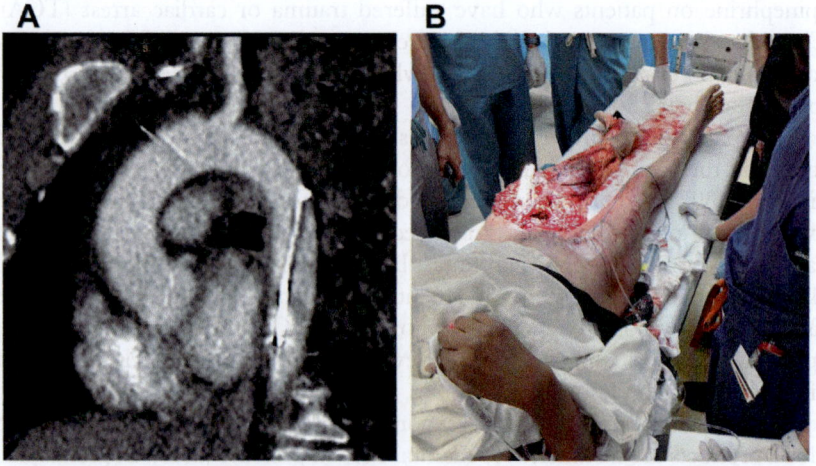

Fig. 1. (A) REBOA catheter visualized under CT scan. (B) REBOA catheter in situ.

associated with direct cardiac injury, tamponade, or hemo-pneumothorax that might benefit from open exploration, whereas REBOA might be the more suitable approach when trauma is solely below the diaphragm. According to the corrected results of the first meta-analysis, REBOA is more effective than RT (odds ratio [OR] 0.38; 95% CI 0.20–0.74) [44]. Amputations, hematomas, and pseudoaneurysms were among the adverse effects. REBOA has improved survival in severely wounded trauma patients in all trials where it has been compared to RT, although these findings may be biased since the research included only the most severely injured patients who were in cardiac arrest and underwent RT as a result.

In a recent systematic review, REBOA and RT were compared for their efficacy in treating noncompressible thoracic hemorrhage. The published meta-analysis comparing the 2 therapies revealed that REBOA reduced the risk of hospital mortality by 0.80 (95% CI 0.68–0.95) and enhanced overall survival compared to RT, although only observational studies were found. According to another meta-analysis, the relative risk was 0.81 [0.68–0.97] [45,46]. Despite the fact that RT may achieve aortic occlusion faster than REBOA, this does not always equate to improved outcomes. Although cardiac compressions during REBOA are slower than during open massage, they are less susceptible to interruption. It is likely that these persistent cardiac compressions contribute to improved outcomes after REBOA installation by aiding in the maintenance of cerebral perfusion in hypotensive patients. The fact that RT was performed in higher-risk patients in this review highlights the lack of specific indications for using REBOA in trauma patients.

TRAUMATIC BRAIN INJURY
Intracranial pressure monitoring

Patients who sustain TBI with associated intracranial hypertension (ICH) have been found to have a poor clinical prognosis. The principles of ICP monitoring include guiding therapies to limit or reduce ICH and to optimize cerebral perfusion pressure (CPP) (Table 1 for treatment strategies). Although invasive continuous ICP monitoring has been considered the standard of care for patients with severe TBI, there is conflicting evidence as to whether it is associated with improved outcomes [47]. In the largest retrospective study to date investigating ICP monitoring for severe TBI, data obtained from the American College of Surgeons Trauma Quality Improvement Program (TQIP) from 2009 to 2011 demonstrated that there is a strong correlation between the use of ICP monitoring with reduced in-hospital mortality [47]. Based on multiple observational studies, invasive ICP monitoring can be used as a guide in the "staircase approach" to escalating treatment for TBI management shown in Table 1, with aggressive therapy reserved for refractory ICH [48].

Reduced in-hospital and 2-week post-injury mortality may be achieved with ICP monitoring, as recommended by the Brain Trauma Foundation [49]. Previously it was recommended to strive for an ICP of less than 20 mm Hg and a

Table 1
Treatment strategies

Categories	Interventions
Supportive care & measures to avoid secondary brain injury	• Standard trauma care • Hemorrhage control • Adequate resuscitation and administration of blood products • Elevation of the head of bed • Analgesics/sedatives • Fluid and electrolyte management • Avoidance of hyponatremia • Prevention of hyperpyrexia • Treatment of hyper/hypoglycemia • Supplemental oxygen to maintain oxygen saturation >90% and Po_2 >60 mm Hg. • Normocarbic ventilation (Pco_2 35–40 mm Hg) • Correction of coagulopathy • Early delivery of nutrition (preferentially enteral) • Treatment of infections
Tier 1	• Additional analgesia/sedation • Cerebrospinal fluid drainage
Tier 2	• Hyperosmolar therapy • Neuromuscular paralysis
Tier 3	• High-dose barbiturates • High-dose propofol
Rescue strategies	• Decompressive craniectomy • Experimental therapies

From Alam HB, Vercruysse G, Martin M, et al. Western Trauma Association critical decisions in trauma: Management of intracranial hypertension in patients with severe traumatic brain injuries. J Trauma Acute Care Surg. 2020;88(2):345-351.

CPP of 50 to 70 mm Hg in all potentially reversible patients with severe TBI and an abnormal computed tomography (CT) scan [50]. Although an ICP or CPP-based strategy should be established individually in combination with an examination of whether cerebral autoregulation is maintained, there is presently no level 1 evidence to support specific ICP or CPP target objectives using therapeutic interventions [50].

Although the role of intraoperative ICP monitoring has been shown to facilitate early and aggressive interventions for ICH and serve as an early prognostic indicator, more studies are required to determine the optimal ICP and CPP thresholds for the treatment of patient with severe TBI [51]. The application of continuous ICP monitoring in the perioperative setting may be considered on a case-by-case basis. The use of ICP monitoring varies across clinical sites but should be strongly considered as it may be associated with reduced 6-month mortality in patients with severe TBI [52].

Use of hyperosmolar agents

Although hyperosmolar agents play a role in lowering ICP, there is insufficient evidence to support a specific recommendation or use of a specific agent for patients with severe TBI as the effects on clinical outcomes are inconclusive [53]. Although mannitol at doses of 0.25 g/kg to 1 g/kg has been considered the gold standard and shown to be effective in significantly reducing ICP, it is associated with clinically important adverse effects including renal failure, worsening cerebral edema, hypotension, heart failure, and hypovolemia which may impact resuscitation in patients with TBI [54]. A systematic review revealed that when comparing mannitol to other ICP-lowering agents, treatment with mannitol may have improved mortality rates compared to that with phenobarbital but had worse mortality rates compared to hypertonic saline [55].

Boone and Shi suggested that currently, clinicians have increased the use of hypertonic saline to improve ICP among patients as it is not only effective but also does not compromise hemodynamics [56,57]. Hypertonic saline works by increasing the oxygenation and blood flow of the cerebral vasculature [56–58]. It was found through a recent meta-analysis that even though hypertonic saline is associated with better outcomes, reduced ICP, decreased mortality rate, and higher CPP values after 30 to 60 minutes of infusion termination, it also showed minimal impact on pressure variables 90 to 120 minutes after termination of infusion. Similarly, it did not show any impact on higher levels of ICP after a day of use [59].

When it comes to the appropriate concentration of hypertonic saline, a range between 3% and 23.4% is suggested for the treatment of increased ICP. However, it is suggested in a systematic review that with therapeutic bolus ranging between 1.4 and 2.5 mL/kg, a 3% concentration is optimal for the improvement of CPP and ICP [60,61]. Multicenter RCTs are necessary for determining standardized guidelines and optimal hyperosmolar therapy for traumatic head injury cases.

Blood transfusion goals

Individuals in critical condition with TBI and anemia are at an increased risk for secondary brain injury as a result of cerebral tissue hypoxia. There is a high probability that blood transfusion complications will increase the risk of both mortality and morbidity. Red blood cell transfusion has been found to have a detrimental effect on mortality, functional outcomes, intensive care unit (ICU) duration of stay, and brain autoregulation [62]. Although there is a strong recommendation for a hemoglobin (Hg) transfusion threshold below 7 g/dL in some critically ill trauma patients, there is inadequate evidence to support this guideline in patients with TBI (see Table 1) [63].

A more liberal transfusion strategy, using a Hg trigger of 10 g/dL, was associated with an elevated risk of developing cerebral hemorrhage and thromboembolic events compared to a more restrictive transfusion method [64]. Because of the small number of research studies investigating the influence of red blood cell transfusion on outcomes for patients with TBI, the recommendations for administering blood transfusions are variable. The American Society of Anesthesiologists recommends limiting the number of transfusions to prevent negative neurologic and cardiovascular consequences when a patient's hemoglobin level is higher than 8 g/dL and their hematocrit is greater than 25% [65].

Most emergency medicine and intensive care subspecialties agree that a restrictive transfusion strategy with a Hg target of 7 to 9 g/dL is the optimal treatment (Table 2) [66,67]. Instead of assessing whether a patient needs a blood transfusion based on a Hg trigger, clinicians should consider the patient's intravascular volume status, cardiopulmonary comorbidities, and trend in Hg levels. A comprehensive evaluation of the patient's state and the underlying

Table 2
Transfusion strategies in traumatic brain injury

	Transfusion Thresholds	Neurotrauma Specific Transfusion Strategies for TBI
American Association of Blood Banks (AABB) 2016	Hg ≤ 7 g/dL for hemodynamically stable hospitalized patients Hg ≤ 8 g/dL for orthopedic, cardiac patients	7–10 g/dL for hemodynamically stable patients, 8 g/dL for orthopedic trauma and cardiovascular disease
American Red Cross 2017	Hg ≤ 7 g/dL for critically ill trauma patients	Maintain Hg > 7 g/dL for patients with hemorrhagic shock or on mechanical ventilation
American Society of Anesthesiologists	Hg ≤ 6 g/dL Restrictive strategy Hg 6–10 g/dL	Recommend massive transfusion protocol with higher ratios of plasma and platelets to packed red blood cells
Brain Trauma Foundation 2017	No recommendation	No recommendations
British Committee of Standards in Haematology 2012	Restrictive strategy Hg 7–9 g/dL	Maintain Hg > 9 g/dL in patients with evidence of cerebral ischemia or TBI Maintain Hg 8–9 g/dL in patients with subarachnoid hemorrhage
Eastern Association for the Surgery of Trauma	No recommendation	Consider transfusion threshold > 7 g/dL
Task Force for Advanced Bleeding Care in Trauma (European guidelines)	Restrictive strategy Hg 7–9 g/dL	Limit crystalloids; maintain mean arterial pressure (MAP) >80
Western Trauma Association Critical Decisions in Trauma	No recommendation	No recommendation

cause of the bleeding or cardiac arrest is necessary when considering restrictive transfusion in the management of TCA. It may be essential to employ more restrictive transfusion techniques to achieve hemostasis and restore perfusion in some patients; however, this must be evaluated against the risks of inadequate oxygen supply and tissue hypoxia. The conservative approach to improve patient outcomes in TCA is to involve specialists in trauma care, transfusion medicine, and intensive care in a multidisciplinary effort. Given the paucity of studies assessing the effects of red blood cell transfusion on outcomes in patients with TBI and suffering from TCA, there remains a wide variability in transfusion guidelines.

Role of therapeutic hypothermia

Early investigations of a few extraordinary recoveries highlighted the potential benefits of hypothermia in avoiding subsequent brain injury [68]. By artificially decreasing a patient's body temperature quickly after an injury, early prophylactic hypothermia can aid in reducing inflammation, tissue damage, and subsequent brain impairment in injured individuals. Animal models have revealed that hypothermia slows cellular metabolism and reduces the damage produced by ischemia. The efficacy of this method in the treatment of trauma victims is still under discussion, despite its widespread use.

Clinical studies exploring the use of early preventative hypothermia in trauma patients have produced contradictory results. Initially, it was believed that prophylactic hypothermia would enhance long-term neurologic outcomes by reducing the brain's metabolic rate, blood flow, inflammatory mediators, and biochemical processes [69,70]. Recent research indicates that prophylactic hypothermia has no discernible effect on ICH and does not enhance neurologic outcomes at 6 months in patients with severe TBI [71,72]. According to the most recent guidelines from the Brain Trauma Foundation, preventive hypothermia during early (within 2.5 hours) and short-term (within 48 hours) therapy for patients with diffuse brain injury is not recommended to improve outcomes [49]. Those hospitalized with TBI and unintentional hypothermia had a considerably greater likelihood of death during their hospital stay [73].

Systematic trials on the use of therapeutic hypothermia at targeted temperatures (32°C–33°C) and for longer durations (at least 24–48 hours) have proven a reduction in mortality and a decrease in the chance of adverse neurologic outcomes when the treatment is delivered [74,75]. Those with moderate to severe brain damage may benefit from therapeutic hypothermia as a potential treatment for traumatic brain injury. In a 2014 RCT published in the *New England Journal of Medicine*, it was discovered that early preventative hypothermia improved mortality and functional results in patients with TBI. However, there is insufficient data to support therapeutic hypothermia for broad usage and these beneficial results may only apply to a minority of individuals [76].

According to a large-scale study, therapeutic hypothermia did not reduce the risk of death from TBI although a smaller study suggested that certain patients may have benefited more from therapeutic management than its preventative

use [77]. The utility of therapeutic hypothermia in TBI continues to be controversial, as are the optimal temperature range, timing, and duration of therapy.
Some studies indicate that therapeutic hypothermia increases the chance of
complications such as pneumonia, coagulopathy, and electrolyte abnormalities.
More research is necessary to determine the optimal patient selection criteria,
timing, and duration of therapy to reduce the possibility of secondary brain
damage [78].

Decompressive craniectomy

The Brain Trauma Foundation currently recommends ICP monitoring for patients with TBI with a Glasgow Coma Scale (GCS) score of 9, despite the fact
that many patients with TBI did not have DC prior to having their ICP
measured. In numerous randomized controlled trials including patients with
TBI, DC has been compared to standard medical treatment [79]. It was

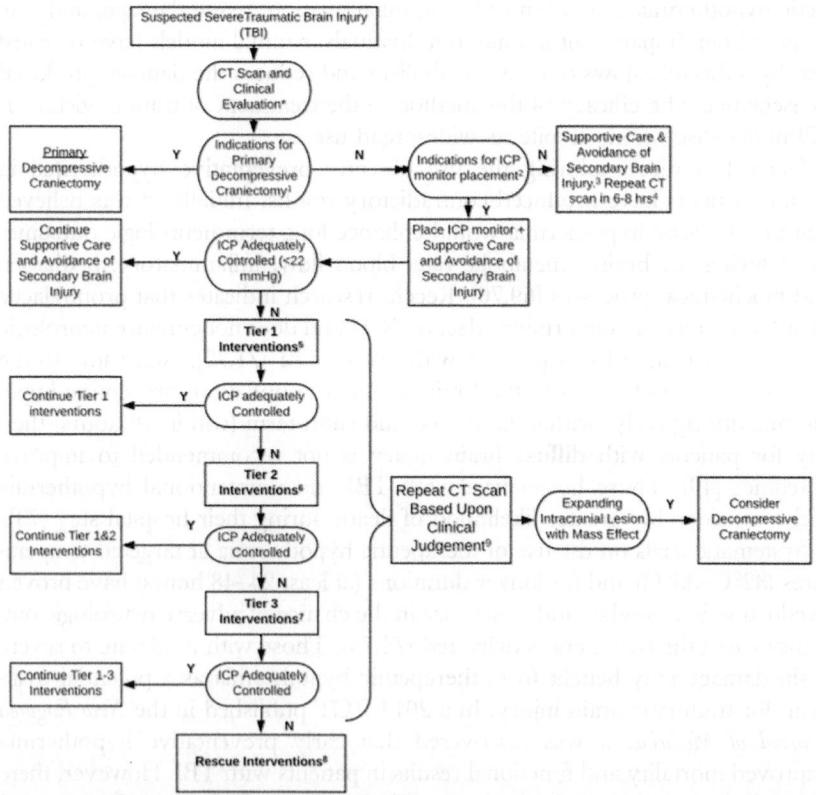

Fig. 2. An algorithm for the management of increased ICP in patients with severe TBI. (*From*
Alam HB, Vercruysse G, Martin M, et al. Western Trauma Association critical decisions in
trauma: Management of intracranial hypertension in patients with severe traumatic brain injuries. J Trauma Acute Care Surg. 2020;88(2):345-351.)

discovered that patients with axonal injury or extensive TBI had a decreased probability of acquiring dementia than those with more limited lesions. Many studies have been conducted on the utility of DC for those who have suffered significant traumatic head injuries and difficulty managing intracranial bleeding. DC has been shown to significantly lower ICP and increase CPP in the first 24 hours after damage, 48 hours after damage, and immediately after surgery [80].

According to the DECRA trial which looked at the effectiveness of DC within 72 hours of the injury for mild to severe refractory ICH in patients with diffuse TBI, early DC lowered ICP and length of ICU stay but was associated with increased adverse outcomes [81,82]. Medically intervened patients fared better than those who underwent early bifrontal DC on the Extended Glasgow Outcome Scale (GOS-E) 6 months after treatment.

In the more current RESCUEicp trial, patients with TBI with refractory ICH (ICP>25 mm Hg) were randomly assigned to undergo DC as the last-resort treatment or to continue medication therapy. DC was associated with decreased death, increased rates of vegetative state, and adverse disability outcomes based on GOS-E scores at 6 months [83]. Despite the numerous inconsistencies between the studies, the results of both indicate that DC, either unilaterally or bilaterally, as a form of salvage therapy for individuals with severe ICH who have not responded to other treatments, results in significantly lower mortality rates but an increase in the impairments caused by the condition (Fig. 2) [84]. In contrast to other multicenter cohort studies undertaken in Europe, the United Kingdom, and Australia, the findings of this study are contradictory [85]. In the most recent Brain Trauma Foundation treatment guidelines, these findings have bolstered the rationale for secondary DC.

SUMMARY

Various unsettled approaches to practice exist due to the absence of standardization in trauma anesthesia care. To clarify best practices and optimize patient outcomes, these topics require continuing research and discussion. Management of hemodynamic instability in trauma patients using vasoactive medications requires further review. The same holds true with intubation and the management of patients with TBI. Although intubation via rapid sequence is a frequent practice, the benefits of cricoid pressure or low-pressure ventilation BMV are not conclusive. When it comes to intubation for trauma patients, the creation of evidence-based guidelines is crucial for improving patient outcomes. Recent evidence suggests a moderately conservative transfusion strategy, specific indications for therapeutic hypothermia, and selective use of decompressive craniectomy may be beneficial in the management of acute TBI cases.

DISCLOSURE

The authors have nothing to disclose.

References

[1] Kauvar DS, Lefering R, Wade CE. Impact of haemorrhage on trauma outcome: an overview of epidemiology, clinical presentations, and therapeutic considerations. J Trauma 2006;60(6):S3–11.

[2] Committee on Trauma American College of Surgeons. Collaborative clinical services. In: Resources for optimal care of the injured patient. Chicago: American College of Surgeons; 2014. p. 76–87.

[3] Subcommittee TLS, American College of Surgeons Committee on Trauma. J Trauma Acute Care Surg 2018;108–16.

[4] Olasveengen TM, Mancini ME, Perkins GD, et al. Adult basic life support. Resuscitation 2020;156–64.

[5] Zhao KL, Herrenkohl M, Paulsen M, et al. Trauma Surg Acute Care Open 2019;1:4-10.

[6] Carney N, Totten AM, Cheney T, et al. Prehospital Airway Management: A systematic review. Prehosp Emerg Care 2021;26(5):716–27.

[7] Jabre P, Penaloza A, Pinero D, et al. Effect of bag-mask ventilation vs endotracheal intubation during cardiopulmonary resuscitation on neurological outcome after out-of-hospital cardiorespiratory arrest. JAMA 2018;319(8):779.

[8] Bell S, Pennington E, Hill J, et al. Prehospital Airway Management. J Paramedic Pract 2022;14(2):51–3.

[9] Gleason JM, Christian BR, Barton ED. Nasal Cannula Apneic Oxygenation Prevents Desaturation During Endotracheal Intubation: An Integrative Literature Review. West J Emerg Med 2018;19(2):403–11.

[10] Trivedi DJ, Bass GA, Forssten MP, et al. The significance of direct transportation to a trauma center on survival for severe traumatic brain injury. Eur J Trauma Emerg Surg 2022;48(4): 2803–11.

[11] Hristovska A-M, Duch P, Allingstrup M, et al. Efficacy and safety of sugammadex versus neostigmine in reversing neuromuscular blockade in adults. Cochrane Database Syst Rev 2017;9:1–10.

[12] Tran DTT, Newton EK, Mount VAH, et al. Rocuronium versus succinylcholine for rapid sequence induction intubation. Cochrane Database Syst Rev 2015;(10):1–8.

[13] Wahlen BM, El-Menyar A, Asim M, et al. Rapid sequence induction (RSI) in trauma patients: Insights from healthcare providers. World J Emerg Med 2019;10(1):19–26.

[14] Curley JM, Ciceri DP, Culp WC. Sugammadex administration to facilitate timely neurologic examination in the traumatic brain injury patient. Neurocritical Care 2020;32(3):880–2.

[15] Clancy M. In patients with head injuries who undergo rapid sequence intubation using succinylcholine, does pretreatment with a competitive neuromuscular blocking agent improve outcome? A literature review. Emerg Med J 2001;18(5):373–5.

[16] Lanier WL, Milde JH, Michenfelder JD. Cerebral stimulation following succinylcholine in dogs. Anesthesiology 1986;64(5):551–9.

[17] Cottrell JE. Succinylcholine and intracranial pressure. Anesthesiology 2018;129(6): 1159–62.

[18] Patanwala AE, Erstad BL, Roe DJ, et al. Succinylcholine is associated with increased mortality when used for rapid sequence intubation of severely brain injured patients in the emergency department. Pharmacotherapy 2016;36(1):57–63.

[19] Sellick BA. Cricoid pressure to control regurgitation of stomach contents during induction of Anæsthesia. Lancet 1961;278(7199):404–6.

[20] Andruszkiewicz P, Zawadka M, Kosińska A, et al. Measurement of cricoid pressure force during simulated Sellick's manoeuvre. Anaesthesiol Intensive Ther 2017;49(4):283–7.

[21] Landsman I. Cricoid pressure: indications and complications. Paediatr Anaesth 2004;14(1):43–7.

[22] Birenbaum A, Hajage D, Roche S, et al. IRIS Investigators Group. Effect of Cricoid Pressure Compared With a Sham Procedure in the Rapid Sequence Induction of Anesthesia: The IRIS Randomized Clinical Trial. JAMA Surg 2019;154(1):9–17.

[23] Frerk C, Mitchell VS, McNarry AF, et al. Difficult airway society 2015 guidelines for management of unanticipated difficult intubation in adults. Br J Anaesth 2015;115(6):827–48.

[24] Zdravkovic M, Rice MJ, Brull SJ. The clinical use of cricoid pressure: First, do no harm. Anesth Analg 2019;132(1):261–7.

[25] Soar J, Nolan JP, Bottiger BW, et al. European resuscitation council guidelines for resuscitation 2015: section 3. Adult advanced life support. Resuscitation 2015;95:100–47.

[26] Piepho T, Cavus E, Noppens R, et al. S1 guidelines on airway management: a guideline of the German society of anesthesiology and intensive care medicine. Anaesthesist 2015;64(1):27–40.

[27] Maremanda KR, Jayaram K, Durga P. Comparison of intubation conditions between Airtraq, McGrath video laryngoscopes, and Macintosh under conditions of simulated trauma airway and rapid sequence induction intubation. The Journal of Emergency Medicine. J Emerg Med 2023;S0736-4679(22):797–801.

[28] Luna GK, Pavlin EG, Kirkman T, et al. Hemodynamic effects of external cardiac massage in trauma shock. J Trauma 1989;29(10):1430–3.

[29] Millin MG, Galvagno SM, Khandker SR, et al. Withholding and termination of resuscitation of adult cardiopulmonary arrest secondary to trauma: resource document to the joint NAEMSP-ACSCOT position statements. J Trauma Acute Care Surg 2013;75(3):459–67.

[30] Glober NK, Tainter CR, Abramson TM, et al. A simple decision rule predicts futile resuscitation of out-of-hospital cardiac arrest. Resuscitation 2019;142:8–13.

[31] Barnard EB, Sandbach DD, Nicholls TL, et al. Prehospital determinants of successful resuscitation after traumatic and non-traumatic out-of-hospital cardiac arrest. Emerg Med J 2019;36(6):333–9.

[32] Ohlén D, Hedberg M, Martinsson P, et al. Characteristics and outcome of traumatic cardiac arrest at a level 1 trauma centre over 10 years in Sweden. Scand J Trauma Resusc Emerg Med 2022;30(1):54–7.

[33] Lalande E, Burwash-Brennan T, Burns K, et al. Is point-of-care ultrasound a reliable predictor of outcome during traumatic cardiac arrest? A systematic review and meta-analysis from the SHoC investigators. Resuscitation 2021;167:128–36.

[34] Watts S, Smith JE, Gwyther R, et al. Closed chest compressions reduce survival in an animal model of haemorrhage-induced traumatic cardiac arrest. Resuscitation 2019;140:37–42.

[35] Bradley MJ, Bonds BW, Chang L, et al. Open chest cardiac massage offers no benefit over closed chest compressions in patients with traumatic cardiac arrest. J Trauma Acute Care Surg 2016;81(5):849–54.

[36] Evans CC, Petersen A, Meier EN, et al. Resuscitation Outcomes Consortium Investigators. Prehospital traumatic cardiac arrest: Management and outcomes from the resuscitation outcomes consortium registry-trauma and PROPHET registries. J Trauma Acute Care Surg 2016;81(2):285–93.

[37] Atiksawedparit P, Rattanasiri S, McEvoy M, et al. Effects of prehospital adrenaline administration on out-of-hospital cardiac arrest outcomes: a systematic review and meta-analysis. Crit Care 2014;18(4):463–9.

[38] Wongtanasarasin W, Thepchinda T, Kasirawat C, et al. Treatment Outcomes of Epinephrine for Traumatic Out-of-hospital Cardiac Arrest: A Systematic Review and Meta-analysis. J Emerg Trauma Shock 2021;14(4):195–200.

[39] Perkins GD, Ji C, Deakin CD, et al. A randomized trial of epinephrine in out-of-hospital cardiac arrest. N Engl J Med 2018;379:711–21.

[40] Aoki M, Abe T, Oshima K. Association of prehospital epinephrine administration with survival among patients with traumatic cardiac arrest caused by traffic collisions. Sci Rep 2019;9:1–7.

[41] Gupta B, Garg N, Ramachandran R. Vasopressors: Do they have any role in hemorrhagic shock? J Anaesthesiol Clin Pharmacol 2017;33(1):3–8.

[42] Seamon MJ, Haut ER, Van Arendonk K, et al. An evidence-based approach to patient selection for emergency department thoracotomy: A practice management guideline from the

Eastern Association for the Surgery of Trauma. J Trauma Acute Care Surg 2015;79(1): 159–73.

[43] Burlew C, Cothren EE, Moore D, et al. Western Trauma Association critical decisions in trauma: resuscitative thoracotomy. J Trauma Acute Care Surg 2012;73(6):1359–63.

[44] Castellini G, Gianola S, Biffi A, et al. Italian National Institute of Health guideline working group on Major Trauma. Resuscitative endovascular balloon occlusion of the aorta (REBOA) in patients with major trauma and uncontrolled haemorrhagic shock: a systematic review with meta-analysis. World J Emerg Surg 2021;16(1):41.

[45] Manzano NR, Naranjo MP, Foianini E, et al. A meta-analysis of resuscitative endovascular balloon occlusion of the aorta (REBOA) or open aortic cross-clamping by resuscitative thoracotomy in non-compressible torso hemorrhage patients. World J Emerg Surg 2017;14(12):30–5.

[46] Khalid S, Khatri M, Siddiqui MS, et al. Resuscitative Endovascular Balloon Occlusion of Aorta Versus Aortic Cross-Clamping by Thoracotomy for Noncompressible Torso Hemorrhage: A Meta-Analysis. J Surg Res 2022;270:252–60.

[47] Alali AS, Fowler RA, Mainprize TG, et al. Intracranial pressure monitoring in severe traumatic brain injury: results from the American College of Surgeons Trauma Quality Improvement Program. J Neurotrauma 2013;30(20):1737–46.

[48] Anania P, Battaglini D, Miller JP, et al. Escalation therapy in severe traumatic brain injury: how long is intracranial pressure monitoring necessary? Neurosurg Rev 2021;44: 2415–23.

[49] Carney N, Totten AM, O'Reilly C, et al. Brain Trauma Foundation. Guidelines for the management of severe traumatic brain injury, fourth edition. Neurosurg 2016;1:1–10.

[50] Hawthorne C, Piper I. Monitoring of intracranial pressure in patients with traumatic brain injury. Front Neurol 2014;5:121.

[51] Tsai TH, Huang TY, Kung SS, et al. Intraoperative intracranial pressure and cerebral perfusion pressure for predicting surgical outcome in severe brain traumatic injury. Kaohsiung J Med Sciences 2013;29(10):540–6.

[52] Robba C, Graziano F, Rebora P, et al. Intracranial pressure monitoring in patients with acute brain injury in the intensive care unit (SYNAPSE-ICU): an international, prospective observational cohort study. Lancet Neurol 2021;20(7):548–58.

[53] Gu J, Huang H, Huang Y, et al. Hypertonic saline or mannitol for treating elevated intracranial pressure in traumatic brain injury: a meta-analysis of randomized controlled trials. Neurosurg Rev 2019;42(2):499–509.

[54] Tenny S, Patel R, Thorell W. Mannitol. In: StatPearls Internet. Treasure Island: StatPearls Publishing. Updated 2022. Available at: https://www.ncbi.nlm.nih.gov/books/ NBK470392. Accessed on Feb 4, 2023.

[55] Wakai A, McCabe A, Roberts I, et al. Mannitol for acute traumatic brain injury. Cochrane Database Syst Rev 2013;8:1–8.

[56] Boone MD, Oren-Grinberg A, Robinson TM, et al. Mannitol or hypertonic saline in the setting of traumatic brain injury: What have we learned? Surg Neurol Int 2015;6:177.

[57] Shi J, Tan L, Ye J, et al. Hypertonic saline and mannitol in patients with traumatic brain injury: a systematic and meta-analysis. Medicine 2020;99(35):1–10.

[58] Shackford SR, Zhuang J, Schmoker J. Intravenous fluid tonicity: effect on intracranial pressure, cerebral blood flow, and cerebral oxygen delivery in focal brain injury. J Neurosurg 1992;76(1):91–8.

[59] Han C, Yang F, Guo S, et al. Hypertonic saline compared to mannitol for the management of elevated intracranial pressure in traumatic brain injury: a meta-analysis. Front Surg 2022;8: 765–84.

[60] Susanto M, Riantri I. Optimal dose and concentration of hypertonic saline in traumatic brain injury: a systematic review. Medeni Med J 2022;37(2):203–11.

[61] Kochanek PM, Adelson PD, Rosario BL, et al. Comparison of intracranial pressure measurements before and after hypertonic saline or mannitol treatment in children with severe traumatic brain injury. JAMA Netw Open 2022;5(3):1–12.

[62] Salim A, Hadjizacharia P, DuBose J, et al. Role of anemia in traumatic brain injury. J Am Coll Surg 2008;207(3):398–406.

[63] East JM, Viau-Lapointe J, McCredie VA. Transfusion practices in traumatic brain injury. Curr Opin Anaesthesiol 2018;31(2):219–26.

[64] Vedantam A, Yamal JM, Rubin ML, et al. Progressive hemorrhagic injury after severe traumatic brain injury: effect of hemoglobin transfusion thresholds. J Neurosurg 2016;125(5):1229–34.

[65] Practice Guidelines for Perioperative Blood Management: an updated report by the American Society of Anesthesiologists Task Force on Perioperative Blood Management. Anesthesiology 2015;122:241–75.

[66] Napolitano LM, Kurek S, Luchett FA, et al. American College of Critical Care Medicine of the Society of Critical Care Medicine the Eastern Association for the Surgery of Trauma Practice Management Workgroup. Clinical practice guideline: Red blood cell transfusion in adult trauma and critical care. Crit Care Med 2009;37(12):3124–57.

[67] Hebert P, Wells G, Blajchman M, et al. A multicenter, randomized, controlled clinical trial of transfusion requirements in critical care. N Eng J Med 1999;340(6):409–17.

[68] Gilbert M, Busund R, Skagseth A, et al. Resuscitation from accidental hypothermia of 13.7 degrees C with circulatory arrest. Lancet 2000;355:375–6.

[69] Marion DW, Penrod LE, Kelsey SF, et al. Treatment of traumatic brain injury with moderate hypothermia. N Engl J Med 1997;336(8):540–6.

[70] Crossley S, Reid J, McLatchie R, et al. A systematic review of therapeutic hypothermia for adult patients following traumatic brain injury. Crit Care 2014;18(2):R75.

[71] Cooper DJ, Nichol AD, Bailey M, et al. Effect of early sustained prophylactic hypothermia on neurologic outcomes among patients with severe traumatic brain injury: The POLAR Randomized Clinical Trial. JAMA 2018;320(21):2211–20.

[72] Kim J, Lee SH, Hur JW, et al. Current prophylactic hypothermia for intracranial hypertension after traumatic brain injury. J Neurointensive Care 2020;3(2):29–32.

[73] Rösli D, Schnüriger B, Candinas D, et al. The impact of accidental hypothermia on mortality in trauma patients overall and patients with traumatic brain injury specifically: s systematic review and meta-analysis. World J Surg 2020;44:4106–17.

[74] McIntyre LA, Fergusson DA, Hébert PC, et al. Prolonged therapeutic hypothermia after traumatic brain injury in adults: a systematic review. JAMA 2003;289(22):2992–9.

[75] Fox JL, Vu EN, Doyle-Waters M, et al. Prophylactic hypothermia for traumatic brain injury: a quantitative systematic review. Can J Emerg Med 2010;12(4):355–64.

[76] Shaefi S, Mittel AM, Hyam JA, et al. Hypothermia for severe traumatic brain injury in adults: Recent lessons from randomized controlled trials. Surg Neurol Int 2016;28(7):103.

[77] Chen H, Wu F, Yang P, et al. A meta-analysis of the effects of therapeutic hypothermia in adult patients with traumatic brain injury. Crit Care 2019;23:396.

[78] Dietrich WD, Bramlett HM. Therapeutic hypothermia and targeted temperature management in traumatic brain injury: clinical challenges for successful translation. Brain Res 2016;1640:94–103.

[79] Kolias AG, Adams H, Timofeev I, et al. Decompressive craniectomy following traumatic brain injury: developing the evidence base. Br J Neurosurg 2016;30(2):246–50.

[80] Bor-Seng-Shu E, Figueiredo EG, Amorim RL, et al. Decompressive craniectomy: a meta-analysis of influences on intracranial pressure and cerebral perfusion pressure in the treatment of traumatic brain injury. J Neurosurg 2012;117(3):589–96.

[81] Jo K, Joo WI, Yoo DS, et al. Clinical Significance of Decompressive Craniectomy Surface Area and Side. J Korean Neurosurg Soc 2021;64(2):261–70.

[82] Cooper DJ, Rosenfeld JV, Murray L, et al. Decompressive craniectomy in diffuse traumatic brain injury. N Engl J Med 2011;364(16):1493–502.

[83] Hutchinson PJ, Kolias AG, Timofeev IS, et al. Trial of Decompressive Craniectomy for Traumatic Intracranial Hypertension. N Engl J Med 2016;375(12):1119–30.

[84] Gantner D, Wiegers E, Bragge P, et al. Decompressive craniectomy practice following traumatic brain injury in comparison with randomized trials: harmonized, multi-center cohort studies in Europe, the United Kingdom, and Australia. J Neurotrauma 2022;39(12): 860–9.

[85] Alam HB, Vercruysse G, Martin M, et al. Western Trauma Association Critical Decisions in Trauma Committee: Management of intracranial hypertension in patients with severe traumatic brain injuries. J Trauma Acute Care Surg 2020;88(2):345–51.

Advances in Anesthesia 41 (2023) 163–178

ADVANCES IN ANESTHESIA

Perioperative Concerns in the Patient with History of Alcohol Use

Ivet T. Cordoba Torres, MD[a], Eslam A. Fouda, MD[a],
Myrna Eliann Reinhardt, MD[b], Fouad G. Souki, MD, MS[a],*

[a]Department of Anesthesia, Jackson Memorial Hospital, University of Miami, 1611 Northwest 12th Avenue, DTC 318, Miami, FL, 33136, USA; [b]Albany Medical College, 43 New Scotland Avenue, Albany, NY 12208, USA

Keywords
• Anesthesia • Alcohol use disorder • Heavy alcohol use • Risky alcohol use
• Chronic alcohol use • Perioperative • Perianesthetic

Key points
- Alcohol use is prevalent in society and in patients presenting for surgery.
- Alcohol use is associated with significant multisystem effects leading to increased postoperative complications.
- Anesthesiologists should be aware of the physiologic changes and potential complications associated with alcohol consumption and formulate a suitable anesthetic plan.

INTRODUCTION

Alcohol is widely consumed in the United States, with 85% of adults having tried it in their lifetime and 70% having consumed it in the past year. According to the 2021 National Survey on Drug Use and Health, 1 in 5 adults reported binge drinking and 1 in 15 reported heavy drinking in the past month, whereas 1 in 9 had alcohol use disorder (AUD) in the past year [1].

Excessive alcohol use has been linked to a range of health conditions and is responsible for a significant number of deaths and disabilities globally. The World Health Organization attributes 5% of all global annual deaths to alcohol. In the United States, alcohol-related causes account for more than 140,000 deaths annually, making it the fourth leading preventable cause of death

*Corresponding author. E-mail address: fsouki@med.miami.edu

https://doi.org/10.1016/j.aan.2023.06.004
0737-6146/23/© 2023 Elsevier Inc. All rights reserved.

behind tobacco, poor diet, and physical inactivity [2,3]. Among hospitalized and surgical patients, alcohol use is prevalent, with 8% to 88% of surgical patients having alcohol-related conditions depending on the surgical subspecialty (bariatric, vascular, thoracic, otolaryngology) [4–8]. A history of alcohol use is associated with a 2 to 4 times higher risk of postoperative complications, including pneumonia, wound infections, delirium, acute renal failure, blood transfusion, liver complications, cerebrovascular accidents, myocardial infarctions, deep venous thrombosis, prolonged hospital stay, readmission to hospital, admission to the intensive care unit (ICU), and death [9–11].

Given the prevalence of alcohol use, related diseases, and associated morbidity and mortality in surgical patients, it is crucial that anesthesiologists identify and understand the management of these patients. Here, the authors review the perioperative concerns and management of the patient with history of alcohol use.

DEFINITIONS AND CATEGORIES OF ALCOHOL USE

Alcohol consumption has various definitions and categories, including the Diagnostic and Statistical Manual of Mental Disorders, Fifth Edition classification of AUD, which replaces the terms alcohol abuse and alcohol dependence (Table 1) [12,13]. AUD is characterized by a problematic pattern of alcohol use that leads to impairment or distress and is diagnosed based on the presence of 2 out of 11 symptoms during the same 12-month period [14].

PHYSIOLOGIC CHANGES RELATED TO ALCOHOL USE

Because of the high prevalence of alcohol-related diseases, anesthesiologists often encounter patients with chronic effects of alcohol on various organ

Table 1
Definitions and categories of alcohol consumption

Sensible alcohol consumption	Per day limited to 2 drinks or less for men and 1 drink or less for women[a]
Binge drinking	≥ 5 drinks for men or ≥ 4 drinks for women within 2 h
	Leads to a blood alcohol concentration ≥ 0.08%
Heavy drinking	> 4 drinks on any day or > 14 drinks per week for men
	> 3 drinks on any day or > 7 drinks per week for women
Risky alcohol use	Includes binge drinking, heavy drinking, or any use by pregnant women or those younger than 21 years
Alcohol use disorder	Having 2 out of 11 criteria defined by the DSM-V
Unhealthy drinking/Alcohol misuse	Binge drinking, risky alcohol use, heavy alcohol use, or alcohol use disorder

[a] In the United States a standard drink contains approximately 14 g of alcohol.
Abbreviation: DSM-V, Diagnostic and Statistical Manual of Mental Disorders, Fifth Edition.

systems (Fig. 1). Unhealthy alcohol use can lead to numerous comorbidities varying in severity and frequency. Hospitalized patients with AUD were found to have alcohol-related diagnosis in 33.6% of mild, 70.9% of moderate, and 97.8% of severe cases [5].

Cardiovascular system

There is a complex association between alcohol consumption and cardiovascular conditions [15]. Unhealthy alcohol users have up to 5 times more cardiac complications in the postoperative period compared with nondrinkers [16].

Alcoholic cardiomyopathy

Chronic alcohol consumption can increase reactive oxygen species levels, causing oxidative stress and various cardiac dysfunctions, including myocyte disarray, sarcoplasmic reticulum dysfunction, altered intracellular calcium hemostasis, mitochondrial dysfunction, and contractility disruption [17,18]. Heavy alcohol consumption is linked to up to 40% of cardiomyopathy cases [19]. Patients with alcohol-related cardiomyopathy may present with heart failure symptoms, a dilated left ventricle, normal or reduced left ventricular (LV) wall thickness, and a reduced LV ejection fraction [20]. Thiamine deficiency can also lead to a high-output cardiac failure (wet beriberi) due to vasodilatation and decreased vascular resistance [21].

Cardiac arrhythmias

Heavy alcohol consumption can increase the risk of abnormal heart rhythms both acutely and chronically by disrupting the cardiac intrinsic conductive system. Unhealthy alcohol users may experience postdrink rhythm irregularities, such as premature contractions, atrial fibrillation, and ventricular tachycardia,

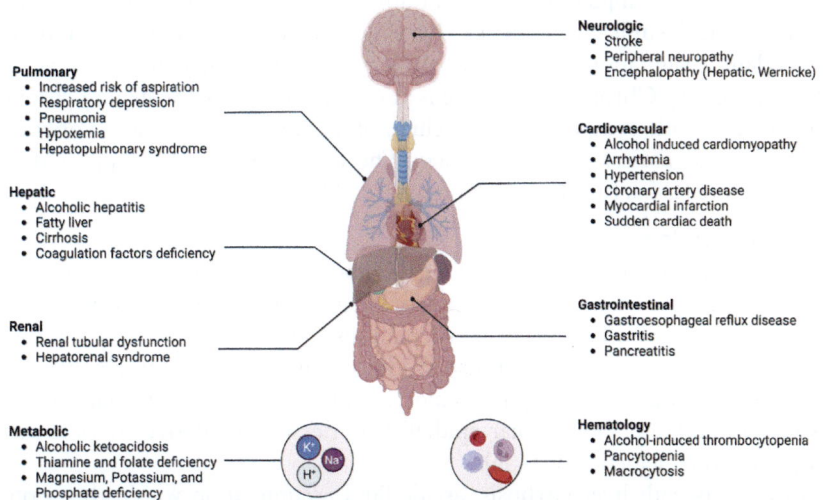

Fig. 1. Effect of alcohol on the human body. (Created with BioRender.com.)

even without clinical heart disease [22]. These arrhythmias can lead to sudden cardiac death, especially in the context of binge drinking [23]. Multiple factors favor arrhythmogenesis in alcoholic patients, including structural changes in the cardiac muscle due to alcohol-related cardiomyopathy, electrolyte disturbances (hypokalemia, hypomagnesemia), prolonged QT interval, altered calcium ion movement, and excessive adrenergic stimulation and vagal activity [24,25].

Hypertension
Alcohol consumption can cause hypertension by disrupting endothelial cells, decreasing nitric oxide availability, and increasing plaque buildup in arteries. Other mechanisms include increasing intracellular calcium levels, altering arterial-vascular function, activating the sympathetic nervous system, and releasing stress hormones [26].

Coronary artery disease
Studies have extensively examined the link between alcohol consumption and coronary artery disease (CAD), showing a J-shaped relationship. Generally, alcohol intake of less than 2 drinks per day is associated with a reduction in CAD risk, whereas heavy alcohol consumption is linked to a greater risk [27,28].

Gastrointestinal system
Alcohol is a significant cause of liver disease, leading to hepatic steatosis, inflammation, and oxidative stress, which can result in hepatocellular injury, alcoholic hepatitis, and irreversible alcoholic cirrhosis [29,30]. Decompensated liver disease can lead to various complications, such as portal hypertension, ascites or hydrothorax, variceal bleeding, chronic gastritis, synthetic dysfunction, coagulopathy, thrombocytopenia, hepatic encephalopathy, bacterial infections, and acute kidney injury. Coagulation abnormalities are common in patients with hepatic insufficiency due to the synthetic dysfunction of vitamin K–dependent coagulation factors, which is worsened in patients with active alcohol use [31]. Chronic alcohol use is also a major cause of acute and chronic pancreatitis, with symptoms that include abdominal pain, nausea, vomiting, anorexia, and pancreatic insufficiency. The diagnosis may be supported by elevated levels of serum lipase and amylase [32].

Pulmonary system
Chronic alcohol use weakens the lungs' immunity to infections by disrupting the mucociliary system and macrophage function and increasing airway colonization by harmful bacteria [33]. Alcohol also impairs airway protective reflexes, increasing the risk of aspiration pneumonia. Heavy alcohol use doubles the odds of developing acute respiratory distress syndrome due to its direct effects on the alveolar epithelial barrier and oxidative stress caused by glutathione depletion [34–36].

In patients with liver cirrhosis, ascitic fluid accumulation within the peritoneal cavity reduces vital and functional residual capacities, increasing the risk of atelectasis, tachypnea, and dyspnea. Hepatopulmonary syndrome, affecting

4% to 19% of patients with cirrhosis, is characterized by reduced pulmonary vascular resistance and intrapulmonary shunts, resulting in hypoxemia [37,38]. These conditions compromise the lungs' ability to function correctly and increase the risk of respiratory complications.

Renal system

Electrolyte and trace element imbalances are common during alcohol consumption and withdrawal due to alcohol's effect on Na+/K + ATPase, leading to reduced glucose reabsorption and phosphate excretion [39]. Moreover, hypophosphatemia, hypomagnesemia, hypocalcemia, hypokalemia, and hyponatremia can be further exacerbated by gastrointestinal losses and poor dietary intake, such as beer-based diet [40–42]. These imbalances can lead to complications such as cardiac dysrhythmias, respiratory failure, or rhabdomyolysis. Hypocalcemia and hypokalemia may not be corrected until the underlying magnesium deficiency is addressed.

Metabolic

Up to 80% of patients with AUD suffer from thiamine deficiency due to inadequate dietary intake, decreased absorption, and high caloric value of alcohol [43,44]. Thiamine deficiency can lead to Wernicke encephalopathy, which may go undiagnosed in up to 75% to 80% of cases, and progress to Wernicke-Korsakoff syndrome, characterized by memory loss, amnesia, and confabulation [45]. Because it can be difficult to diagnose these patients, thiamine should be given to all patients with AUD. Alcoholic ketoacidosis is another condition that occurs in chronic alcoholic patients due to malnourishment and increased hormone and ketone production [46]. Diabetic ketoacidosis should be excluded before diagnosing alcoholic ketoacidosis in patients with a history of diabetes [47].

Hematology

Chronic alcohol use can cause various hematologic complications, including anemia, leukopenia, and thrombocytopenia [48,49]. Alcohol intake decreases fibrinogen, factor VII, and von Willebrand factor levels and increases fibrinolysis by increasing tissue plasminogen activator activity [50]. Anemia can result from toxic effects on red blood cells, chronic gastrointestinal bleeding or inflammation, folate deficiency, or hypersplenism [51]. Macrocytosis is commonly observed in individuals with excessive alcohol intake and folate or cobalamin deficiency [52]. Leukopenia may occur due to similar factors that cause anemia, but it is usually mild and reversible with alcohol cessation. Alcohol-induced thrombocytopenia is reported in about 25% of hospitalized alcohol users due to bone marrow depression or direct toxic effects on platelets that accelerate their degradation. These complications increase the risk of postoperative bleeding and infections [49,53].

Neurologic system

Alcohol users commonly experience neuropathies (autonomic, compression) and myopathy due to alcohol toxicity and nutritional deficiencies [54]. AUD is also associated with dementia and cognitive impairment in 50% to 80% of cases, which may affect a patient's ability to comply with perioperative treatment [55]. Evidence suggests that 1 to 2 drinks per day may not affect the number of stroke events or may slightly reduce it, but higher daily alcohol intake increases the risk of all stroke events [56].

Preoperative evaluation

The management of patients with chronic alcohol use before surgery can be challenging due to comorbidities and alcohol withdrawal syndrome. To achieve the best outcomes, it is essential to address these issues before elective surgery. Enhanced recovery after surgery protocols recommend 4 weeks of preoperative abstinence for alcohol users [57]. During the perioperative period, intravenous thiamine is typically given at a dose of 100 mg/day for 3 to 5 days to prevent Wernicke-Korsakoff syndrome. Moreover, patients with alcoholic liver disease may require vitamin K, clotting factors, fresh frozen plasma, or platelets to correct coagulopathy.

History

The American Society of Anesthesiologists physical status classification system considers alcohol consumption as a risk factor and assigns patients a perioperative risk score based on the extent of their alcohol use. Patients who are social alcohol drinkers are given a score of 2, whereas unhealthy alcohol users are given a score of 3, equivalent to moderate/severe disease [58].

Establishing and confirming the extent of alcohol use (frequency, amount, duration) and any negative effects on the body through history-taking, physical examination, and laboratory evaluations are crucial. Previous perioperative complications (bleeding, infections, respiratory issues, delirium) related to alcohol use, alcohol withdrawal symptoms, and psychiatric diagnosis should also be assessed. Attentive perioperative management of patients with a history of alcohol use can positively affect the hospital course and decrease related complications [59].

Screening and diagnosis

Preoperative screening for alcohol use is crucial in identifying patients at increased risk for surgical complications [60]. Patients are usually comfortable answering questions about their alcohol use before surgery, especially when presented in a straightforward, nonjudgmental manner [61].

Anesthesiologists can incorporate screening tools for unhealthy alcohol use into routine preoperative assessments, but alcohol use is frequently overlooked due to lack of awareness of screening practices, how to assess alcohol use, and where to access information [62].

Several instruments are available to screen for unhealthy alcohol consumption that may be appropriate for use in the perioperative period:

- Single item screening
- Alcohol Use Disorders Identification Test-Consumption (AUDIT-C)
- Alcohol Use Disorders Identification Test (AUDIT)
- CAGE (Cut down, Annoyance by criticism, Feeling guilty, and Eye-opener)

Single-item alcohol screening questions are brief and require no scoring [63,64]. One example validated in primary care, "How many times in the past year have you had five (four for women) or more drinks in a day?". When the response is greater than 0 then the test is positive with 82% sensitive and 79% specific for unhealthy alcohol use. Following a positive screening for unhealthy alcohol use, patients should be assessed for the quantity, frequency, recency of alcohol use, and AUD, including physical dependence and alcohol withdrawal syndrome. The AUDIT-C is a validated questionnaire for screening unhealthy alcohol use or AUD before surgery that consists of the first 3 questions of the full 10-item AUDIT, and a score greater than 5 in the year before surgery has been associated with increased postoperative complications (Box 1) [61,65–67]. The CAGE questionnaire is not recommended for screening because questions are not sensitive for detecting the full spectrum of unhealthy alcohol use, but it can be useful for quickly finding out if someone who screens positive on a single-item screening question has a more severe problem [68].

Alcohol interventions before surgery
The perioperative period is an opportunity to affect long-term health by capitalizing on the motivation of patients to engage in positive behavior change.

Box 1: AUDIT-C questionnaire

1. How often did you have a drink containing alcohol in the past year?
   0. Never
   1. Monthly or less
   2. 2 to 4 times a month
   3. 2 to 3 times a week
   4. Daily or almost daily
2. How many drinks containing alcohol did you have on a typical day when you were drinking in the past year?
   0. 1 or 2
   1. 3 or 4
   2. 5 or 6
   3. 7, 8, or 9
   4. 10 or more
3. How often did you have 6 or more drinks on one occasion in the past year?
   0. Never
   1. Less than monthly
   2. Monthly
   3. Weekly
   4. Daily or almost daily

* Positive result score: men ≥4, woman ≥3.

Patients prefer interventions that focus on alcohol use from a surgical health optimization standpoint rather than addiction [61].

Alcohol cessation interventions have been proved effective in reducing alcohol intake before and after surgery, reversing adverse physiologic alcohol effects, reducing surgical complications, and preventing severe consequences of AUD. Two weeks of abstinence can improve some alcohol-related organ dysfunction, but at least 4 weeks of preoperative alcohol abstinence has been recommended to achieve reductions in postoperative complications [59,69]. Abstinence for 4 weeks can improve immunity and the body's stress response to surgery, reduce postoperative arrhythmias, improve LV function and ejection fraction, and reverse prolonged bleeding time during the perioperative period [70,71].

Preoperative interventions can be brief or intensive. Brief interventions include advice based on motivational interviewing techniques, with or without pharmacologic strategies. They aim to reduce alcohol intake or achieve alcohol cessation and are typically less than an hour in length, can be as brief as 5 min, and can be delivered by a variety of medical staff [72]. Intensive interventions, which can last from 4 to 8 weeks, aim to achieve complete alcohol cessation before surgery and prevention of withdrawal symptoms through a combination of pharmacologic regimens (disulfiram, chlordiazepoxide, B vitamins), psychosocial methods (interview, motivational counseling, recommendations), and follow-up by experienced staff [69].

Physical examination

Discrepancies between physical examination and history may indicate inaccurate ingestion history, recreational drug use, or a prolonged time between exposure and examination. Mental status, appearance, and vital signs are useful for assessment, with features such as tachycardia, tremors, and a smell of alcohol indicating alcohol use. Patients may seem sober despite high alcohol blood levels due to tolerance from chronic alcohol use [73]. Documentation of cognitive baseline, anxiety/restlessness, and existing weakness due to neuropathy or myopathy is needed for postoperative comparisons, regional anesthesia use, assessing positional injuries, or detecting early alcohol withdrawal. Examination of the cardiovascular system should assess hypertension, arrhythmias, and signs of cardiac failure. Chest auscultation and pulse oximetry should be performed to detect respiratory failure due to aspiration pneumonitis or cardiogenic pulmonary edema. Abdominal pain, nausea, jaundice, or ascites could be signs of pancreatitis or liver cirrhosis, with portal hypertension related to chronic alcohol consumption. A history of bruising or gum/nose bleeds may indicate thrombocytopenia and coagulopathy from advanced liver disease.

Laboratory and ancillary studies

Laboratory investigation for patients with alcohol use before surgery should include complete blood count, electrolyte panel, creatinine, liver function tests (bilirubin, coagulation studies), and liver enzymes. A rapid serum glucose concentration should be obtained in all suspected cases of heavy alcohol use who present for emergent surgery. Elevated g-glutamyl transpeptidase and alkaline phosphatase levels can indicate alcoholic liver disease. An aspartate transaminase/alanine transaminase ratio greater than 2 can also indicate alcoholic liver disease. Arterial blood gas and serum lactate measurements may be necessary in patients with acid-base or respiratory disturbances. Chest radiography is important in patients with adventitious lung sounds or hypoxia [74]. Preoperative electrocardiogram is useful in identifying rhythm abnormalities or ischemic changes, and echocardiogram is indicated if there is a history or clinical signs of impaired cardiac function, particularly alcoholic cardiomyopathy [75].

Intraoperative management

Attention to affected organ systems, hemostasis, and effects of unhealthy alcohol use on surgical stress, anesthesia, and analgesia may prevent the development of complications and improve postsurgical outcomes. Before induction, stress should be inhibited with benzodiazepines and opioids [59]. Anxiety can be an early sign of alcohol withdrawal syndrome, and prophylactic treatment with benzodiazepines is recommended in surgical patients with continued unhealthy alcohol use to prevent withdrawal symptoms [74]. Disulfiram, which is used as a deterrent to alcohol consumption but has various side effects, can reduce the plasma clearance of benzodiazepines, resulting in a prolonged effect. Underlying cardiac disease due to alcohol use can impair the heart's ability to cope with increased demands, leading to dysrhythmias (atrial fibrillation) and acute coronary syndrome.

Large bore intravenous access, monitoring of arterial blood gases, and pulmonary function may be necessary. Rapid sequence induction is recommended due to delayed gastric emptying and reflux disease associated with acute or chronic alcohol ingestion [76]. Propofol is generally well tolerated in patients with stable cardiovascular systems, but etomidate or ketamine may be preferred in hemodynamically unstable patients associated with alcohol use [73].

The anesthetic and analgesic requirements for patients with alcohol use vary depending on the duration of alcohol use, degree of intoxication, and liver disease. In patients with acute intoxication, elective surgery should be postponed until the alcohol effect subsides. However, emergent surgery in such patients requires lower anesthetic doses due to the additive central nervous system depression caused by alcohol [77–79]. Intravenous or inhalation agents can lead to hemodynamic instability in patients with preexisting alcoholic cardiomyopathy, heart failure, dehydration, or a diminished adrenocortical response to stress. Doses of induction agents such as propofol should be decreased or substituted with other agents (etomidate, ketamine). During maintenance of anesthesia, volatile agents should be carefully titrated using bispectral index because the minimum alveolar concentration requirements are typically lower than those for nonintoxicated patients [80–82].

In chronic alcohol users, increased anesthesia requirements for induction and maintenance are anticipated due to ethanol enzyme induction and cross-tolerance [74,83–87]. This increased requirement of anesthetics might lead to more hemodynamic instability, particularly with volume depletion and cardiac insufficiency. Anesthesiologists should anticipate these challenges and be prepared to manage them accordingly.

Patients with alcoholic liver dysfunction have an increased volume of distribution and delayed metabolism, leading to exaggerated and prolonged effects of anesthetic drugs. Effective doses of propofol and opioids could be increased, and larger doses of nondepolarizing muscle relaxants may be needed. Neuromuscular blocking agents should be titrated using a quantitative peripheral nerve stimulator monitor due to affected onset, metabolism, and duration of action in liver insufficiency [74]. Drugs with minimal or nonhepatic metabolism, such as cis-atracurium or remifentanil, are recommended; this will help to minimize the potential for drug accumulation and prolongation of drug effects in patients with alcoholic liver disease.

Postoperative care

Alcohol use increases the risk of various postoperative complications, and surgical patients with a history of alcohol use should be closely monitored for withdrawal symptoms, infections, cerebral, hematological, metabolic, and cardiovascular complications during the perioperative period to reduce the risk of complications and mortality [9,71,74,87].

Alcohol use is an independent risk factor for postoperative delirium, which can be reduced by careful pain management, adequate oxygenation, and metabolic correction. Neuroleptic drugs such as haloperidol, chlorpromazine, risperidone, or olanzapine are preferred to benzodiazepines for treating delirium when alcohol withdrawal is not the primary cause [74]. Agitation due to alcohol withdrawal may be wrongly attributed to postoperative pain, use of restraints, medications, or continued pulmonary intubation [87]. Postoperative patient disposition should consider surgery-related criteria, patient's health status, and preoperative interventions. Early communication with surgical teams and ICU admission for alcohol-related issues can enhance outcomes and minimize potential complications. Sensitivity to pain varies widely depending on the degree of alcohol use, and underdosing or overdosing of pain medicine is a possibility [73]. Chronic alcohol users may require high doses of opioids, and naltrexone should be discontinued 48 to 72 hours before surgery [88–90]. Multimodal postoperative pain management plans, including acetaminophen, nonsteroidal antiinflammatory drugs, local anesthesia, dexmedetomidine, steroids, and ketamine, could be effective in managing pain [91]. However, acetaminophen use should be limited in patients with chronic alcohol use due to the possibility of acute hepatic failure, with even moderate therapeutic doses [92].

Alcohol withdrawal syndrome

Patients with a history of heavy alcohol consumption are at a higher risk of physiologic dependence and alcohol withdrawal syndrome (AWS), with an estimated incidence of 50% [93]. Risk factors for developing complicated AWS include a history of delirium tremens, seizures during alcohol cessation trial, and concurrent substance use disorder or mental health condition. Several scales can be used to identify individuals at risk of developing AWS [94].

Table 2
Alcohol withdrawal syndrome

Syndrome	Symptoms	Onset after last drink
Mild withdrawal	• Autonomic hyperactivity (tachycardia, tremor, hypertension, hyperreflexia, nausea, vomiting, sweating) • Psychological (anxiety, restlessness, sleep disturbance) • Intact mental status	6–12 h
Hallucinations	• Occurs in 2%–8% • Transient visual, auditory, and/or tactile hallucinations	12–24 h
Seizures	• 10% of symptomatic individuals • Generalized tonic-clonic seizures	24–48 h
Delirium tremens	• Occurs in 30% of patients having withdrawal seizures • Severe confusion, disorientation, and/or hallucinations • Severe autonomic hyperactivity • Increased risk in patients with thrombocytopenia • Fatal if not treated	48–72 h

Symptoms of AWS can start within 6 to 24 hours after alcohol cessation and last up to 2 weeks. They range from mild tremors to severe electrolyte abnormalities, hemodynamic instability, and seizures, and early correction of metabolic and hemodynamic abnormalities, nutrition, and hydration are important starting points in management (Table 2) [95].

Prevention and treatment of withdrawal symptoms should be initiated as soon as the patient has abstained from alcohol because withdrawal symptoms may develop before the patient is completely sober. Symptom-triggered withdrawal prophylaxis guidelines using benzodiazepines and haloperidol can decrease the development of withdrawal syndromes. Alpha 2 agonists such as clonidine and dexmedetomidine are recommended as adjunct therapy for hyperactivity and anxiety symptoms that are not controlled with benzodiazepines alone and for patients in the ICU experiencing resistant alcohol withdrawal symptoms. The Clinical Institute Withdrawal Assessment of Alcohol Scale-Revised can be used to assess alcohol withdrawal treatment and guide benzodiazepine dosing [95].

SUMMARY

Alcohol use is prevalent among patients undergoing surgery and is linked to worse postoperative outcomes. It is essential for anesthesiologists to identify patients with a history of unhealthy alcohol use and consider the negative multisystem impact of alcohol. Adequate preoperative evaluation, optimization, and management strategies can help mitigate the risks associated with alcohol use during the perioperative period. These strategies include alcohol cessation interventions, personalized anesthetic management, and postoperative care plans with close monitoring for complications such as alcohol withdrawal syndrome.

CLINICS CARE POINTS

- Preoperative screening for unhealthy alcohol use is crucial for identifying patients at increased risk for surgical complications.
- At least 4 weeks of preoperative alcohol abstinence is recommended to reverse adverse physiologic alcohol effects and achieve reductions in postoperative complications.
- Due to varying anesthetic requirements and increased postoperative complications, patients with unhealthy alcohol use will require personalized anesthetic management and postoperative care plans.

DISCLOSURE

The authors have nothing to disclose.

References

[1] The NSDUH report. Rockville, Md. :Office of Applied Studies, Substance Abuse and Mental Health Services Administration, Dept. of Health & Human Services. Accessed March, 30, 2023.

[2] Esser MB, Leung G, Sherk A, et al. Estimated Deaths Attributable to Excessive Alcohol Use Among US Adults Aged 20 to 64 Years, 2015 to 2019. JAMA Netw Open 2022;5(11): e2239485.

[3] CDC. Alcohol and Public Health: Alcohol-Related Disease Impact. https://nccd.cdc.gov/ DPH_ARDI/Default/Report.aspx?T=AAM&P=612EF325-9B55-442B-AE0C- 789B06E3A8D5&R=C877B524-834A-47D5-964D-158FE519C894&M=DB4DAAC0- C9B3-4F92-91A5-A5781DA85B68&F=&D. Accessed March, 30, 2023.

[4] Wakeman SE, Herman G, Wilens TE, et al. The prevalence of unhealthy alcohol and drug use among inpatients in a general hospital. Subst Abus 2020;41(3):331–9.

[5] Martin M, Clement J, Defries T, et al. Prevalence and Characteristics of Hospitalizations with Unhealthy Alcohol Use in a Safety-Net Hospital from 2016 to 2018. J Gen Intern Med 2022;37(12):3211–3.

[6] Fernandez AC, Waljee JF, Gunaseelan V, et al. Prevalence of Unhealthy Substance Use and Associated Characteristics Among Patients Presenting for Surgery. Ann Surg 2022; https:// doi.org/10.1097/SLA.0000000000005767.

[7] Ungur AL, Neumann T, Borchers F, et al. Perioperative Management of Alcohol Withdrawal Syndrome. Visc Med 2020;36(3):160–6.

[8] Courtney R, Gupta D, Gould GS. The Australasian Professional Society on Alcohol and other Drugs' submission to the consultation draft National Tobacco Strategy 2022-2030. Drug Alcohol Rev 2023;42(3):507–12.

[9] White CA, Quinones A, Tang JE, et al. A national analysis of the effect alcohol use disorder has on short-term complications and readmissions following total shoulder arthroplasty. J Orthop 2023;35:13–7.

[10] Rolfzen ML, Mikulich-Gilbertson SK, Natvig C, et al. Association between alcohol use disorder and hospital outcomes in colectomy patients - A retrospective cohort study. J Clin Anesth 2022;78:110674.

[11] Kulshrestha S, Bunn C, Gonzalez R, et al. Unhealthy alcohol and drug use is associated with an increased length of stay and hospital cost in patients undergoing major upper gastrointestinal and pancreatic oncologic resections. Surgery 2021;169(3):636–43.

[12] NIAAA. National Institute on Alcohol Abuse and Alcoholism. What Is A Standard Drink? https://www.niaaa.nih.gov/alcohols-effects-health/overview-alcohol-consumption/what-standard-drink#:~:text=In%20the%20United%20States%2C%20one,which%20is%20about%2040%25%20alcohol. Accessed April, 16 2023.

[13] CDC. Planning and Implementing Screening and Brief Intervention for Risky Alcohol Use. https://www.cdc.gov/ncbddd/fasd/documents/alcoholsbiimplementationguide.pdf.

[14] NIAAA. National Institute on Alcohol Abuse and Alcoholism. Alcohol Use Disorder: A Comparison Between DSM–IV and DSM–5. https://www.niaaa.nih.gov/publications/brochures-and-fact-sheets/alcohol-use-disorder-comparison-between-dsm. Accessed April, 16 2023.

[15] Piano MR. Alcohol's Effects on the Cardiovascular System. Alcohol Res 2017;38(2):219–41.

[16] Tonnesen H, Kehlet H. Preoperative alcoholism and postoperative morbidity. Br J Surg 1999;86(7):869–74.

[17] Capasso JM, Li P, Guideri G, et al. Myocardial mechanical, biochemical, and structural alterations induced by chronic ethanol ingestion in rats. Circ Res 1992;71(2):346–56.

[18] Zhang RH, Gao JY, Guo HT, et al. Inhibition of CYP2E1 attenuates chronic alcohol intake-induced myocardial contractile dysfunction and apoptosis. Biochim Biophys Acta 2013;1832(1):128–41.

[19] Guzzo-Merello G, Segovia J, Dominguez F, et al. Natural history and prognostic factors in alcoholic cardiomyopathy. JACC Heart Fail 2015;3(1):78–86.

[20] Piano MR, Phillips SA. Alcoholic cardiomyopathy: pathophysiologic insights. Cardiovasc Toxicol 2014;14(4):291–308.

[21] Lei Y, Zheng MH, Huang W, et al. Wet beriberi with multiple organ failure remarkably reversed by thiamine administration: A case report and literature review. Medicine (Baltim) 2018;97(9):e0010.

[22] Greenspon AJ, Stang JM, Lewis RP, et al. Provocation of ventricular tachycardia after consumption of alcohol. N Engl J Med 1979;301(19):1049–50.

[23] Larsson SC, Drca N, Wolk A. Alcohol consumption and risk of atrial fibrillation: a prospective study and dose-response meta-analysis. J Am Coll Cardiol 2014;64(3):281–9.

[24] Habuchi Y, Furukawa T, Tanaka H, et al. Ethanol inhibition of $Ca2+$ and $Na+$ currents in the guinea-pig heart. Eur J Pharmacol 1995;292(2):143–9.

[25] Mandyam MC, Vedantham V, Scheinman MM, et al. Alcohol and vagal tone as triggers for paroxysmal atrial fibrillation. Am J Cardiol 2012;110(3):364–8.

[26] Marchi KC, Muniz JJ, Tirapelli CR. Hypertension and chronic ethanol consumption: What do we know after a century of study? World J Cardiol 2014;6(5):283–94.

[27] Mostofsky E, Chahal HS, Mukamal KJ, et al. Alcohol and Immediate Risk of Cardiovascular Events: A Systematic Review and Dose-Response Meta-Analysis. Circulation 2016;133(10):979–87.

[28] Leong DP, Smyth A, Teo KK, et al. Patterns of alcohol consumption and myocardial infarction risk: observations from 52 countries in the INTERHEART case-control study. Circulation 2014;130(5):390–8.

[29] Friedman LS. Surgery in the patient with liver disease. Trans Am Clin Climatol Assoc 2010;121:192–204, ; discussion 205.

[30] Patel R, Mueller M. Alcoholic liver disease. In: StatPearls internet. Treasure Island (FL): StatPearls Publishing; 2023 Available from: https://www.ncbi.nlm.nih.gov/books/NBK546632/.

[31] Shah NL, Intagliata NM, Northup PG, et al. Procoagulant therapeutics in liver disease: a critique and clinical rationale. Nat Rev Gastroenterol Hepatol 2014;11(11):675–82.

[32] Lankisch PG, Apte M, Banks PA. Acute pancreatitis. Lancet 2015;386(9988):85–96.

[33] Mehta AJ, Guidot DM. Alcohol abuse, the alveolar macrophage and pneumonia. Am J Med Sci 2012;343(3):244–7.

[34] Simou E, Leonardi-Bee J, Britton J. The Effect of Alcohol Consumption on the Risk of ARDS: A Systematic Review and Meta-Analysis. Chest 2018;154(1):58–68.

[35] Burnham EL, Brown LA, Halls L, et al. Effects of chronic alcohol abuse on alveolar epithelial barrier function and glutathione homeostasis. Alcohol Clin Exp Res 2003;27(7):1167–72.

[36] Jensen JS, Fan X, Guidot DM. Alcohol causes alveolar epithelial oxidative stress by inhibiting the nuclear factor (erythroid-derived 2)-like 2-antioxidant response element signaling pathway. Am J Respir Cell Mol Biol 2013;48(4):511–7.

[37] Schenk P, Fuhrmann V, Madl C, et al. Hepatopulmonary syndrome: prevalence and predictive value of various cut offs for arterial oxygenation and their clinical consequences. Gut 2002;51(6):853–9.

[38] Garcia-Tsao G, Sanyal AJ, Grace ND, et al. Prevention and management of gastroesophageal varices and variceal hemorrhage in cirrhosis. Hepatology 2007;46(3):922–38.

[39] Adewale A, Ifudu O. Kidney injury, fluid, electrolyte and acid-base abnormalities in alcoholics. Niger Med J 2014;55(2):93–8.

[40] Adams C. Anaesthetic implications of acute and chronic alcohol abuse. South Afr J Anaesth Analg 2010;16(3):42–9.

[41] Baj J, Flieger W, Teresiński G, et al. Magnesium, Calcium, Potassium, Sodium, Phosphorus, Selenium, Zinc, and Chromium Levels in Alcohol Use Disorder: A Review. J Clin Med 2020;9(6):1901.

[42] Ouellette L, Michel K, Riley B, et al. Beer potomania: Atypical cause of severe hyponatremia in older alcoholics. Am J Emerg Med 2018;36(7):1303.

[43] Harper C. Thiamine (vitamin B1) deficiency and associated brain damage is still common throughout the world and prevention is simple and safe. Eur J Neurol 2006;13(10): 1078–82.

[44] Pruckner N, Baumgartner J, Hinterbuchinger B, et al. Thiamine Substitution in Alcohol Use Disorder: A Narrative Review of Medical Guidelines. Eur Addict Res 2019;25(3):103–10.

[45] Day E, Bentham P, Callaghan R, et al. Thiamine for Wernicke-Korsakoff Syndrome in people at risk from alcohol abuse. Cochrane Database Syst Rev 2004;1:Cd004033.

[46] Suzuki K, Tamai Y, Urade S, et al. Alcoholic ketoacidosis that developed with a hypoglycemic attack after eating a high-fat meal. Acute Med Surg 2014;1(2):109–14.

[47] McGuire LC, Cruickshank AM, Munro PT. Alcoholic ketoacidosis. Emerg Med J 2006;23(6): 417–20.

[48] Tønnesen H. Alcohol abuse and postoperative morbidity. Dan Med Bull 2003;50(2): 139–60.

[49] Silczuk A, Habrat B. Alcohol-induced thrombocytopenia: Current review. Alcohol 2020;86: 9–16.

[50] Salem RO, Laposata M. Effects of alcohol on hemostasis. Am J Clin Pathol 2005;123(Suppl): S96–105.

[51] Latvala J, Parkkila S, Niemelä O. Excess alcohol consumption is common in patients with cytopenia: studies in blood and bone marrow cells. Alcohol Clin Exp Res 2004;28(4): 619–24.

[52] Medici V, Halsted CH. Folate, alcohol, and liver disease. Mol Nutr Food Res 2013;57(4): 596–606.

[53] Trevejo-Nunez G, Kolls JK, de Wit M. Alcohol Use As a Risk Factor in Infections and Healing: A Clinician's Perspective. Alcohol Res 2015;37(2):177–84.

[54] Julian T, Glascow N, Syeed R, et al. Alcohol-related peripheral neuropathy: a systematic review and meta-analysis. J Neurol 2019;266(12):2907–19.

[55] Bernardin F, Maheut-Bosser A, Paille F. Cognitive impairments in alcohol-dependent subjects. Front Psychiatry 2014;5:78.

[56] Ronksley PE, Brien SE, Turner BJ, et al. Association of alcohol consumption with selected cardiovascular disease outcomes: a systematic review and meta-analysis. BMJ 2011;342: d671.

[57] Jankowski CJ. Preparing the Patient for Enhanced Recovery After Surgery. Int Anesthesiol Clin 2017;55(4):12–20.

[58] Doyle DJ, Hendrix JM, Garmon EH. American Society of Anesthesiologists Classification. In: StatPearls. Treasure island (FL). StatPearls Publishing; 2023.

[59] Tønnesen H, Nielsen PR, Lauritzen JB, et al. Smoking and alcohol intervention before surgery: evidence for best practice. Br J Anaesth 2009;102(3):297–306.

[60] Rubinsky AD, Sun H, Blough DK, et al. AUDIT-C alcohol screening results and postoperative inpatient health care use. J Am Coll Surg 2012;214(3):296–305.e291.

[61] Fernandez AC, Guetterman TC, Borsari B, et al. Gaps in alcohol screening and intervention practices in surgical healthcare: a qualitative study. J Addict Med 2021;15(2):113–9.

[62] Fernandez AC, Claborn KR, Borsari B. A systematic review of behavioural interventions to reduce preoperative alcohol use. Drug Alcohol Rev 2015;34(5):508–20.

[63] Smith PC, Schmidt SM, Allensworth-Davies D, et al. A single-question screening test for drug use in primary care. Arch Intern Med 2010;170(13):1155–60.

[64] Smith PC, Schmidt SM, Allensworth-Davies D, et al. Primary care validation of a single-question alcohol screening test. J Gen Intern Med 2009;24(7):783–8.

[65] Tønnesen H, Faurschou P, Ralov H, et al. Risk reduction before surgery. The role of the primary care provider in preoperative smoking and alcohol cessation. BMC Health Serv Res 2010;10:121.

[66] Rubinsky AD, Bishop MJ, Maynard C, et al. Postoperative risks associated with alcohol screening depend on documented drinking at the time of surgery. Drug Alcohol Depend 2013;132(3):521–7.

[67] Fernandez AC, Chapman L, Ren TY, et al. Preoperative alcohol interventions for elective surgical patients: Results from a randomized pilot trial. Surgery 2022;172(6):1673–81.

[68] Maisto SA, Saitz R. Alcohol use disorders: screening and diagnosis. Am J Addict 2003;12(s1):s12–25.

[69] Egholm JW, Pedersen B, Møller AM, et al. Perioperative alcohol cessation intervention for postoperative complications. Cochrane Database Syst Rev 2018;11(11):Cd008343.

[70] Tonnesen H, Rosenberg J, Nielsen HJ, et al. Effect of preoperative abstinence on poor postoperative outcome in alcohol misusers: randomised controlled trial. BMJ 1999;318(7194): 1311–6.

[71] Kip MJ, Neumann T, Jugel C, et al. New strategies to detect alcohol use disorders in the preoperative assessment clinic of a German university hospital. Anesthesiology 2008;109(2): 171–9.

[72] McQueen J, Howe TE, Allan L, et al. Brief interventions for heavy alcohol users admitted to general hospital wards. Cochrane Database Syst Rev 2009;3.

[73] Fox CJ, Liu H, Kaye AD. The anesthetic implications of alcoholism. Int Anesthesiol Clin 2011;49(1):49–65.

[74] Chapman R, Plaat F. Alcohol and anaesthesia. Cont Educ Anaesth Crit Care Pain 2009;9(1):10–3.

[75] Spies CD, Sander M, Stangl K, et al. Effects of alcohol on the heart. Curr Opin Crit Care 2001;7(5):337–43.

[76] Chen SH, Wang JW, Li YM. Is alcohol consumption associated with gastroesophageal reflux disease? J Zhejiang Univ - Sci B 2010;11(6):423–8.

[77] Gould R, Lindenbaum L, Rogers WK, et al. Anesthesia for patients with substance use disorder or acute intoxication. In: Post TW, editor. UpToDate. 2023. Available at: www.uptodate.com 2023. Accessed April 16, 2023.

[78] Wolfson B, Freed B. Influence of alcohol on anesthetic requirements and acute toxicity. Anesth Analg 1980 Nov;59(11):826–30.

[79] Garfield JMMD, Bukusoglu CPhD. Propofol and ethanol produce additive hypnotic and anesthetic effects in the mouse. Anesth Analg 1996;83(1):156–61.

[80] Müller J, Plöchl W, Mühlbacher P, et al. Ethanol reduces the minimum alveolar concentration of sevoflurane in rats. Sci Rep 2022;12(1):280.

[81] Gerstman MD, Merry AF, McIlroy DR, et al. Acute alcohol intoxication and bispectral index monitoring. Acta Anaesthesiol Scand 2015;59(8):1015–21.

[82] Oliveira CR, Bernardo WM, Nunes VM. Benefit of general anesthesia monitored by bispectral index compared with monitoring guided only by clinical parameters. Systematic review and meta-analysis. Braz J Anesthesiol 2017;67(1):72–84.

[83] Rottenberg H, Waring A, Rubin E. Tolerance and cross-tolerance in chronic alcoholics: reduced membrane binding of ethanol and other drugs. Science 1981;213(4507):583–5.

[84] Tsuchiya H. Anesthetic effects changeable in habitual drinkers: Mechanistic drug interactions with neuro-active indoleamine-aldehyde condensation products associated with alcoholic beverage consumption. Med Hypotheses 2016;92:62–6.

[85] Fassoulaki A, Farinotti R, Servin F, et al. Chronic alcoholism increases the induction dose of propofol in humans. Anesth Analg 1993 Sep;77(3):553–6.

[86] Liang C, Chen J, Gu W, et al. Chronic alcoholism increases the induction dose of propofol. Acta Anaesthesiol Scand 2011 Oct;55(9):1113–7.

[87] Gordon AJ. Identification and management of unhealthy alcohol use in the perioperative period. In: Post TW, editor. UpToDate. 2023. Available at: www.uptodate.com 2023. Accessed April 16, 2023.

[88] Vickers AP, Jolly A. Naltrexone and problems in pain management. BMJ 2006;332(7534): 132–3.

[89] Kao SC, Tsai HI, Cheng CW, et al. The association between frequent alcohol drinking and opioid consumption after abdominal surgery: A retrospective analysis. PLoS One 2017;12(3):e0171275.

[90] St Haxholdt O, Krintel JJ, Johansson G. Pre-operative alcohol infusion. The need for analgesic supplementation in chronic alcoholics. Anaesthesia 1984;39(3):240–5.

[91] Echeverria-Villalobos M, Stoicea N, Todeschini AB, et al. Enhanced Recovery After Surgery (ERAS): A Perspective Review of Postoperative Pain Management Under ERAS Pathways and Its Role on Opioid Crisis in the United States. Clin J Pain 2020;36(3):219–26.

[92] Louvet A, Ntandja Wandji LC, Lemaître E, et al. Acute Liver Injury With Therapeutic Doses of Acetaminophen: A Prospective Study. Hepatology 2021 May;73(5):1945–55.

[93] Goodson CM, Clark BJ, Douglas IS. Predictors of severe alcohol withdrawal syndrome: a systematic review and meta-analysis. Alcohol Clin Exp Res 2014;38(10):2664–77.

[94] Wood E, Albarqouni L, Tkachuk S, et al. Will This Hospitalized Patient Develop Severe Alcohol Withdrawal Syndrome?: The Rational Clinical Examination Systematic Review. JAMA 2018;320(8):825–33.

[95] The ASAM Clinical Practice Guideline on Alcohol Withdrawal Management. J Addict Med 2020;14(3S Suppl 1):1–72.

Advances in Anesthesia 41 (2023) 179–204

ADVANCES IN ANESTHESIA

Diagnosis and Treatment of New-Onset Perioperative Atrial Fibrillation

Robert J. McCusker, DO[1], Jonathan Wheelwright, DO[2], Travis J. Smith, MD[3], Conrad S. Myler, MD[*], Elizabeth Sinz, MD, MEd, FCCM, FSSH

Anesthesiology, Penn State Health, Hershey, PA, USA

Keywords
- Postoperative atrial fibrillation • Paroxysmal atrial fibrillation
- Silent atrial fibrillation • Dysrhythmia • Cardioversion • Defibrillation
- Antiarrhythmic • Case cancellation

Key points

- The incidence of atrial fibrillation (AF) increases with age and comorbidities. Patients with newly diagnosed AF should be assessed for underlying causes that should be managed before surgery.
- Postoperative AF is common, particularly following cardiac, thoracic, and abdominal surgeries, and is associated with longer hospital stays and worse outcomes.
- Most episodes of postoperative AF are self-limited regardless of the treatment approach.
- Patients with new-onset unstable AF should undergo direct current cardioversion if it is likely that the AF is causing the instability.
- Vasopressor selection can significantly impact patients' incidence of AF, with vasopressin appearing least predisposing.

[1]Present address: 460 Douglas Road, Hummelstown, PA 17036.
[2]Present address: 3998 Sumner Drive, Harrisburg, PA 17109.
[3]Present address: 585 Lovell Ct., Hummelstown, PA 17036.

[*]Corresponding author. 876 Zurich Drive, Hummelstown, PA 17036. *E-mail address:* cmyler@pennstatehealth.psu.edu

https://doi.org/10.1016/j.aan.2023.06.007

INTRODUCTION
Epidemiology
With a prevalence estimated between 3 and 6 million, atrial fibrillation (AF) is the most common sustained dysrhythmia in the United States. [1], and prevalence is projected to increase to 12.1 million by the year 2050 [2,3]. The likelihood of a clinician encountering a patient with silent AF (SAF), defined as asymptomatic or subclinical AF detected only by monitoring, in the preoperative period is quite high, with approximately 25% to 33% of patients diagnosed with new-onset AF (NOAF) presenting as SAF [4,5].

Postoperative AF (POAF) is a common, clinically relevant complication which occurs in 20% to 65% of patients after cardiac surgery [6–9], 10% to 30% after noncardiac thoracic surgery [10], and 0.5% to 15% after noncardiac non-thoracic surgery [11,12], with abdominal procedures having the highest risk of noncardiac, non-thoracic surgeries [13]. About 3% of patients undergoing other major noncardiac surgeries develop clinically significant POAF while hospitalized [14].

The underlying mechanisms causing POAF are not fully understood. Often it will arise 2 to 4 days postoperatively. Contributing factors seem to include inflammation, sympathetic activation, and cardiac ischemia, which combine to trigger AF in vulnerable patients [10].

Risk factors
Given the multifactorial nature of AF, the risk factors for the development of POAF can be both patient-related (often mirroring the risk factors for the development of AF in the general population) and surgery-specific [15]. The single most important non-modifiable risk factor for POAF is age, with a sharp inflection point after the age of 65 years [16]. Additional risk factors are included in Table 1.

POAF can also be triggered by potentially self-limiting medical events, such as acute alcohol intoxication, hyperthyroidism, sepsis, pneumonia, or acute myocardial infarction (MI) [17–19].

Related morbidity and mortality
AF is associated with an increase in both short- and long-term morbidity and mortality [20,21]. Patients with AF are at an increased risk of perioperative stroke, heart failure, morbidity, and mortality [22,23] with the risk of 30-day perioperative mortality in one series reaching 6.4%, including 5.7% for those with a history of AF undergoing even minor surgical procedures[23].

Although NOAF can be detrimental for any patient, there are several conditions where it may be particularly problematic. The loss of atrial contraction may markedly decrease cardiac output, particularly when diastolic ventricular filling is impaired by mitral stenosis, systemic or pulmonary hypertension, hypertrophic cardiomyopathy, or restrictive cardiomyopathy [24,25]. In patients undergoing Transcatheterl Aortic Valve Replacement (TAVR), those with NOAF have a twofold higher risk of mortality and heart failure compared

Table 1
Risk factors for developing atrial fibrillation

Surgical Risk Factors	Patient Risk Factors
Cardiac surgery (especially valve surgery, CABG)	Age > 65 y
Longer time on cardiopulmonary bypass	History hypertension
Thoracic surgery	History paroxysmal AF
Abdominal surgery	Obesity
Vascular surgery	History of ischemic heart disease
	Obstructive sleep apnea
	Chronic renal failure
	Rheumatic heart disease
Non-case-specific surgical factors	Male sex
Sympathetic stimulation	COPD
Hypoxemia	Diabetes mellitus
Intraoperative hypotension	Heart failure
Electrolyte derangements	Left ventricular hypertrophy
	Increased left atrial volume
	Elevated B-type natriuretic peptide (BNP)
	Withdrawal of chronic beta blockade
	Withdrawal of chronic angiotensin converting enzyme (ACE) inhibitors

Risk factors associated with POAF. A more exhaustive list is included in references. [1–16]

with those in sinus rhythm [26,27]. Thus, is it particularly important to avoid AF in these populations.

POAF typically occurs at 2 to 4 days postoperatively, and episodes are generally self-limited [10,21,28]. However, POAF has also been associated with higher mortality, longer length of hospital stay, and higher costs [29,30], so strategies are needed to help prevent and treat it.

MANAGEMENT GOALS

The general goals remain consistent whether a patient with NOAF is encountered in a preoperative anesthesia clinic, the pre-op holding area, the operating room (OR), the recovery room, or the intensive care unit (ICU). The primary goals are to assure adequate end-organ perfusion while minimizing complications, particularly thromboembolic events. Secondary goals include identifying and optimizing comorbidities that may be contributing to AF.

Atrial fibrillation diagnosed in preoperative clinic

Early identification of AF in the preoperative clinic allows for coordination with primary care physicians and cardiologists to determine AF chronology, and diagnose, evaluate, and optimize contributing comorbidities such as ischemic heart disease, hypertension, heart failure, valvular disease, diabetes, alcohol

Table 2
Recommended tests or studies on initial evaluation of the patient with atrial fibrillation [3]

Test	Clinical Rationale and/or Implication
ECG	Establish diagnosis; assess for additional conduction abnormalities or evidence of comorbidities, that is, atrial or ventricular hypertrophy or ischemia
Chest radiography	Identify possible cardiopulmonary source that is, pneumonia, chronic obstructive pulmonary disease (COPD), cardiomegaly
Complete blood count	Identify comorbid conditions, that is, severe anemia or infection
Complete metabolic profile	Identify electrolyte, hepatic, or endocrine comorbidities
Echocardiogram	Evaluate size, structure, and function of the heart, its valves and great vessels; identify presence of pericardial or valvular pathologies. Additionally, TEE is the most sensitive and specific technique to detect LA thrombi as a potential source of systemic embolism in AF.
Thyroid stimulating hormone	Identify hyperthyroidism
Polysomnography	Indicated if the history and examination are suspicious for obstructive sleep apnea

abuse, thyroid disorders, and disorders of the lung and pleura [31] before surgery.

In 2014, the American College of Cardiology and the American Heart Association established guidelines on evaluation and management recommendations for the patient with AF [32] summarized in Table 2, with focused update in 2019 [33]. The highlights of the updates most applicable to anesthesiologists are presented in Table 3. The recommendations address diagnosis, evaluation, lab and imaging studies, as well as risk stratification tools for embolic events and provide guidance when selecting rate versus rhythm control strategies for patients with AF. Most recommendations were derived from outpatient AF evaluation and management, with a paucity of data regarding the perioperative setting. Thus, the guidelines are most applicable in patients with AF in the pre-op clinic, with uncertain generalizability to the remainder of the perioperative period.

The initial evaluation of the patient with new AF involves a focused history, obtaining the approximate date of onset, precipitating factors, frequency and duration of episodes, descriptive characteristics, and associated symptoms such as palpitations, dizziness, angina, or dyspnea. Unfortunately, much of this information may be unavailable when AF is diagnosed in the preoperative clinic.

Focused cardiovascular examination investigates signs of heart failure or murmurs that may indicate valvular AF. The most recent American Heart Association (AHA) guideline emphasizes differentiating between valvular and non-valvular AF [34], which is important when determining which anticoagulant

Table 3
Critical changes pertinent to the practicing anesthesiologist addressed in the 2019 Atrial Fibrillation Focused Update [17]

Clinical Item	2014 Clinical Guideline	2019 Focused Update	Rationale	Potential Anesthetic Implications
Oral anticoagulants recommended for non-valvular AF	Warfarin or non-vitamin K oral antagonists (NOACs)	NOACs recommended OVER warfarin	Shorter half-lives, more predictable clinical response that does not require frequent laboratory testing, risk of major bleeding is lower	Half-lives range between 5 and 15 h compared with 20–60 h for warfarin; NOACs do not require routine laboratory testing.
Reversal agent for dabigatran	No prior recommendations	Idarucizumab	Monoclonal antibody reverses dabigatran anticoagulation	Rapidly binds dabigatran and normalization of activated partial thromboplastin time (aPTT) within 30 minutes
Reversal agent for NOACs	No prior recommendations	Andexanet alfa	Recombinant modified factor Xa protein, sequesters FXa inhibitors	~90% reduction in rivaroxaban and apixaban activity within 2 minutes. Time to medication reconstitution may be longer than prothrombin complex concentrates.
Left atrial appendage occlusion	No prior recommendations	Percutaneous LAA occlusion may be considered in patients with AF where anticoagulation is contraindicated	New FDA approval of the Watchman device demonstrated less hemorrhagic strokes than patients taking warfarin	Additional procedure anesthesiologists may be involved in providing care.

(continued on next page)

Table 3
(continued)

Clinical Item	2014 Clinical Guideline	2019 Focused Update	Rationale	Potential Anesthetic Implications
AF catheter ablation	No prior recommendations	Catheter-directed isolation of the pulmonary vein and or ectopic foci may be considered as a component of heart failure therapy in select patients.	May be reasonable to pursue in patients with resistive AF and HFrEF to reduce mortality and HF hospitalizations.	Procedure may confer benefit to a narrow cardiac population.
Bridging anticoagulation for patients on warfarin	Updated level of evidence	Bridging anticoagulation of warfarin is unnecessary except for patients with mechanical heart valves and those deemed to be at high thromboembolic risk	BRIDGE trial demonstrated non-inferior arterial thromboembolism prevention and decreased risk of major bleeding compared with those bridged with heparin	Only patients deemed to be at high embolic stroke risk and those with mechanical heart valves should be bridged with heparin before surgery.

Strategy for Anticoagulation Initiation in New-Onset Perioperative AFIB

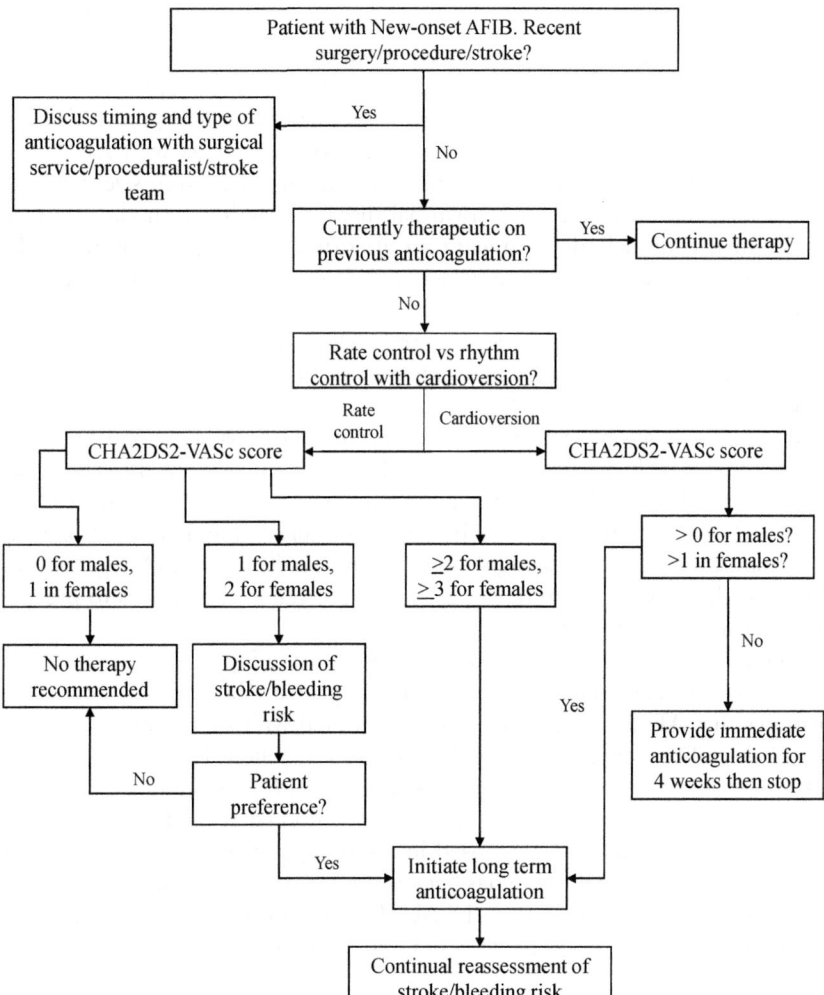

Strategy for Anticoagulation Initiation in New-Onset Perioperative AFIB

Fig. 1. Anticoagulation in atrial fibrillation.

a patient should receive. A summary diagram of recommended anticoagulation in AF is presented in Fig. 1.

The gold standard for diagnosis of AF is the electrocardiogram (EKG) [32]. AF is identified as a disorganized, irregular atrial activation with a loss of coordinated atrial contraction (fibrillation waves) and an irregularly irregular ventricular rate owing to variable conduction [35]. Accessing previous EKGs may provide a baseline and help to determine a prior history of AF while providing clues for contributing causes of AF such as atrial or ventricular hypertrophy indicative of hypertensive heart disease, Q waves indicative of a prior MI, or evidence of prior electrical conduction system diseases.

Although routine preoperative chest x-ray and echocardiography are not recommended for all patients, complete transthoracic echocardiogram (TTE) is recommended as part of the initial evaluation of all patients with AF [32] to assess for structural abnormalities, valvular heart disease, atrial size, left ventricular size and function, and pericardial disease, together with chest radiography when clinical findings suggest an abnormality [32]. The timing of the TTE may depend on procedural urgency, including potential deferral to postoperative or outpatient follow-up.

When new AF is diagnosed in the pre-op clinic, it is essential to coordinate with the patient's cardiologist regarding anticoagulation and whether perioperative bridging will be required.

Although transesophageal echocardiography (TEE) is more sensitive and specific than TTE for detecting thrombus, particularly in the left atrial appendage (LAA) [36–39], it is not generally required in the assessment of patients with AF who are otherwise hemodynamically stable. For select patients in whom therapeutic anticoagulation is contraindicated, LAA ligation, or closure with the Watchman device may provide viable alternatives to prevent thromboembolic complications.

When an ischemic etiology is suspected as contributing to the cause of AF, a patient may benefit from stress testing [40]. A growing body of evidence demonstrates that AF associated with MI is associated with significantly increased risk of mortality compared with either AF or MI alone [41].

One challenge with the recent increase in telehealth preoperative evaluations is that patients with SAF who could be diagnosed in clinic, and fully evaluated preoperatively, are instead diagnosed in the preoperative holding area on the day of surgery. Although there has been some early work on the ability of consumer wearable devices to identify AF [42], routine incorporation into telehealth pre-anesthesia assessments is not yet common.

Goals for atrial fibrillation diagnosed immediately preoperatively

Although the AHA recommendations on evaluation of AF can be applicable and helpful when AF is diagnosed in the pre-op clinic, they fail to fully address some common clinical situations frequently encountered by anesthesiologists. Chief among these is the evaluation of AF diagnosed in the preoperative holding area on the scheduled day of surgery.

The current recommendation that new-onset arrhythmias should prompt investigation into underlying causes is well justified when considering the serious and treatable nature of many precipitating causes. However, given the high prevalence of SAF, it is inappropriate to cancel every procedure in a patient with AF discovered immediately preoperatively until full evaluation can be completed. In Fig. 2, we proposed a stepwise approach for the preoperative assessment and

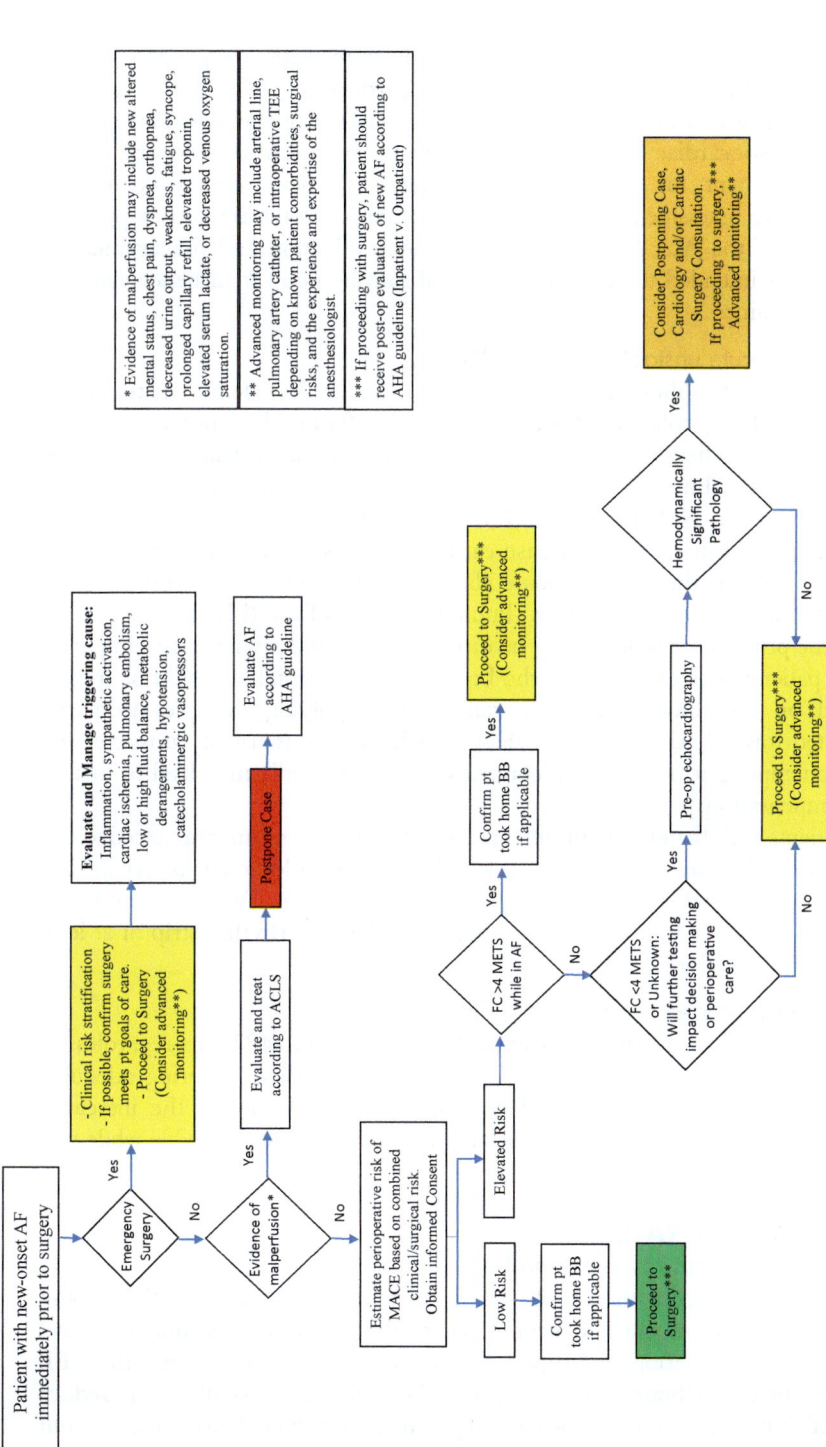

Fig. 2. Stepwise approach to assessment of newly diagnosed atrial fibrillation immediately preoperatively.

management of newly diagnosed AF in the immediate preoperative setting, inspired by the 2014 American College of Cardiology (ACC)/AHA Guideline on Perioperative Cardiovascular Evaluation and Management of Patients Undergoing Noncardiac Surgery figure, "Stepwise approach to perioperative cardiac assessment for CAD" [40]. Although this new framework for the preoperative assessment and management of AF lacks the rigorous supporting evidence of the ACC/AHA guideline on the evaluation and management of CAD, it is intended to serve as a practical starting point until better evidence can be obtained.

Goals for acute unstable atrial fibrillation

It is essential to differentiate stable versus unstable AF. Hemodynamic instability includes systolic blood pressure less than 90 mm Hg, altered mental status, cardiac ischemia, or severely decompensated heart failure due to the underlying rhythm [40]. The acute loss of atrial systole and onset of rapid ventricular rates in NOAF often lead to decreased cardiac output and hemodynamic compromise, in which case cardioversion is the initial treatment [25]. AF may also be the result of acute illness including other causes of shock hypovolemia, hemorrhage, sepsis, Pulmonary Embolism (PE), and so forth, and the primary treatment must be directed at the underlying cause. In particular, patients with chronic AF who become acutely unstable should be treated based on the underlying cause rather than applying therapies primarily directed toward AF. In these patients, cardioversion is usually unsuccessful, and attempting to rate control compensatory tachycardia may lead to further decompensation.

Patients with hemodynamically unstable AF should not undergo elective surgery. Probable causes and modifiable risk factors should be evaluated and addressed while stabilizing heart rate and blood pressure. Diagnosis should be confirmed with a 12-lead electrocardiogram (ECG) or rhythm strip of at least 30-second duration.

Goals for postoperative acute atrial fibrillation

Most cases of POAF return to a sinus rhythm after 24 to 48 hours regardless of treatment strategy [43]. Thus, in addition to the goal of assuring adequate perfusion above, goals should focus on prevention to avoid the increased cost, morbidity, and mortality associated with AF whenever possible while preventing treatment-related complications.

TREATMENT STRATEGIES

Rate control versus rhythm control

Probably the simplest modifiable risk factor to reduce the rates of POAF is to assure patients on chronic beta blocker (BB) therapy, continue their BB throughout the perioperative period if possible, or if not, resume their BB within 48 to 96 hours after surgery [8,44]. Intraoperative BBs can reduce POAF/flutter [45] and ventricular arrhythmias in high-risk patients, without increased risk hypotension and bradycardia [46]. BB should not be routinely initiated immediately before surgery due to the increased risk of mortality and stroke [47].

Regarding the choice between rate and rhythm control, the current consensus favors rate control for the initial management of hemodynamically stable patients.[150,151] In the outpatient setting, as many as 25% to 62% of cases of NOAF presented with mildly symptomatic or asymptomatic paroxysmal AF [48], and many patients spontaneously convert to sinus rhythm. A similar strategy is often instituted in the acute inpatient setting by administering rate controlling medications in hemodynamically stable AF with rapid ventricular response (RVR) to target a rate between 80 and 100 beats per minute. The second reason for the historical preference for rate control over rhythm control is the AFFIRM and RACE trials, which demonstrated similar mortality and stroke outcomes between the two strategies [49,50].

This paradigm has recently been challenged by the EAST-AFNET4 trial which demonstrated less death, stroke, or serious adverse events at 1 and 5 year follow-up in patients considered high risk for a cardiovascular event assigned to the rhythm control group [51].

For patients who fail to respond to rate control therapy but remain hemodynamically stable, rhythm control may be attempted [52]. Amiodarone is the most frequently used option in the inpatient setting [9,15,24]. In patients with decompensated heart failure or ejection fraction less than 35%, amiodarone may be preferable to BB or CCB, as it has less negative inotropic effects [24,52]. Manufacturer instructions recommend intravenous amiodarone be administered through central venous access due to the risk of tissue necrosis in cases of extravasation. When this is not practical, administration via extended dwell peripheral catheter has been found to decreased phlebitis and interruptions in drug therapy [53].

Cardioversion

Patients experiencing inadequate systemic perfusion, inadequate rate control, or refractory hemodynamic compromise suspected to be secondary to AF should receive urgent R-wave synchronized direct-current electrical cardioversion (DCCV) [9,15,24,54] regardless of their anticoagulation status. If the patient is conscious, sedation should be provided to minimize the sympathetic surge that may accompany DCCV. Airway equipment and personnel should be readily available. AF generally requires higher voltages than superventricular tachycardia (SVT) or A-flutter to achieve cardioversion [55,56]. Evaluation and treatment of potential triggers should be addressed, as this may aid in prevention and resolution of the arrhythmia.

For hemodynamically stable patients with AF, non-pharmacologic rhythm control may be accomplished by AF ablation [57,58] or cardioversion in select patients. Both have the potential benefit of improving cardiac output through restoration of coordinated atrial contraction. Cardioversion is seldom used immediately preoperatively, as most protocols recommend oral anticoagulation (OAC) for at least 3 weeks before cardioversion, and 4 weeks after, with a considerable risk of AF recurrence (see Fig. 1). If timing prohibits this approach, loading a patient with either a DOAC or heparin combined with the use of TEE rule out thrombus in the LAA is another option.

There are several pharmacologic agents that may aid in cardioversion. Magnesium may aid spontaneous conversion to normal sinus rhythm, thus reducing the need for anti-arrhythmic medications and electrical cardioversion procedures [59,60]. Ibutilide has been shown to achieve higher success rates at restoring sinus rhythm when used before cardioversion [24,43]. It can be associated with ventricular arrhythmias, including sustained polymorphic ventricular tachycardia, and requires close rhythm monitoring for at least 4 hours after administration. It is contraindicated in patients with QT prolongation, hypokalemia, and heart failure with reduced ejection fraction (HFrEF) [43]. Vernakalant was approved in 2010 by the European Medicines Agency for cardioversion of NOAF of 3 days or less in cardiac surgical patients as well as cardioversion of other AF less than 7 days in duration but is not currently approved for use in ultrasound (US) [43].

Anesthetic considerations

A general approach to the intraoperative management of the patient with new AF is presented in Fig. 3.

Volatile anesthetics do not differ from total intravenous anesthesia with respect to AF risk. Desflurane is associated with increased sympathetic stimulation and potential for arrhythmias and may reasonably be avoided, as other sympathomimetics mentioned above, in high-risk patients [15].

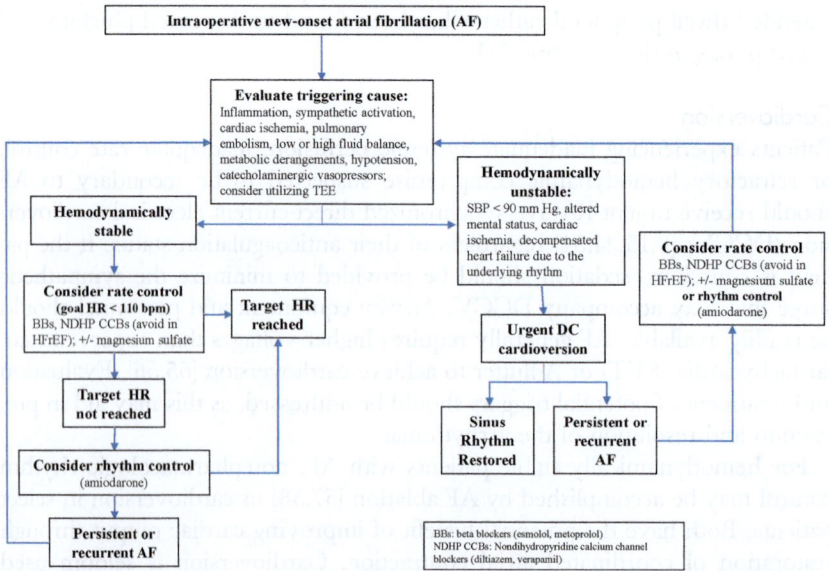

Fig. 3. Intraoperative atrial fibrillation treatment algorithm.

Reducing sympathetic stimulation and avoiding parasympathetic antagonism may be beneficial in helping prevent POAF. Although ketamine has
not been linked to POAF, it increases sympathetic activity which may predis-
pose patients at risk of POAF [15]. Anticholinergic medications such as atro-
pine and glycopyrrolate cause tachycardia and may precipitate dysrhythmias
[15]. Therefore, the use of sugammadex for neuromuscular blockade reversal
may be preferable in high-risk patients.

Metabolic abnormalities such as acidosis, hypomagnesemia, hypokalemia,
and cardiac ischemia should be assessed and treated [15,25,61,62]. If a central
line was recently inserted, catheter position should be confirmed as catheter tip
irritation can precipitate AF [15].

Hemodynamic support
Vasopressor choice can also influence POAF occurrence. Vasopressin is associated with less AF in septic surgical and nonsurgical patient when compared
with catecholamine-based vasopressors such as norepinephrine [63]. The
earlier use of vasopressin to limit or decrease catecholamine-based vasopressors
may be preferred in patients with strong risk factors for developing POAF
[15,63,64]. Although we do not yet have trials evaluating comparative rates
of AF in patients receiving angiotensin II, as a non-catecholamine vasopressor
without significant beta agonism, one would expect it to be among the vasopressors less predisposing to AF. Phenylephrine induces a reflex bradycardia
and has been effective in suppressing focal AF [15] and may have some effect
in helping achieve rate control in AF with RVR [65]. When compared with
norepinephrine, phenylephrine provided only a modest reduction in heart
rate [66].

Epinephrine is associated with higher heart rates and increased myocardial
oxygen consumption as compared with norepinephrine [67]. Epinephrine
and dopamine exhibit chronotropic effects that can lead to increased atrial
ectopic discharges, potentially triggering new AF, and the incidence of
arrhythmia does not seem to vary significantly different between them [25,67].

Dobutamine facilitates atrioventricular (AV) conduction, and some studies
have shown arrhythmias to be more common with dobutamine than milrinone
in patients with cardiogenic shock [68]. However, recent studies have shown no
difference in mortality, atrial, or ventricular arrhythmias between the two [69].

Advanced monitors include arterial lines, pulmonary artery catheters, or
TEE can be used to guide therapies depending on the anesthesiologist's abilities
and preference. TEE can help assess for acute MI and guide fluid management,
among other things [15,24,70,71]. Arterial waveform analysis such as stroke
volume variation and pulse pressure variation is unreliable as indicators of patient volume status in patients with AF due to their variable diastolic filling time
and should not be used in this patient population.

Anticoagulation
Every patient with AF should be evaluated for anticoagulation, given the risk
thrombotic complications, particularly stroke, in patient with AF. The

congestive heart failure, hypertension, age, diabetes mellitus, prior stroke or TIA or thromboembolism, vascular disease, age, sex category (CHA_2DS_2-VASc) scoring system [33,34,58,72–74] is the most frequently used (Table 4).

For patients with valvular atrial fibrillation (AFIB) (especially if a mechanical valve is present), warfarin is often the agent of choice. This may require perioperative bridging [34,57]. Regardless, patients should be referred to an anticoagulation clinic and the decision to start or not start anticoagulation can be continually reassessed in follow-up. Antiplatelet monotherapy is considered inadequate for stroke prevention and may even pose a risk of harm, particularly in elderly patients with AF [57]. On the other hand, dual antiplatelet therapy carries a bleeding risk comparable to OAC therapy [57]. Therefore, antiplatelet therapy should not be administered for stroke prevention in AF patients.

Therapeutic anticoagulation has been shown to decrease the risk of stoke but increase the risk of bleeding complications which are of heightened concern in the immediate postoperative period. Current guidelines recommend beginning therapeutic anticoagulation as soon as practical following cardioversion [34,57,73,75]. This should always be discussed with the surgical team before initiation given the risk of bleeding in the postoperative patient. Ongoing trials are in process to guide long-term anticoagulation after both noncardiac (ASPIRE-AF) and cardiac surgery (PACES). Patient situation and informed consent must also be considered. Multiple studies have found that even in patients cardioverted with a duration of AF less than 48 hours, those without anticoagulation were at significantly increased risk of a thromboembolic event in the next 30 days, up to fivefold higher risk than therapeutically anticoagulated patients [76,77]. Thus, it is essential to communicate the cardioversion and the need for anticoagulation to the team caring for the patient postoperatively. Cardiology consultation is often indicated not only for management of anticoagulation but also to establish follow-up for the patient with new AF.

Table 4
CHA_2DS_2-VASc score for atrial fibrillation stroke risk [17]

Criterion	Point Assignment[a]
Age	$<65 = 0$; $65–74 = 1$;$>/ = 75 = 2$
Sex	Male $= 0$; Female $= 1$
History of congestive heart failure	No $= 0$; Yes $= 1$
History of hypertension	No $= 0$; Yes $= 1$
History of a transient ischemic attack, stroke, or thromboembolism	No $= 0$; Yes $= 2$
History of vascular disease (prior MI, peripheral arterial disease [PAD], aortic plaque)	No $= 0$; Yes $= 1$
History of diabetes	No $= 0$; Yes $= 1$

[a]A CHA_2DS_2-VASc score of 2 or greater is an indication to consider oral anticoagulants.
Ref[6–9,14,15,18,32,33,43,108,129–134].

Anticoagulation is so critically important to the patient with AF that documentation of a CHA_2DS_2-VASc score and anticoagulation use at discharge are now being identified as inpatient care quality indicators by the AHA [78].

Left atrial appendage ablation
In patients where anticoagulation is contraindicated, an alternative means of embolic stroke prevention should be considered. Because the primary source of thromboembolism in AF is the LAA, surgical options of reducing stroke while avoiding long-term anticoagulation consist of the percutaneous WATCHMAN device or surgical closure of the LAA. In reviewing the 5 year follow-up from the PREVAIL and PROTECT AF trials, Reddy and colleagues found the WATCHMAN device to be efficacious in preventing stroke while being associated with a reduction in major life-threatening bleeding compared with long-term anticoagulation [79]. This device may be a viable option before elective surgery to eliminate the need for perioperative anticoagulation in patients whose only indication for anticoagulation is AF.

The main drawbacks of open surgical closure of the LAA over a transcatheter approach are the more invasive procedure and the incidence of incomplete LAA closure, with estimates ranging as high as 40% [80]. Neither the WATCHMAN device nor LAA closure does anything to improve the potential adverse hemodynamic effects related to the loss of atrial kick in AF.

Post-op atrial fibrillation prevention
In cardiac surgery, there is clear evidence that BB initiation preoperatively decreases POAF [81]. This is supported by multiple society guidelines [57,73,82].

Both hypovolemia and hypervolemia are risk factors for POAF [83,84] that may be addressed throughout the perioperative period. A significant "U-shaped" association between intraoperative net fluid balance and early atrial tachyarrhythmia recurrence has been demonstrated among patients undergoing the Cryo-Maze procedure [85]. Patients with NOAF tend to have significantly more positive fluid balance on the day of surgery and postoperative days 1 and 2 as well as a higher rate of dialysis and hospital mortality [86].

Results of intraoperative intravenous magnesium administration for reduction of POAF have been mixed [43,45,61]. The routine use of magnesium therapy for POAF prophylaxis is not recommended [87,88], although there is benefit in patients with contraindications to BBs and amiodarone [89,90]. There is significant heterogeneity regarding the optimal timing and dosage of magnesium [91]. A total load of 30 to 60 mmol/L of Mg may be preferable as well as continued Mg administration for greater than 24 hour postoperatively [91].

Although no clear threshold for replacement exists, patients with potassium levels less than 3.5 mg/dL have demonstrated an increased risk of developing arrhythmias [15,61,62].

Pharmacologic prophylaxis with amiodarone, BBs, steroids, statins, and colchicine has demonstrated mixed results in reducing the incidence of POAF after surgery [24,43,45,92–97], unfortunately without improving morbidity or mortality [94,98,99]. Intravenous and oral amiodarone have been shown to be equivalent in the prevention of POAF [100]. If using amiodarone, patients should be adequately loaded. A load of 5000 mg versus 3000 mg has been shown to be equally effective [101].

Trials of POAF prophylaxis with glucocorticoids, statins, and polyunsaturated fatty acids after cardiac surgery have been mixed and their use in not presently recommended by major society guidelines [57,73,82,102].

Several antioxidants have also been studied for POAF prevention in cardiac surgery. A few small clinical trials suggested that vitamin D supplementation may reduce POAF [103] in vitamin D deficient patients after coronary artery bypass graft (CABG). N-acetylcysteine, L-carnitine, and vitamins C and E have all shown somewhat promising results but require further investigation before endorsement [43,104]. Although levosimendan has some antioxidant properties, studies have found either no difference or an increase in NOAF with prophylactic use [43].

In cardiac surgery specifically, there is not significant benefit in the use of calcium channel blockers (CCBs) for the use of POAF prophylaxis [99]. Sotalol has been used for effective POAF prophylaxis [89], although it has not been shown to be superior to other BBs and was associated with an increased risk of hemodynamic instability [105], electrolyte disturbances, acute kidney injury (AKI), and QT prolongation [106] with a higher discontinuation rate compared with other BBs [89,107].

Many patients undergoing noncardiac thoracic surgery will benefit from POAF prophylaxis [99,108,109]. The initiation of new therapies for POAF prophylaxis after noncardiac thoracic surgery should be considered after stratification of patient and surgical risk factors (ie, pleurodeses vs wedge resections vs lobectomy). A 2022 systematic review revealed that BBs are the most effective treatment for preventing POAF after thoracic surgery [109]. In patients who cannot tolerate BB therapy, although not as effective, amiodarone has also been shown to decrease the risk of POAF without increasing risk and can be considered a safe alternative [87,109–112].

The evidence for using other anti-arrhythmic drugs (propafenone, procainamide, flecainide, dofetilide, ranolazine, vernakalant) for POAF prophylaxis is sparse making then only useful in particular patient populations until further randomized control trials are done [99]. These drugs in themselves can also be pro-arrhythmogenic and can cause hemodynamic instability [99].

NSAIDs have been considered for their anti-inflammatory properties. Studies have been limited due to the increased risk of renal failure, bleeding risk, and particularly with the COX-2 inhibitors, myocardial ischemia, or infarction [43].

Preoperative, intraoperative, or early postoperative use of non-dihydropyridine CCBs was associated with a significant decrease in supraventricular arrhythmias, but there was an increase in adverse effects such as increased AV blocks and low cardiac output syndrome. Use for prophylaxis is therefore limited and not currently recommended [43].

When used for prophylaxis, digoxin actually trended toward an increased incidence of POAF [45,113] and may cause an increase in mortality[99].

Non-pharmacologic methods have also been used in cardiac surgery in attempts to prevent POAF. Prophylactic overdrive atrial pacing after cardiac surgery improves intra-atrial conduction, preventing triggering events such as premature atrial contractions or atrial refractoriness [43]. Bi-atrial pacing is recommend over LA or RA pacing for POAF prophylaxis [89,94]. Right ventricular (RV) pacing in a VVI mode is associated with higher incidence of AF, mitral regurgitation, and left atrial enlargement. Non-VVI-based pacing has demonstrated lower incidence of NOAF [114,115]. Patients with left bundle branch area pacing (dual-chamber PPM) has less NOAF compared with those with RV pacing [115].

The routine use of prophylactic pacing is limited by the potential risks associated with placement or removal of temporary pacing wires, such as mediastinal infection and damage to coronary grafts or atriotomy sites potentially resulting in tamponade [43].

Prophylactic interventions such as LAA amputation and pulmonary vein isolation have been studied and may be effective, but to imposed cost and operative risk, the routine use is discouraged [9,43].

Performing a posterior pericardiotomy allows pericardial fluid to drain out of the pericardial space. This decreases the accumulation of pericardial effusions, which may be a trigger for AF and supraventricular tachyarrhythmias [43,116,117]. Routine posterior pericardiotomy has been limited due to potential for compression of bypass grafts or cardiac herniation [43]. Recent studies have demonstrated safety and high efficacy of the posterior pericardiotomy in reducing the incidence of POAF after cardiac surgery[116,117].

Another area that may warrant additional investigation is the use of regional anesthesia. A preoperative unilateral stellate ganglion block has shown to be effective in reducing the incidence of intraoperative and postoperative AF [118,119]. More research is needed before this can be recommended.

Post-op atrial fibrillation treatment
The general approach to NOAF includes starting with intravenous (IV) BBs, until a rate less than 110 bpm is achieved [9,15,25,40,52,120]. In patients with heart failure, a target of less than 80 bpm may be beneficial [121]. Using a short-acting BB may be preferable to determine the patient's clinical response [15,122–124]. Non-dihydropyridine CCB can be used in patients who have contraindications to or in conjunction with BB [43]. If used in patients with HFrEF great care should be taken with non-dihydropyridine CCBs due to their negative inotropic effects [125].

The AFFIRM study demonstrated that BBs were able to achieve overall rate control as the primary drug in 70% of patients, whereas CCBs only achieved rate control in 54% of patients [126]. Of note, these are generally contraindicated in patients with an accessory pathway, second- or third-degree AV blockade, and sick sinus syndrome [43]. An individualized approach using incremental low-dose BB or CCB therapy, closely monitoring a patient's clinical response, while simultaneously identifying and correcting triggers of AF, is advisable [15,52]. If a third agent is required, digoxin or amiodarone can be considered [57,73,82,108].

Digoxin provides a useful option for rate control in patients unable to tolerate the negative inotropy of BB and CCB, though it has a slower onset of action and may be less effective for rate control in high catecholaminergic states [15,43]. It acts synergistically with other rate control agents such as BB or CCB [15,24,43,52].

Digoxin has a narrow therapeutic index as compared with other agents and is renally cleared. As renal function is often compromised in the perioperative period, along with electrolyte disturbances, digoxin should generally be considered in the perioperative setting only when other pharmacologic options have been exhausted [15,43]. It requires frequent checks of plasma concentrations to avoid toxicity in patients with significant renal impairment [15,43].

Magnesium affects ion channel activity to decrease cardiac automaticity and prolong atrioventricular (AV) node refractoriness [25]. In patients who are not responding adequately to rate controlling medications, but remain hemodynamically stable, magnesium sulfate works synergistically with other AV nodal blockers [127,128]. It can contribute to hypotension if administered too quickly. Given magnesium's overall low side effect profile, it is a reasonable adjunct [25].

SUMMARY

The incidence of AF increases with age and comorbidities. Patients with newly diagnosed AF should be assessed for underlying causes that should be managed before surgery.

POAF is common, particularly following cardiac, thoracic, and abdominal surgeries, and is associated with longer hospital stays and worse outcomes.

Most episodes of POAF are self-limited regardless of the treatment approach.

Patients with new-onset unstable AF should undergo direct current cardioversion if it is likely that the AF is causing the instability.

Vasopressor selection can significantly impact patients' incidence of AF, with vasopressin appearing least predisposing.

KEY REFERENCES (HYPERLINKED TO ARTICLES)

2014 AHA/ACC/Heart Rhythm Society (HRS) guideline for the management of patients with atrial fibrillation: A report of the American College of Cardiology/American Heart Association Task Force on Practice Guidelines and the Heart Rhythm Society.

2019 AHA/ACC/HRS focused update of the 2014 AHA/ACC/HRS guideline for the management of patients with atrial fibrillation: A Report of the American College of Cardiology/American Heart Association Task Force on Clinical Practice Guidelines and the Heart Rhythm Society.

2014 ACC/AHA guideline on perioperative cardiovascular evaluation and management of patients undergoing noncardiac surgery: executive summary: A report of the American College of Cardiology/American Heart Association Task Force on practice guidelines.

CLINICS CARE POINTS

- Treatment of new-onset perioperative AF should focus on management of the precipitating conditions.
- Patients with new-onset unstable AF should undergo synchronized direct current cardioversion
- In patients with AF with RVR, beta blockers are more likely to achieve adequate rate control than calcium channel blockers
- Most episodes of new onset post operative AF are self limited regardless of the treatment approach.

DISCLOSURE

The authors have nothing to disclose.

References

[1] Kornej J, Börschel CS, Benjamin EJ, et al. Epidemiology of Atrial Fibrillation in the 21st Century: Novel Methods and New Insights. Circ Res 2020;127(1):4–20.

[2] Schnabel RB, Yin X, Gona P, et al. 50 year trends in atrial fibrillation prevalence, incidence, risk factors, and mortality in the Framingham Heart Study: a cohort study. Lancet 2015;386(9989):154–62.

[3] Miyasaka Y, Barnes ME, Gersh BJ, et al. Secular trends in incidence of atrial fibrillation in Olmsted County, Minnesota, 1980 to 2000, and implications on the projections for future prevalence. Circulation 2006;114(2):119–25.

[4] Dilaveris PE, Kennedy HL. Silent atrial fibrillation: epidemiology, diagnosis, and clinical impact. Clin Cardiol 2017;40(6):413–8.

[5] Denas G, Battaggia A, Fusello M, et al. General population screening for atrial fibrillation with an automated rhythm-detection blood pressure device. Int J Cardiol 2021;322: 265–70.

[6] Choi HJ, Seo EJ, Choi JS, et al. Perioperative risk factors for new-onset postoperative atrial fibrillation among patients after isolated coronary artery bypass grafting: A retrospective study. J Adv Nurs 2022;78(5):1317–26.

[7] Robert R, Porot G, Vernay C, et al. Incidence, Predictive Factors, and Prognostic Impact of Silent Atrial Fibrillation After Transcatheter Aortic Valve Implantation. Am J Cardiol 2018;122(3):446–54.

[8] Muehlschlegel JD, Burrage PS, Ngai JY, et al. Society of Cardiovascular Anesthesiologists/ European Association of Cardiothoracic Anaesthetists Practice Advisory for the Management of Perioperative Atrial Fibrillation in Patients Undergoing Cardiac Surgery. Anesth Analg 2019;128(1):33–42.

[9] Axtell AL, Moonsamy P, Melnitchouk S, et al. Preoperative predictors of new-onset prolonged atrial fibrillation after surgical aortic valve replacement. J Thorac Cardiovasc Surg 2020;159(4):1407–14.

[10] Dobrev D, Aguilar M, Heijman J, Guichard JB, Nattel SA-O. Postoperative atrial fibrillation: mechanisms, manifestations and management. (1759-5010 (Electronic))

[11] Kanji S, Williamson DR, Yaghchi BM, et al. Epidemiology and management of atrial fibrillation in medical and noncardiac surgical adult intensive care unit patients. J Crit Care 2012;27(3):326.e1–8.

[12] Bedford JP, Nuffield Department of Clinical Neurosciences UoO, John Radcliffe Hospital, Way Headley, Headington Oxford, et al. New-onset atrial fibrillation in intensive care: epidemiology and outcomes. European Heart Journal Acute Cardiovascular Care 2022;11(8):620–8.

[13] Rühlmann F, Tichelbäcker T, Mackert AF, et al. Incidence, Associated Risk Factors, and Outcomes of Postoperative Arrhythmia After Upper Gastrointestinal Surgery. JAMA Netw Open 2022;5(7):e2223225.

[14] Bhave PD, Goldman LE, Vittinghoff E, et al. Incidence, predictors, and outcomes associated with postoperative atrial fibrillation after major noncardiac surgery. Am Heart J 2012;164(6):918–24.

[15] Karamchandani K, Khanna AK, Bose S, et al. Atrial Fibrillation: Current Evidence and Management Strategies During the Perioperative Period. Anesth Analg 2020;130(1): 2–13.

[16] Amar D, Zhang H, Leung DH, et al. Older age is the strongest predictor of postoperative atrial fibrillation. Anesthesiology 2002;96(2):352–6.

[17] Lopes LA, Agrawal DK. Post-Operative Atrial Fibrillation: Current Treatments and Etiologies for a Persistent Surgical Complication. J Surg Res 2022;5(1):159–72.

[18] Polanczyk CA, Goldman L, Marcantonio ER, et al. Supraventricular arrhythmia in patients having noncardiac surgery: clinical correlates and effect on length of stay. Ann Intern Med 1998;129(4):279–85.

[19] Joshi KK, Tiru M, Chin T, et al. Postoperative atrial fibrillation in patients undergoing non-cardiac non-thoracic surgery: A practical approach for the hospitalist. Hosp Pract 2015;43(4):235–44.

[20] Albini A, Vincenzo Livio M, Marco V, et al. Long-term outcomes of postoperative atrial fibrillation following non cardiac surgery: A systematic review and metanalysis. Eur J Intern Med 2021; https://doi.org/10.1016/j.ejim.2020.12.018.

[21] Bessissow A, Khan J, Devareaux PJ, Alvarz-Garcia J, et al. Postoperative atrial fibrillation in non-cardiac and cardiac surgery: an overview. J Thromb Haemostasis : JTH 2015; https://doi.org/10.1111/jth.12974.

[22] Prasada S, Desai MY, Saad M, et al. Preoperative Atrial Fibrillation and Cardiovascular Outcomes After Noncardiac Surgery. J Am Coll Cardiol 2022;79(25):2471–85.

[23] van Diepen S, Bakal JA, McAlister FA, et al. Mortality and readmission of patients with heart failure, atrial fibrillation, or coronary artery disease undergoing noncardiac surgery: an analysis of 38 047 patients. Circulation 2011;124(3):289–96.

[24] January CT, Wann LS, Calkins H, et al. 2019 AHA/ACC/HRS Focused Update of the 2014 AHA/ACC/HRS Guideline for the Management of Patients With Atrial Fibrillation: A Report of the American College of Cardiology/American Heart Association Task Force on Clinical Practice Guidelines and the Heart Rhythm Society. J Am Coll Cardiol 2019;74(1):104–32.

[25] Bosch NA, Cimini J, Walkey AJ. Atrial Fibrillation in the ICU. Chest 2018;154(6): 1424–34.

[26] Mentias A, Saad M, Girotra S, et al. Impact of Pre-Existing and New-Onset Atrial Fibrillation on Outcomes After Transcatheter Aortic Valve Replacement. JACC Cardiovasc Interv 2019;12(21):2119–29.

[27] Okuno T, Hagemeyer D, Brugger N, et al. Valvular and Nonvalvular Atrial Fibrillation in Patients Undergoing Transcatheter Aortic Valve Replacement. JACC Cardiovasc Interv 2020;13(18):2124–33.

[28] Lee JK, George JK, Andrew DK, et al. Rate-control versus conversion strategy in postoperative atrial fibrillation: trial design and pilot study results. Card Electrophysiol Rev 2003;7(2); https://doi.org/10.1023/a:1027428003609.

[29] Almassi GH, Hawkins RB, Bishawi M, et al. New-onset postoperative atrial fibrillation impact on 5-year clinical outcomes and costs. J Thorac Cardiovasc Surg 2021;161(5): 1803–10.e3.

[30] Filardo G, Ailawadi G, Pollock BD, et al. Postoperative atrial fibrillation: Sex-specific characteristics and effect on survival. J Thorac Cardiovasc Surg 2020;159(4):1419–25.e1.

[31] Lip GY, Watson T. Atrial fibrillation (acute onset). BMJ Clin Evid 2008;2008.

[32] January CT, Wann LS, Alpert JS, et al. AHA/ACC/HRS guideline for the management of patients with atrial fibrillation: a report of the American College of Cardiology/American Heart Association Task Force on Practice Guidelines and the Heart Rhythm Society. J Am Coll Cardiol 2014;64(21):e1–76.

[33] January CT, Wann LS, Calkins H, et al. AHA/ACC/HRS focused update of the 2014 AHA/ACC/HRS guideline for the management of patients with atrial fibrillation: A Report of the American College of Cardiology/American Heart Association Task Force on Clinical Practice Guidelines and the Heart Rhythm Society. Heart Rhythm 2019;16(8): e66–93.

[34] January CT, Wann LS, Calkins H, et al. AHA/ACC/HRS Focused Update of the 2014 AHA/ACC/HRS Guideline for the Management of Patients With Atrial Fibrillation: A Report of the American College of Cardiology/American Heart Association Task Force on Clinical Practice Guidelines and the Heart Rhythm Society in Collaboration With the Society of Thoracic Surgeons. Circulation 2019;140(2):e125–51.

[35] Longo DL, Harrison TR. Harrison's principles of internal medicine. 18th edition. McGraw-Hill; 2012.

[36] Hwang JJ, Chen JJ, Lin SC, et al. Diagnostic accuracy of transesophageal echocardiography for detecting left atrial thrombi in patients with rheumatic heart disease having undergone mitral valve operations. Am J Cardiol 1993;72(9):677–81.

[37] Manning WJ, Weintraub RM, Waksmonski CA, et al. Accuracy of transesophageal echocardiography for identifying left atrial thrombi. A prospective, intraoperative study. Ann Intern Med 1995;123(11):817–22.

[38] Bunch TJ, Day JD. Examining the risks and benefits of transesophageal echocardiogram imaging during catheter ablation for atrial fibrillation. Circ Arrhythm Electrophysiol 2012;5(4):621–3.

[39] Ruiz J, Kandah F, Ganji M, et al. A rare sighting: left atrial appendage thrombus seen on transthoracic echocardiogram. J Geriatr Cardiol 2021;18(3):238–9.

[40] Fleisher LA, Fleischmann KE, Auerbach AD, et al. 2014 ACC/AHA guideline on perioperative cardiovascular evaluation and management of patients undergoing noncardiac surgery: executive summary: a report of the American College of Cardiology/American Heart Association Task Force on practice guidelines. Developed in collaboration with the American College of Surgeons, American Society of Anesthesiologists, American Society of Echocardiography, American Society of Nuclear Cardiology, Heart Rhythm Society, Society for Cardiovascular Angiography and Interventions, Society of Cardiovascular Anesthesiologists, and Society of Vascular Medicine Endorsed by the Society of Hospital Medicine. J Nucl Cardiol 2015;22(1):162–215.

[41] Podolecki T, Lenarczyk R, Kowalczyk J, et al. Significance of Atrial Fibrillation Complicating ST-Segment Elevation Myocardial Infarction. Am J Cardiol 2017;120(4):517–21.

[42] Perez MV, Mahaffey KW, Hedlin H, et al. Large-Scale Assessment of a Smartwatch to Identify Atrial Fibrillation. N Engl J Med 2019;381(20):1909–17.

[43] Burrage PS, Low YH, Campbell NG, et al. New-Onset Atrial Fibrillation in Adult Patients After Cardiac Surgery. Current Anesthesiology Reports 2019;9(2):174–93.

[44] Couffignal C, Amour J, Ait-Hamou N, et al. Timing of β-Blocker Reintroduction and the Occurrence of Postoperative Atrial Fibrillation after Cardiac Surgery: A Prospective Cohort Study. Anesthesiology 2020;132(2):267–79.

[45] Oesterle A, Weber B, Tung R, et al. Preventing Postoperative Atrial Fibrillation After Noncardiac Surgery: A Meta-analysis. Am J Med 2018;131(7):795–804.e5.

[46] Blessberger H, Lewis SR, Pritchard MW, et al. Perioperative beta-blockers for preventing surgery-related mortality and morbidity in adults undergoing cardiac surgery. Cochrane Database Syst Rev 2019;9(9):CD013435.

[47] Devereaux PJ, Yang H, Yusuf S, et al. Effects of extended-release metoprolol succinate in patients undergoing non-cardiac surgery (POISE trial): a randomised controlled trial. Lancet 2008;371(9627):1839–47.

[48] Lip GY, Hee FL. Paroxysmal atrial fibrillation. QJM 2001;94(12):665–78.

[49] Wyse DG, Waldo AL, DiMarco JP, et al. A comparison of rate control and rhythm control in patients with atrial fibrillation. N Engl J Med 2002;347(23):1825–33.

[50] Hagens VE, Crijns HJ, Van Veldhuisen DJ, et al. Rate control versus rhythm control for patients with persistent atrial fibrillation with mild to moderate heart failure: results from the RAte Control versus Electrical cardioversion (RACE) study. Am Heart J 2005;149(6): 1106–11.

[51] Kirchhof P, Camm AJ, Goette A, et al. Early Rhythm-Control Therapy in Patients with Atrial Fibrillation. N Engl J Med 2020;383(14):1305–16.

[52] Smith H, Yeung C, Gowing S, et al. A review and analysis of strategies for prediction, prevention and management of post-operative atrial fibrillation after non-cardiac thoracic surgery. J Thorac Dis 2018;10(Suppl 32):S3799–808.

[53] Woods C, Hughes P, Wood M, et al. Improved Patient Safety and Quality Outcomes With Amiodarone Infusions. J Nurs Care Qual 2022;37(2):130–4.

[54] Dalia AA, Kuo A, Vanneman M, et al. Anesthesiologists Guide to the 2019 AHA/ACC/ HRS Focused Update for the Management of Patients With Atrial Fibrillation. J Cardiothorac Vasc Anesth 2020;34(7):1925–32.

[55] Andrew SS, Kasper GL, Peter T, et al. Maximum-fixed energy shocks for cardioverting atrial fibrillation. Eur Heart J 2020;41(5).

[56] Glover BM, Walsh SJ, McCann CJ, et al. Biphasic energy selection for transthoracic cardioversion of atrial fibrillation. The BEST AF Trial. Heart (British Cardiac Society) 2008;94(7); https://doi.org/10.1136/hrt.2007.120782.

[57] Hindricks G, Potpara T, Dagres N, et al. 2020 ESC Guidelines for the diagnosis and management of atrial fibrillation developed in collaboration with the European Association for Cardio-Thoracic Surgery (EACTS): The Task Force for the diagnosis and management of atrial fibrillation of the European Society of Cardiology (ESC) Developed with the special contribution of the European Heart Rhythm Association (EHRA) of the ESC. Eur Heart J 2021;42(5); https://doi.org/10.1093/eurheartj/ehaa612.

[58] Laura D, Jonatha PB, Liam OB, et al. Treatment strategies for new onset atrial fibrillation in patients treated on an intensive care unit: a systematic scoping review. Crit Care 2021;25(1); https://doi.org/10.1186/s13054-021-03684-5.

[59] Gilardi E, Pomero F, Ravera E, et al. Intravenous Magnesium Sulfate Reduces the Need for Antiarrhythmics during Acute-Onset Atrial Fibrillation in Emergency and Critical Care. J Clin Med 2022;(19):11; https://doi.org/10.3390/jcm11195527.

[60] Cacioppo F, Reisenbauer D, Herkner H, et al. Association of Intravenous Potassium and Magnesium Administration With Spontaneous Conversion of Atrial Fibrillation and Atrial Flutter in the Emergency Department. JAMA Netw Open 2022;5(10):e2237234.

[61] Rafaqat S, Rafaqat S, Khurshid H, et al. Electrolyte's imbalance role in atrial fibrillation: Pharmacological management. International Journal of Arrhythmia 2022;23(1):15.

[62] Farah R, Nassar M, Aboraya B, et al. Low serum potassium levels are associated with the risk of atrial fibrillation. Acta Cardiol 2021;76(8):887–90.

[63] Hajjar LA, Vincent JL, Barbosa Gomes Galas FR, et al. Vasopressin versus Norepinephrine in Patients with Vasoplegic Shock after Cardiac Surgery: The VANCS Randomized Controlled Trial. Anesthesiology. Jan 2017;126(1):85–93.

[64] McIntyre WF, Um KJ, Alhazzani W, et al. Association of Vasopressin Plus Catecholamine Vasopressors vs Catecholamines Alone With Atrial Fibrillation in Patients With Distributive Shock: A Systematic Review and Meta-analysis. JAMA 2018;319(18):1889–900.

[65] Haiduc M, Radparvar S, Aitken SL, et al. Does Switching Norepinephrine to Phenylephrine in Septic Shock Complicated by Atrial Fibrillation With Rapid Ventricular Response Improve Time to Rate Control? J Intensive Care Med 2021;36(2):191–6.

[66] Law AC, Bosch NA, Peterson D, et al. Comparison of Heart Rate After Phenylephrine vs Norepinephrine Initiation in Patients With Septic Shock and Atrial Fibrillation. Chest 2022;162(4):796–803.

[67] Levy B, Clere-Jehl R, Legras A, et al. Epinephrine Versus Norepinephrine for Cardiogenic Shock After Acute Myocardial Infarction. J Am Coll Cardiol 2018;72(2):173–82.

[68] Lewis TC, Aberle C, Altshuler D, et al. Comparative Effectiveness and Safety Between Milrinone or Dobutamine as Initial Inotrope Therapy in Cardiogenic Shock. J Cardiovasc Pharmacol Ther 2019;24(2):130–8.

[69] Mathew R, Di Santo P, Hibbert B. Milrinone as Compared with Dobutamine in the Treatment of Cardiogenic Shock. Reply. N Engl J Med 2021;385(22):2108–9.

[70] Pontes JPJ, Dos Santos AT, Salgado Filho MF. [Transesophageal echocardiography in perioperative period guiding the decision making during hemodynamic instability due to atrial fibrillation]. Braz J Anesthesiol 2019;69(1):82–6.

[71] Fayad A, Shillcutt SK. Perioperative transesophageal echocardiography for non-cardiac surgery. Can J Anaesth 2018;65(4):381–98.

[72] Lane DA, Lip GY. Use of the CHA(2)DS(2)-VASc and HAS-BLED scores to aid decision making for thromboprophylaxis in nonvalvular atrial fibrillation. Circulation 2012;126(7): 860–5.

[73] Jason GA, Atul V, Lbrent M, et al. Focused Update of the Canadian Cardiovascular Society Guidelines for the Management of Atrial Fibrillation. Can J Cardiol 2018;34(11); https:// doi.org/10.1016/j.cjca.2018.08.026.

[74] Ghaith A, Mohamed Z, Yasar S, et al. Anticoagulation management of post-cardiac surgery new-onset atrial fibrillation. Cleve Clin J Med 2022;89(6); https://doi.org/10. 3949/ccjm.89a.21003.

[75] Malik E, Michelle S, Ahmed A, et al. Anticoagulant Use and the Risk of Thromboembolism and Bleeding in Postoperative Atrial Fibrillation After Noncardiac Surgery. Can J Cardiol 2021;37(3); https://doi.org/10.1016/j.cjca.2020.08.023.

[76] Garg A, Khunger M, Seicean S, et al. Incidence of Thromboembolic Complications Within 30 Days of Electrical Cardioversion Performed Within 48 Hours of Atrial Fibrillation Onset. JACC Clin Electrophysiol 2016;2(4):487–94.

[77] Airaksinen KE, Grönberg T, Nuotio I, et al. Thromboembolic complications after cardioversion of acute atrial fibrillation: the FinCV (Finnish CardioVersion) study. J Am Coll Cardiol 2013;62(13):1187–92.

[78] Heidenreich PA, Estes NAM, Fonarow GC, et al. 2020 Update to the 2016 ACC/AHA Clinical Performance and Quality Measures for Adults With Atrial Fibrillation or Atrial Flutter: A Report of the American College of Cardiology/American Heart Association Task Force on Performance Measures. Circ Cardiovasc Qual Outcomes 2021;14(1): e000100.

[79] Reddy VY, Doshi SK, Kar S, et al. 5-Year Outcomes After Left Atrial Appendage Closure: From the PREVAIL and PROTECT AF Trials. J Am Coll Cardiol 2017;70(24):2964–75.

[80] Kanderian AS, Gillinov AM, Pettersson GB, et al. Success of surgical left atrial appendage closure: assessment by transesophageal echocardiography. J Am Coll Cardiol 2008;52(11):924–9.

[81] Norhayati MN, Shaiful Bahari I, Zaharah S, et al. Metoprolol for prophylaxis of postoperative atrial fibrillation in cardiac surgery patients: systematic review and meta-analysis. BMJ Open 2020;10(10); https://doi.org/10.1136/bmjopen-2020-038364.

[82] January CT, Wann LS, Alpert JS, et al. AHA/ACC/HRS guideline for the management of patients with atrial fibrillation: a report of the American College of Cardiology/American Heart Association Task Force on practice guidelines and the Heart Rhythm Society. Circulation 2014;130(23):e199–267.

[83] Goulden CJ, Hagana A, Ulucay E, et al. Optimising risk factors for atrial fibrillation post-cardiac surgery. Perfusion 2022;37(7):675–83.

[84] Schnaubelt S, Pilz A, Koller L, et al. The impact of volume substitution on post-operative atrial fibrillation. Eur J Clin Invest 2021;51(5):e13456.

[85] Minami K, Kabata D, Kakuta T, et al. U-Shaped Association Between Intraoperative Net Fluid Balance and Risk of Postoperative Recurrent Atrial Tachyarrhythmia Among Patients Undergoing the Cryo-Maze Procedure: An Observational Study. J Cardiothorac Vasc Anesth 2021;35(8):2392–6.

[86] Todorov H, Janssen I, Honndorf S, et al. Clinical significance and risk factors for new onset and recurring atrial fibrillation following cardiac surgery - a retrospective data analysis. BMC Anesthesiol 2017;17(1):163.

[87] Mohamed K, Ahmed EAA, Wael GA, et al. A comparative study between amiodarone and magnesium sulfate as antiarrhythmic agents for prophylaxis against atrial fibrillation following lobectomy. J Anesth 2013;27(1).

[88] Terzi A, Furlan G, Chiavacci P, et al. Prevention of atrial tachyarrhythmias after non-cardiac thoracic surgery by infusion of magnesium sulfate. Thorac Cardiovasc Surg 1996;44(6); https://doi.org/10.1055/s-2007-1012041.

[89] Burgess DC, MJ Kilborn, Keech AC. Interventions for prevention of post-operative atrial fibrillation and its complications after cardiac surgery: a meta-analysis. Eur Heart J 2006;27(23); https://doi.org/10.1093/eurheartj/ehl272.

[90] Bakhsh M, Abbas S, Hussain RM, Ali khan S, et al. Role of magnesium in preventing postoperative atrial fibrillation after coronary artery bypass surgery. J Ayub Med Coll Abbottabad : JAMC (J Assoc Med Can) 2009;21(2).

[91] JL Fairley, Zhang L, Glassford NJ, et al. Magnesium status and magnesium therapy in cardiac surgery: A systematic review and meta-analysis focusing on arrhythmia prevention. J Crit Care 2017;42doi; https://doi.org/10.1016/j.jcrc.2017.05.038.

[92] Chen MJ, Bala A, Huddleston JI, et al. Statin use is associated with less postoperative cardiac arrhythmia after total hip arthroplasty. Hip Int 2019;29(6):618–23.

[93] Dvirnik N, Belley-Cote EP, Hanif H, et al. Steroids in cardiac surgery: a systematic review and meta-analysis. Br J Anaesth 2018;1471–6771, (Electronic)).

[94] Arsenault KA, Yusuf AM, Crystal E, et al. Interventions for preventing post-operative atrial fibrillation in patients undergoing heart surgery. Cochrane Database Syst Rev 2013;(1): 2013; https://doi.org/10.1002/14651858.CD003611.pub3.

[95] Carsen L, Manish B, Mahmoud T, et al. Colchicine for primary prevention of atrial fibrillation after open-heart surgery: Systematic review and meta-analysis. Int J Cardiol 2017; https://doi.org/10.1016/j.ijcard.2017.08.039.

[96] Guerra F, Romandini A, Barbarossa A, et al. Ranolazine for rhythm control in atrial fibrillation: A systematic review and meta-analysis. Int J Cardiol 2017;227:284–91.

[97] Zhao H, Chen Y, Mao M, et al. Correction: A meta-analysis of colchicine in prevention of atrial fibrillation following cardiothoracic surgery or cardiac intervention. J Cardiothorac Surg 2022;17(1):285.

[98] BC Z, TY H, QW D, et al. Prophylaxis Against Atrial Fibrillation After General Thoracic Surgery: Trial Sequential Analysis and Network Meta-Analysis. Chest 2017;151(1).

[99] Dobrev D, Aguilar M, Heijman J, et al. Postoperative atrial fibrillation: mechanisms, manifestations and management. ReviewPaper. Nature Reviews Cardiology 2019;16(7): 417–36.

[100] Saurav C, Partha S, Debabrata M, et al. Timing and route of amiodarone for prevention of postoperative atrial fibrillation after cardiac surgery: a network regression meta-analysis. PACE (Pacing Clin Electrophysiol) 2013;(8):36; https://doi.org/10.1111/pace.12140.

[101] Buckley MS, Nolan PE, Slack MK, et al. Amiodarone prophylaxis for atrial fibrillation after cardiac surgery: meta-analysis of dose response and timing of initiation. Pharmacotherapy 2007;27(3); https://doi.org/10.1592/phco.27.3.360.

[102] Khan JA, Laurikka JO, Jarvinen OH, et al. Early postoperative statin administration does not affect the rate of atrial fibrillation after cardiac surgery. Eur J Cardio Thorac Surg 2020;57(6); https://doi.org/10.1093/ejcts/ezz365.

[103] Kara H, Yasim A. Effects of high-dose vitamin D supplementation on the occurrence of postoperative atrial fibrillation after coronary artery bypass grafting: randomized controlled trial. General thoracic and cardiovascular surgery 2020;68(5); https://doi.org/10.1007/s11748-019-01209-0.

[104] Shingu Y, Katoh N, Ooka T, et al. L-Carnitine supplementation for the prevention of postoperative atrial fibrillation in aortic valve surgery. Gen Thorac Cardiovasc Surg 2021;69(11):1460–6.

[105] Mooss AN, Wurdeman RL, Sugimotto JT, et al. Amiodarone versus sotalol for the treatment of atrial fibrillation after open heart surgery: the Reduction in Postoperative Cardiovascular Arrhythmic Events (REDUCE) trial. Am Heart J 2004;148(4); https://doi.org/10.1016/j.ahj.2004.04.031.

[106] Chung MK, Schweikert RA, Wilkoff BL, et al. Is hospital admission for initiation of antiarrhythmic therapy with sotalol for atrial arrhythmias required? Yield of in-hospital monitoring and prediction of risk for significant arrhythmia complications. J Am Coll Cardiol 1998;(1):32; https://doi.org/10.1016/s0735-1097(98)00189-2.

[107] Raiten JM, Ghadimi K, Augoustides JG, et al. Atrial fibrillation after cardiac surgery: clinical update on mechanisms and prophylactic strategies. J Cardiothorac Vasc Anesth 2015;29(3); https://doi.org/10.1053/j.jvca.2015.01.001.

[108] Frendl G, Sodickson AC, Chung MK. AATS guidelines for the prevention and management of perioperative atrial fibrillation and flutter for thoracic surgical procedures. J Thorac Cardiovasc Surg 2014;(3):148; https://doi.org/10.1016/j.jtcvs.2014.06.036.

[109] Xiaomei W, Demei Z, Yanxia R, et al. Pharmacological interventions for preventing atrial fibrillation after lung surgery: systematic review and meta-analysis. Eur J Clin Pharmacol 2022;78(11); https://doi.org/10.1007/s00228-022-03383-2.

[110] VanMieghem W, Coolen L, Malysse I, et al. Amiodarone and the development of ARDS after lung surgery. Chest 1994;(6):105; https://doi.org/10.1378/chest.105.6.1642.

[111] Riber LP, Christensen TD, Jensen HK, et al. Amiodarone significantly decreases atrial fibrillation in patients undergoing surgery for lung cancer. Ann Thorac Surg 2012;(2):94; https://doi.org/10.1016/j.athoracsur.2011.12.096.

[112] Tisdale JE, Wroblewski HA, Wall DS, et al. A randomized trial evaluating amiodarone for prevention of atrial fibrillation after pulmonary resection. Ann Thorac Surg 2009;88(3); https://doi.org/10.1016/j.athoracsur.2009.04.074.

[113] Ritchie AJ, Bowe P, Gibbons JR. Prophylactic digitalization for thoracotomy: a reassessment. Ann Thorac Surg 1990;(1):50; https://doi.org/10.1016/0003-4975(90)90094-m.

[114] Said S, Cooper CJ, Alkhateeb H, et al. Incidence of new onset atrial fibrillation in patients with permanent pacemakers and the relation to the pacing mode. Med Sci Monit 2014;20:268–73.

[115] Ravi V, Sharma PS, Patel NR, et al. New-Onset Atrial Fibrillation in Left Bundle Branch Area Pacing Compared With Right Ventricular Pacing. Circ Arrhythm Electrophysiol 2022;15(4):e010710.

[116] Mario G, Tommasao S, Ballman KV, et al. Posterior left pericardiotomy for the prevention of atrial fibrillation after cardiac surgery: an adaptive, single-centre, single-blind, randomised, controlled trial. Lancet (London, England) 2021;398(10316).

[117] Perezgrovas-Olaria R, Chadow D, Lau C, et al. Characteristics of Postoperative Atrial Fibrillation and the Effect of Posterior Pericardiotomy. Ann Thorac Surg 2022; https://doi.org/10.1016/j.athoracsur.2022.11.007.

[118] Ouyang R, Li X, Wang R, et al. [Effect of ultrasound-guided right stellate ganglion block on perioperative atrial fibrillation in patients undergoing lung lobectomy: a randomized controlled trial]. Braz J Anesthesiol 2020;70(3):256–61.

[119] Leftheriotis D, Flevari P, Kossyvakis C, et al. Acute effects of unilateral temporary stellate ganglion block on human atrial electrophysiological properties and atrial fibrillation inducibility. Heart Rhythm 2016;13(11):2111–7.

[120] Van Gelder IC, Groenveld HF, Crijns HJ, et al. Lenient versus strict rate control in patients with atrial fibrillation. N Engl J Med 2010;362(15):1363–73.

[121] Hess PL, Sheng S, Matsouaka R, et al. Strict Versus Lenient Versus Poor Rate Control Among Patients With Atrial Fibrillation and Heart Failure (from the Get With The Guidelines - Heart Failure Program). Am J Cardiol 2020;125(6):894–900.

[122] Matsuishi Y, Mathis BJ, Shimojo N, et al. Evaluating the Therapeutic Efficacy and Safety of Landiolol Hydrochloride for Management of Arrhythmia in Critical Settings: Review of the Literature. Vasc Health Risk Manag 2020;16:111–23.

[123] Milojevic K, Beltramini A, Nagash M, et al. Esmolol Compared with Amiodarone in the Treatment of Recent-Onset Atrial Fibrillation (RAF): An Emergency Medicine External Validity Study. J Emerg Med 2019;56(3):308–18.

[124] Chapalain X, Oilleau JF, Henaff L, et al. Short acting intravenous beta-blocker as a first line of treatment for atrial fibrillation after cardiac surgery: a prospective observational study. Eur Heart J Suppl 2022;24(Suppl D):D34–42.

[125] Kotecha D, Piccini JP. Atrial fibrillation in heart failure: what should we do? Eur Heart J 2015;36(46):3250–7.

[126] Brian O, Rosenfeld LE, Warner AL, et al. The Atrial Fibrillation Follow-up Investigation of Rhythm Management (AFFIRM) study: approaches to control rate in atrial fibrillation. J Am Coll Cardiol 2004;43(7); https://doi.org/10.1016/j.jacc.2003.11.032.

[127] Bouida W, Beltaief K, Msolli MA, et al. Low-dose Magnesium Sulfate Versus High Dose in the Early Management of Rapid Atrial Fibrillation: Randomized Controlled Double-blind Study (LOMAGHI Study). Acad Emerg Med 2019;26(2):183–91.

[128] Onalan O, Crystal E, Daoulah A, et al. Meta-analysis of magnesium therapy for the acute management of rapid atrial fibrillation. Am J Cardiol 2007;99(12):1726–32.

[129] Mathew JP, Fontes ML, Tudor IC, et al. A multicenter risk index for atrial fibrillation after cardiac surgery. JAMA 2004;291(14):1720–9.

[130] Pires LA, Wagshal AB, Lancey R, et al. Arrhythmias and conduction disturbances after coronary artery bypass graft surgery: epidemiology, management, and prognosis. Am Heart J 1995;129(4):799–808.

[131] Seo EJ, Hong J, Lee H-J, et al. Perioperative risk factors for new-onset postoperative atrial fibrillation after coronary artery bypass grafting: a systematic review. BMC Cardiovasc Disord 2021;21(1):418.

[132] Yokota T, Uchino S, Yoshida T, et al. Predictors for sustained new-onset atrial fibrillation in critically ill patients: a retrospective observational study. J Anesth 2018;32(5):681–7.

[133] Krijthe BP, Heeringa J, Kors JA, et al. Serum potassium levels and the risk of atrial fibrillation: the Rotterdam Study. Int J Cardiol 2013;168(6):5411–5.

[134] Khan AM, Lubitz SA, Sullivan LM, et al. Low serum magnesium and the development of atrial fibrillation in the community: the Framingham Heart Study. Circulation 2013;127(1):33–8.

Advances in Anesthesia 41 (2023) 205–224

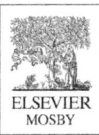

ELSEVIER
MOSBY

ADVANCES IN ANESTHESIA

Perioperative Acute Kidney Injury
Implications, Approach, Prevention

Aditi Balakrishna, MD[1], Jeremy Walco, MD[1],
Frederic T. Billings IV, MD, MSc, Marcos G. Lopez, MD, MS*

Division of Anesthesiology Critical Care Medicine, Department of Anesthesiology, Vanderbilt
University Medical Center, Nashville, TN, USA

Keywords
- Surgery • Acute kidney injury • Anesthesiology • Renal

Key points

- Renal injury is common in the perioperative period and is associated with increased morbidity and mortality. Kidney injury adversely affects other organs.
- Treatment of acute kidney injury is largely supportive and should focus on optimizing hemodynamics and renal perfusion. Timing of renal replacement therapy is controversial but data favor withholding until an absolute indication for dialysis exists.
- Prevention of perioperative renal injury remains a major goal of perioperative care, and the strongest evidence exists for avoiding hypotension, avoiding known nephrotoxins, and maintaining intravascular euvolemia.

INTRODUCTION

Acute kidney injury (AKI) is common in the perioperative period and is associated with increased duration of hospitalization, infection rate, cost, and death [1]. It affects up to 17% of patients undergoing open abdominal surgery and 30% of patients undergoing cardiac surgery [2,3]. The systemic effects of AKI are wide-ranging. Herein, the authors present several important perioperative considerations of AKI including the short- and long-term effects, AKI diagnosis, approaches for limiting and treating AKI, and renal replacement therapy (RRT).

[1]First author contributing equally.

*Corresponding author. 1211 21st Avenue South, Medical Arts Building 422, Nashville, TN 37212. E-mail address: marcos.g.lopez@vumc.org

https://doi.org/10.1016/j.aan.2023.06.005
0737-6146/23/Published by Elsevier Inc.

THE IMPACT OF PERIOPERATIVE ACUTE KIDNEY INJURY

AKI may promote intravascular volume overload, vascular congestion, pulmonary dysfunction, acid-base disturbances, arrhythmia, heart failure, immunosuppression and susceptibility to infection, systemic neurologic dysfunction, and delirium as described later (Fig. 1).

Perioperative AKI reflects impaired glomerular filtration and concomitantly increases the risk for increased vascular congestion, acid-base derangements, and altered electrolyte balance. Each of these increases the risk for congestive heart failure exacerbations (a phenomenon termed type 3 cardiorenal syndrome) and arrhythmia [4]. In the perioperative setting, AKI is associated with increased arrythmia, most commonly atrial fibrillation, and this association may further intensify the risk for cardiac dysfunction. A large retrospective cohort of cardiac surgery patients in Europe found an increased adjusted odds of developing atrial fibrillation of 57% (29%–91%) in patients with AKI, and a large cohort of patients having cardiac surgery in Asia had a 71% (95% confidence interval [CI] 43%–106%) increased adjusted relative risk of developing atrial fibrillation when AKI was present [5,6]. Our understanding of cardiac

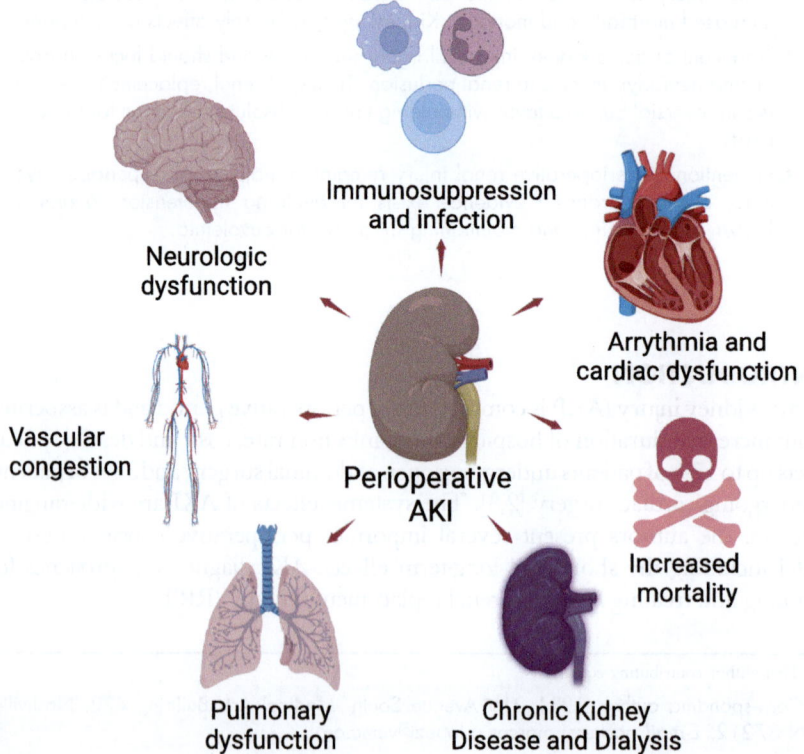

Fig. 1. Acute and chronic effects of acute kidney injury (AKI). (Created with BioRender.com.)

and renal interactions in the perioperative period remains rudimentary, and there remain several potential mechanistic interactions that require further investigation. It is clear, however, that perioperative cardiac and renal dysfunction often occur together and have a synergistic effect on poor patient outcomes.

AKI also increases risk for pulmonary dysfunction related to effects on inflammation, vascular permeability, and pulmonary edema. This pulmonary dysfunction is manifest as longer duration of mechanical ventilation and, in some instances, the need for tracheostomy. Pulmonary dysfunction in the setting of perioperative renal injury is especially evident in cohorts of patients undergoing lung resection surgery or lung transplantation [7–9], but it is also observed in patients undergoing cardiac surgery and neurosurgical procedures [10,11]. Volume overload coupled with pulmonary edema in this setting can be particularly complex to treat because of a decreased or impaired response to diuretic medications and the concern that overaggressive diuresis may exacerbate AKI. Harmful effects of AKI, however, are not limited to those relating to intravascular volume.

AKI predisposes patients to infection likely secondary to immunosuppressive effects. Observational cohort studies of critically ill patients note that a large proportion of patients with AKI subsequently develop infections and sepsis [12]. AKI may induce immunosuppression via altered cytokine signaling, increased inflammation, and altered immune cell function, and these processes contribute to AKI [13,14]. In a large retrospective perioperative cohort of patients in Japan, absolute lymphocyte counts were lower among patients with perioperative AKI, and perioperative AKI was independently associated with subsequent hospitalization for infection [15]. In a cohort of cardiac surgery patients, even the development of mild renal injury, characterized as Kidney Disease Improving Global Outcomes (KDIGO) stage I AKI, was associated with increased postoperative infection and length of hospitalization [16]. These effects may persist even when there is recovery of renal function. In a cohort of patients who had AKI with subsequent renal recovery, odds of infection remained 350% (95% CI, 143%–745%) greater compared with propensity matched controls without AKI [17]. Therefore, perioperative AKI yields an immunosuppressive phenotype and substantially increases subsequent risk of infection to patients with AKI, even in those who have renal recovery after an AKI episode. The absolute underlying cause of these effects is not known but may be from dysregulated inflammation. Similar effects may promote other organ dysfunction in patients with AKI, such as neurologic dysfunction.

AKI promotes both central and peripheral nervous system dysfunction. For example, incidence and severity of AKI are associated with increased odds of delirium in patients undergoing cardiac surgery. In an observational cohort study Kotfis and colleagues noted that odds of delirium measured using the Confusion Assessment Method increased by 140%, 238%, and 873% for patients with KDIGO stage I, stage II, and stage III AKI, respectively, compared with patients without AKI [18]. These brain-kidney dysfunctional interactions likely include effects of uremia and an inability to excrete sufficient metabolic products. The acute effects, however, seem to be different from well-identified sequelae induced by chronic renal dysfunction including encephalopathy, seizure, stroke, movement disorders, and polyneuropathy [19]. In addition to the acute effects of AKI, there also may be longer lasting neurologic impact. In a large retrospective cohort of patients from Taiwan, for example, investigators noted that the development of AKI requiring dialysis is associated with increased long-term risk of dementia compared with those who did not develop AKI [20]. The impact of AKI on neurologic function remains an important area that requires additional investigation so that physicians may prevent additional disability related to AKI.

As investigators have learned about the incidence and impact of AKI, it has become more obvious that patients who develop perioperative AKI are at higher risk of recurrent AKI and long-term worsening of kidney function. Important negative consequences of AKI include increased mortality, development of chronic kidney disease, and increased need for hemodialysis. Mortality for hospitalized surgical patients requiring dialysis as a result of AKI is approximately 50% at 1 year [21]. Even "mild" AKI (ie, KDIGO stage I) is associated with increased mortality, length of hospitalization, and increased cost [22]. Of note, patients with postoperative AKI have worse 10-year survival than patients without AKI even if renal function recovers to normal [21]. A large study of elective major surgery in Canada found that the need for acute dialysis following AKI increased between 1995 and 2009, with much of this increase occurring in patients having cardiac or vascular surgery [23]. The need for RRT is highest in those undergoing cardiac surgery, where rates of dialysis are as high as 4% [24]. Therefore, the chronic impact of severe AKI has increased over time in some populations, and continued efforts to decrease the incidence and severity of AKI and to promote renal recovery are warranted.

Even following severe renal injury, renal recovery is possible. Renal epithelial cells can dedifferentiate, proliferate, and again differentiate to repair injured nephrons, although this process is generally slow and is affected by the severity of the injury [25]. Outcomes following AKI range from complete resolution, partial resolution, resolution with subsequent renal injury, or progression to chronic kidney disease (Fig. 2) [26]. To date, there remain poor indicators to predict renal recovery after AKI—it is typically monitored via return to baseline creatinine values based on the idea that this metric reflects recovered glomerular filtration. There are ongoing efforts to determine additional markers of renal recovery that may aid in determining the effectiveness of therapies aimed at AKI, but the clinical utility of these markers is not yet established.

DIAGNOSIS OF ACUTE KIDNEY INJURY

AKI is commonly underdiagnosed in part because of a lack of universally adopted criteria or routine assessment [27]. Diagnostic criteria for AKI historically and currently rely on changes in urine output and measurement of serum

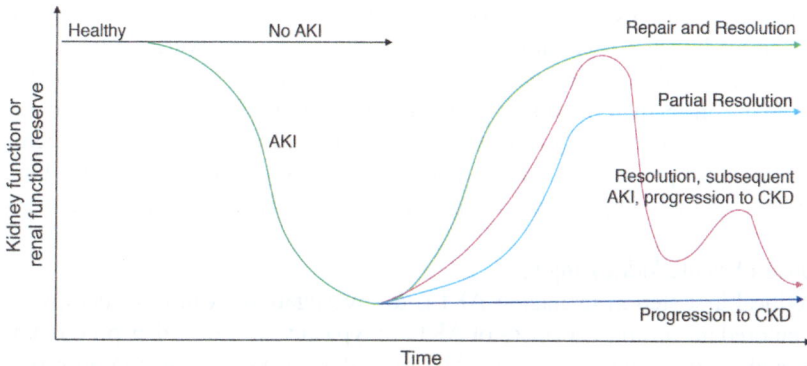

Fig. 2. Outcomes following perioperative acute kidney injury (AKI). CKD, chronic kidney disease. (*From* Billings FT, Lopez MG, Shaw AD. The incidence, risk, presentation, pathophysiology, treatment, and effects of perioperative acute kidney injury. Can J Anaesth. 2021;68(3):409-422.)

creatinine. The KDIGO criteria have become the most routinely used in the study of AKI (Table 1) [28]. AKI may not be readily recognized in the intraoperative period, as it is typically diagnosed 2 to 3 days following surgery, when decreased glomerular filtration leads to an increase in serum creatinine concentration. Urine criteria require a minimum 6 hours of oliguria. Furthermore, common surgical events such as abdominal insufflation or surgical stress–induced syndrome of inappropriate antidiuretic hormone secretion can confound urine criteria, as can commonly administered perioperative medications such as diuretics. Consensus criteria for the diagnosis of AKI are important, however, because they allow for more specific quantification of perioperative AKI and better characterization of the impact of AKI on patient outcomes and effects of treatments aimed at reducing AKI.

TREATMENT OF PERIOPERATIVE RENAL DYSFUNCTION

Once diagnosed, considerations for the management of perioperative AKI depend on its cause, severity, and duration, as well as patient characteristics and comorbidities. The most severe renal injury is managed with hemodialysis,

Table 1
Kidney disease improving global outcomes acute kidney injury criteria

Stage	Serum Creatinine Value	Urine Output
1	1.5–1.9 times baseline creatinine or $\geq$ 0.3 mg/dL increase	<0.5 mL/kg/h for 6–12 h
2	2.0–2.9 times baseline creatinine	<0.5 mL/kg/h for $\geq$12 h
3	3.0 times baseline or increase in serum creatinine to $\geq$4.0 mg/dL or initiation of renal replacement therapy	<0.3 mL/kg/h for $\geq$24 h or anuria for $\geq$12 h

which may be necessary to correct life-threatening consequences including severe electrolyte abnormalities, metabolic acidosis, volume overload, uremia, or toxin accumulation. Hemodialysis is a resource-exhaustive endeavor, however, and many immediate complications and implications for long-term outcomes may result from its use. Furthermore, the optimal timing of initiation of hemodialysis in the perioperative period, as discussed later, remains unclear. Thus, early recognition and predialysis management of AKI is essential.

Cause of acute kidney injury

A critical first step in managing AKI is to investigate the cause so therapy can be tailored accordingly. Causes of AKI are typically categorized as prerenal, intrarenal, or postrenal, relating to AKI secondary to poor perfusion, intrarenal tissue damage or dysfunction, and obstruction in the ureters, bladder, or urethra, respectively. Although convenient, this classification method may not be effective or specific enough to target the pathophysiology or to optimize the management of a patient with AKI. For example, both hypovolemia and impaired cardiac systolic function can lead to prerenal AKI but have opposing optimal treatment strategies. In a recent review of surgical AKI, Zarbock and colleagues address this concern by recommending a paradigm-based approach that is physiology-based [29]. Specifically, instead of classifying AKI as prerenal, intrarenal, or postrenal, the investigators emphasize paradigms such as hepatorenal, cardiorenal, nephrotoxic, sepsis-associated, and obstructive.

Surgery-associated AKI differs from nonsurgical AKI. In the perioperative period, intravascular fluid volume shifts are dynamic, and it requires careful monitoring and physiologic insight to anticipate transitions between resuscitative and mobilization phases. During surgery and the initial resuscitative phase, intravascular volume depletes due to bleeding, evaporative losses, and redistribution into the interstitial space. These volume losses may persist well into the postoperative period and continue to contribute to AKI. Importantly, anesthesiologists are generally unaware of incident AKI in the intraoperative period. AKI frequently is undetected until creatinine increases in the days following surgery. If hypovolemia-induced AKI is recognized early, and intravascular volume is replenished, AKI severity may be diminished, but eventually fluid redistributes from the interstitium back into the intravascular space. At this point, renal dysfunction that was initially effectively managed may worsen or reemerge in the form of volume overload and renal venous congestion [30,31]. In this situation, forced diuresis with medications may be of benefit, but recognition and prediction of when this pathophysiologic transition occurs may be difficult if the cause and potential timing of different renal injuries are not understood [32].

The type and anatomic location of surgery also influences the potential cause and approach to treating AKI. For example, surgery on the renal-genitourinary system may lead to AKI as a result of direct injury. In addition, patients undergoing major abdominal or thoracic surgery may have reduced intraoperative renal perfusion. The RELIEF trial demonstrated that patients undergoing major abdominal surgery with a restrictive intravenous fluid resuscitation strategy had increased kidney injury compared with patients treated with a more liberal fluid resuscitation strategy [33]. Patients undergoing cardiac surgery with cardiopulmonary bypass and cardioplegia may suffer from right ventricular dysfunction, leading to renal venous congestion [31]. Therefore, type of surgery and anatomic location should be considered when determining the cause of AKI to guide treatment.

Intravascular volume and renal perfusion

Management of intravascular volume and perfusion of the kidneys is crucial in the treatment of AKI. Under normal physiologic conditions the kidneys are adequately perfused at a mean arterial pressure (MAP) of 65 mm Hg [34]. This target may need to be higher in patients with increased intraoperative venous pressure, microcirculatory dysfunction, or chronic hypertension. Data on hemodynamic management of AKI in patients with septic shock support the use of vasopressors to avoid hypotension and maintain renal perfusion. In an open-label study, Xu and colleagues assigned patients with septic shock, who had received fluid resuscitation and were requiring norepinephrine, to higher MAP targets titrating norepinephrine from MAP 65 mm Hg to patients' baseline levels [35]. Increased MAP was associated with increased cardiac output, central venous oxygen saturation, small perfused vessel density, and small microvascular flow index. Although these hemodynamic results are encouraging, AKI was not measured in this cohort, so it is unknown if these findings affected AKI. In a multisite, open-label clinical trial, Asfar and colleagues assigned patients with septic shock to an MAP target of 80 to 85 mm Hg or 65 to 70 mm Hg and found in subgroup analyses that in those with chronic hypertension, the higher MAP group had a lower proportion of patients who required RRT [36]. In summary, treatment with vasopressors to at least an MAP of 65 mm Hg or higher is warranted in patients with AKI especially when there is concomitant sepsis or other forms of vasodilatory shock.

Nutrition and hyperglycemia

In addition to optimizing intravascular volume and perfusion pressure, avoidance of hyperglycemia and maintaining adequate nutrition are recommended in the treatment of AKI [37]. In surgical critically ill patients, intensive glycemic control (targeted less than 110 mg/dL) has been associated with decreased severe AKI requiring dialysis [38], but these findings have not been replicated in subsequent trials, and intensive glucose control has been noted to increase mortality, likely secondary to hypoglycemic events [39]. Therefore, most guidelines recommend the avoidance of hyperglycemia, with glucose targets ranging from 140 to 180 to 200 mg/dL in critically ill patients [40,41]. Similarly, surgical patients with renal dysfunction are at high risk of malnutrition and may benefit from targeted energy and protein intake, with a focus on administration of enteral nutrition to reduce risks from parenteral nutrition [42]. Lastly, nutritional formulations must take into consideration the severity of AKI, as volume and electrolytes from nutrition may affect the need for RRT.

Predicting progression of acute kidney injury

There are limited diagnostic tools to determine whether a patient will progress to more severe kidney injury and require RRT. One potential tool is the furosemide stress test. Furosemide, although not an appropriate treatment of AKI unless specifically targeting volume overload or hyperkalemia, may be useful in identifying these patients [26,32]. The furosemide stress test is based on a 2013 study by Chawla and colleagues that demonstrated that patients with mild to moderate AKI who would subsequently develop stage III AKI had significantly lower urine output (<200 mL) in the 6 hours following a 1-time dose of 1.0 to 1.5 mg/kg furosemide [43]. Therefore, the furosemide stress test may be a useful tool for postoperative patients with early signs of renal dysfunction in terms of triage, monitoring, and consideration of RRT.

Renal replacement therapy

RRT may be necessary in the management of severe renal injury. RRT addresses several life-threatening sequelae of renal failure, including severe acidosis, electrolyte derangements, intravascular volume overload, and severe uremia [26]. When there is not an emergent indication for RRT, the timing of initiation of RRT has been a subject of intense study and debate.

The ELAIN trial supports the early use of dialysis in AKI [44]. In this study, 231 critically ill patients were randomly assigned to either RRT within 8 hours of diagnosis of stage II AKI (early) or RRT within 12 hours of AKI stage III development (late). The early RRT group demonstrated lower 90-day mortality, higher proportion of renal function recovery, shorter duration of RRT, shorter duration of mechanical ventilation, and shorter length of hospital stay. Three other recent trials, however, failed to demonstrate significant benefits of early dialysis, although the proportion of patients suffering from perioperative AKI was less [45–47]. In the AKIKI trial, critically ill patients with stage III AKI who required mechanical ventilation, vasopressor infusion, or both were randomly assigned to either immediate RRT or RRT following severe hyperkalemia, metabolic acidosis, pulmonary edema, blood urea nitrogen greater than 112 mg/dL, or oliguria greater than 72 hours (traditional dialysis indication) [45]. There was no difference in 60-day mortality between the groups, and only 51% of patients in the delayed group ever received RRT. The delayed RRT group also had a lower rate of catheter-related bloodstream infections and earlier return of kidney function. In the IDEAL-ICU trial, patients with early septic shock and renal failure were randomly assigned to RRT within 12 hours of diagnosis or RRT after a delay of 48 hours if renal recovery had not occurred [46,48]. The trial was stopped early for futility, and there was no significant difference in death at 90 days between the groups, although only 38% of patients in the delayed group received RRT. Finally, the STARRT-AKI trial randomized 1927 patients to accelerated RRT (within 12 hours of the development of KDIGO stage II or III AKI) versus standard treatment (severe hyperkalemia, metabolic acidosis, hypoxia due to volume overload, and/or AKI lasting >72 hours) [47]. Investigators found no significant difference in survival between accelerated versus standard RRT initiation, and this remained true in a subgroup analysis of surgical patients, although the confidence interval favored increased odds of harm from the accelerated strategy in surgical patients. Furthermore, dependence on RRT at 90 days and adverse events were more common in the group assigned to accelerated RRT. Therefore, although smaller early studies noted some benefit, there is insufficient evidence that early initiation of RRT improves survival in patients with AKI, and early initiation may increase the long-term need for dialysis [49].

Patient and institutional factors often determine the modality of RRT prescribed. Peritoneal dialysis is generally not useful for patients with AKI, as these patients would most likely not have preexisting surgically placed peritoneal catheters for the procedure. Therefore, intermittent hemodialysis or continuous renal replacement therapy (CRRT) remains the mainstay therapy for severe perioperative AKI. Although intermittent hemodialysis is less time-consuming and can correct complications of renal failure more quickly, CRRT is typically reserved for hemodynamically unstable patients [50]. There are multiple modalities of CRRT, including continuous venovenous hemofiltration, continuous venovenous hemodialysis, or a combination of the two. In a 2020 review of prescription of CRRT, Karkar and colleagues contend that modality of RRT should be determined by center and personnel familiarity and comfort because of a lack of demonstrable differences in clinical outcomes for different modalities [50].

In summary, treatment of perioperative AKI is largely supportive and should be targeted at the most likely cause underlying its development. Optimizing intravascular volume and perfusion is the mainstay of treatment, and RRT is the ultimate treatment of severe AKI, but the effect on long-term renal recovery is unclear. Evidence may favor delayed RRT compared with early initiation. Because of the limited therapies to treat AKI, prevention of AKI remains an important perioperative consideration.

PREVENTION OF ACUTE KIDNEY INJURY
Prevention of AKI remains the clinical focus to reduce the impact of AKI, as there has been limited efficacy of interventions aimed at treating AKI. Numerous strategies have been investigated to decrease risk of AKI in the perioperative period. These approaches are summarized later in detail.

Optimizing perfusion to prevent acute kidney injury
Autoregulatory mechanisms within renal vasculature maintain consistent glomerular blood flow across a wide range of perfusion pressures, primarily through vasoconstriction and vasodilation of the afferent arteriole. The renal perfusion autoregulatory curve can shift with chronic hypertension and other comorbid states, making autoregulation less effective at lower blood pressures compared with normal circumstances. At systemic pressures less than lower

limits for effective autoregulation, renal blood flow decreases, and there is increased potential for ischemic injury and decreased glomerular filtration [51]. Accordingly, avoiding inappropriately low systemic pressure has been a target of investigation for AKI prevention. Absolute MAP and systolic blood pressure targets and target blood pressures relative to patients' baseline blood pressures have been examined.

Walsh and colleagues identified intraoperative MAP less than 55 mm Hg as the point at which the risk for AKI increases in noncardiac surgery patients [52]. This finding was also observed by Tang and colleagues, who noted increased AKI risk with more than 10 minutes of intraoperative MAP less than 55 mm Hg [53]. Sun and colleagues examined associations between MAP cutoffs and AKI and noted that AKI occurred with intraoperative MAP less than 60 mm Hg for 11 to 20 minutes and less than 55 mm Hg for greater than 10 minutes, with higher rates of injury associated with longer duration of hypotension in a dose-response type relationship [54].

Examining pressure relative to patients' baseline blood pressure, Futier and colleagues compared an individualized blood pressure management strategy of maintaining systolic pressures within 10% of the patient's baseline versus a "standard" strategy of treating a systolic less than 80 mm Hg or less than 40% of the patient's baseline intraoperatively through 4 hours postoperatively in abdominal surgery. Blood pressure was higher in the individualized blood pressure management strategy, and AKI occurred less frequently [55].

Salmasi and colleagues compared outcomes between patients whose MAP decreased less than 65 mm Hg and those whose MAP decreased 20% below baseline. Similar to previous studies, degree and duration of hypotension were associated with AKI, but neither the absolute threshold nor the relatively decreased threshold treatment affected AKI, supporting the idea that preoperative pressures do not need to dictate intraoperative management [56]. Mathis and colleagues found that AKI risk with hypotension was moderated by baseline risk factors including anemia, baseline glomerular filtration rate, surgery type, American Society of Anesthesiologists Physical Status, and expected anesthetic duration. In their analysis, there was not an association between hypotension and AKI in patients with low baseline risk, but high-risk patients had significant AKI risk even with mild hypotension. In contrast to prior studies, they noted that hypotension less than an absolute threshold was associated with kidney injury, whereas relative hypotension was not in a model validation cohort, although both absolute and relative hypotension thresholds were associated with AKI in the model derivation cohort [57].

Vasoactive medications with activity at the dopamine receptor have also been examined as means of preventing AKI. Fenoldopam is a dopamine-1 agonist that increases renal blood flow and has been hypothesized to be renal protective. In a meta-analysis composed of trials of partial nephrectomy, liver transplant, and cardiac surgery patients, perioperative fenoldopam treatment decreased the incidence of AKI but not the rate of dialysis [58]; this is in contrast to findings from the largest perioperative clinical trial that found no difference in RRT or peak creatinine between fenoldopam and placebo groups and an increased incidence of hypotension in the fenoldopam treatment group [59]. Dopamine has also been examined in critically ill patients. Multiple trials and meta-analyses have demonstrated that dopamine transiently increases urine output but does not prevent AKI or improve renal function [60,61].

Transfusion is another approach to increasing oxygen delivery to the kidney. Liberal versus conservative approaches to blood transfusion have been examined. The Transfusion Requirements in Cardiac Surgery (TRICS) III trial examined effects on renal failure with dialysis as a secondary endpoint by comparing a transfusion threshold of 7.5 g/dL versus 9.5 g/dL hemoglobin during cardiac surgery until intensive care unit (ICU) discharge. Transfusion thresholds did not affect the primary composite outcome of mortality, myocardial infarction, stroke, new-onset renal failure with dialysis, or renal failure as a secondary outcome [62,63]. A prespecified analysis of the TRICS III trial examined less severe grades of kidney injury and also found no evidence that 7.5 g/dL versus 9.5 g/dL hemoglobin transfusion thresholds affect AKI [64].

Optimizing renal perfusion via maintenance of systemic blood pressure may decrease the risk of perioperative AKI. There is not significant evidence for the use of dopamine agonists or blood transfusion to prevent perioperative kidney injury.

Fluid management

Avoiding intravascular hypovolemia via appropriate fluid resuscitation may prevent perioperative AKI. Protocols promoting enhanced recovery of surgical patients include restrictive fluid strategies especially for abdominal surgery patients, with the rationale that fluid restriction may prevent bowel edema and ileus. The RELIEF trial, previously referenced, a large, international pragmatic trial, demonstrated that a restrictive fluid strategy—with a median of 3.7 L intravenous fluids administered in the restrictive therapy group versus 6.1 L in the liberal group during surgery and 24 hours postoperatively—resulted in increased risk of AKI and need for RRT [33]. Additional large clinical trials could further characterize the effect of fluid management on AKI.

With regard to the type of fluid administered, there has been investigation into buffered crystalloid (eg, lactated ringers, plasmalyte) versus normal saline, although perioperative-specific trials are more limited. High volumes of normal saline can lead to hyperchloremic metabolic acidosis and increased serum potassium. Whether balanced or unbalanced chloride-rich solutions affect clinical outcomes has been of particular interest. Two small randomized controlled trials (RCTs) randomized patients to normal saline or a buffered crystalloid for their kidney transplant, during which they received between 20 and 60 cc/kg of the chosen fluid. Although metabolic changes concordant with the fluids administered were seen, there were no significant differences in functional renal outcomes between treatment groups [65,66]. ICU and hospital-based trials have been much larger, but they did not focus solely on the perioperative setting. Young and colleagues did not find a significant difference in AKI risk in a mixed critical care population when using buffered crystalloid versus normal saline [67]. A subsequent, larger pragmatic trial by Semler and colleagues in a mixed critical care population did demonstrate a lower rate of the primary composite outcome of major adverse kidney events (MAKE) including all-cause mortality, renal replacement therapy, and persistent renal dysfunction (creatinine $\geq$ 200% of baseline) in patients who received balanced crystalloids versus normal saline [68]. The adjusted odds for the new receipt of RRT was 10% lower for those who received balanced crystalloids compared with those who received normal saline, but this was not significantly different. A secondary outcome examining days free of RRT, however, was lower in the balanced crystalloid group. This finding was replicated in a study by Bledsoe and colleagues that incorporated education and an electronic health record order-entry substitution to prioritize administration of balanced crystalloids over normal saline to emergency department and hospital inpatients. They found a significant decrease in MAKE at 30 days in the balanced crystalloid group, including a decrease in persistent renal dysfunction and mortality but not the need for dialysis [69].

There has long been interest in albumin as a resuscitative fluid to attenuate kidney injury risk, and it is frequently used to prevent hypotension in patients already undergoing dialysis. Furthermore, hypoalbuminemia is a risk factor for AKI after cardiac surgery [70]. One single-center RCT demonstrated albumin repletion before off-pump coronary artery bypass surgery (CABG), compared with equal volume normal saline, decreased AKI risk [71]. This question has not been robustly investigated in other patient groups. A recent retrospective cohort study suggested perioperative albumin may be associated with higher risk of AKI, severe AKI, positive fluid balance, pulmonary complications, and 30-day mortality in noncardiac surgery. Albumin was most commonly administered during surgeries that required large resuscitation, had higher vasopressor use, and had higher blood losses. Its use increases the likelihood of residual confounding in this study despite propensity matching [72]. There is insufficient evidence to support the routine use of albumin as a resuscitative fluid to reduce AKI risk, although further investigation is warranted.

Medications targeting inflammation

Reducing inflammation is a posited strategy for reducing AKI because AKI is associated with increased renal and systemic markers of inflammation and renal neutrophil infiltration. With regard to efficacy of steroids to reduce AKI, the evidence is mixed. The DECS trial randomized cardiac surgery patients to high-dose dexamethasone or placebo with an endpoint of need for RRT and found overall that dexamethasone decreased RRT, particularly in patients with advanced chronic kidney disease (CKD) [73]. This SIRS trial, however, did not find any effect of perioperative methylprednisolone on AKI [74].

Nonsteroidal antiinflammatory drugs (NSAIDs) are frequently used to treat perioperative pain but are known to contribute to AKI through constriction of the afferent arteriole with subsequent reduction in glomerular filtration rate and a risk for AKI related to interstitial nephritis [75]. The potential for an antiinflammatory benefit on AKI, however, has been investigated. Nussmeier and colleagues found a nonsignificant increase in renal dysfunction and failure in the group that received a cyclooxygenase-2 inhibitor compared with those who received perioperative placebo [76]. Aspirin was investigated in noncardiac surgery patients in the Perioperative Ischemic Evaluation 2 (POISE-2) trial, and in a subgroup analysis, there was a marginal signal for increased AKI that required dialysis in those receiving aspirin [77]. A subgroup analysis, however, did not note a difference in mild AKI with aspirin exposure [78]. Furthermore, the Aspirin and Tranexamic Acid for Coronary Artery Surgery (ATACAS) trial also did not see a difference in AKI risk for patients who continued aspirin perioperatively [79]. Therefore, there is minimal evidence to suggest that NSAIDs reduce risk of perioperative AKI, and in fact there may be an increased risk from this class of medications.

Medications to mitigate oxidative stress

Oxidative stress is independently associated with the development of AKI, and antioxidant treatments such as N-acetylcysteine (NAC), sodium bicarbonate, and statin use as well as practices such as limiting hyperoxygenation have been investigated in the perioperative period to attempt to reduce AKI [80].

NAC is a glutathione precursor and direct antioxidant. In a randomized trial of patients undergoing coronary artery bypass grafting, Burns and colleagues noted no difference in postoperative renal dysfunction between patients who received NAC versus placebo [81]. There was, however, a nonsignificant decrease in the need for RRT, and a post-hoc subgroup analysis of patients with baseline CKD showed a nonsignificant improvement in renal dysfunction with NAC administration. A subsequent trial in cardiac surgical patients showed similar results, with no significant decrease in acute renal failure in patients who received NAC [82]. NAC was also tested in the liver transplant population and was not found to decrease AKI overall. Those patients who had measurable increases in glutathione, however, did show a reduction in AKI [83].

Sodium bicarbonate has been investigated given its ability to alkalinize urine and potentially decrease AKI risk. A meta-analysis of cardiac surgery trials testing this hypothesis concluded that NAC does not affect AKI following cardiac surgery [84].

Hydroxymethylglutaryl-coenzyme A reductase inhibitors (statins) decrease oxidative damage and inflammation in preclinical studies and have been investigated for their potential to reduce AKI. In the Statin-AKI RCT, Billings and colleagues randomly assigned patients receiving cardiac surgery to high-dose perioperative atorvastatin or placebo [85]. The data safety monitoring for the trial recommended a cessation of enrollment of statin-naïve patients due to increased AKI in patients with CKD who were statin-naïve and then recommended stopping the trial for futility given no clinically significant difference in AKI. In a separate clinical trial of perioperative rosuvastatin, Zheng and colleagues found an increase in AKI in patients randomized to rosuvastatin [86]. Perioperative statin therapy does not prevent AKI.

Hyperoxygenation is common during surgery, and in observational studies excess oxygen exposure has been associated with increased AKI [87]; this may be due to increased oxidative stress. A clinical trial comparing intraoperative hyperoxia with normoxia in patients receiving cardiac surgery, however, did not demonstrate that intraoperative oxygenation strategies affect AKI [88]. The intervention was limited to the cardiopulmonary bypass period, leaving some question as to whether hyperoxia throughout the rest of surgery may have had an impact. Similarly, the use of 80% versus 30% inspired oxygen or the use of vitamin C with NAC in major abdominal surgery did not reduce KDIGO criteria AKI, an exploratory outcome in a trial targeting myocardial injury [89]. In this major abdominal surgery cohort, the overall incidence of AKI was less than 0.5%, much lower than is typical for this population, thus it was underpowered to draw conclusions regarding AKI. An ongoing RCT will assess the impact of hyperoxia versus normoxia throughout the entirely of cardiac surgery on AKI and systemic oxidative stress [90].

Ischemic preconditioning

Remote ischemic preconditioning (RIPC) may attenuate systemic ischemia-reperfusion injury [91]. RIPC is typically achieved by inducing a period of temporary ischemia on a limb using an inflatable cuff. Data regarding the efficacy of RIPC in preventing AKI is conflicting. Zarbock and colleagues conducted a small multicenter RCT in high-risk cardiac surgery patients and demonstrated a significantly reduced rate of AKI in patients who received RIPC in the immediate postoperative period and decreased major adverse kidney events at 90 days [92,93]. This effect was also observed in an RCT conducted by Zhou and colleagues in patients undergoing total aortic arch replacement [94]. RIPC was not found to affect AKI in a trial of patients undergoing valvular cardiac surgery [95], and 2 larger multicenter trial in elective cardiac surgery patients by Meybohm and colleagues and Hausenloy and colleagues did not demonstrate any difference in acute renal failure with RIPC [96,97]. The use of propofol as a maintenance anesthetic has been postulated to affect the efficacy of RIPC, as the 2 larger trials used this medication in the maintenance of anesthesia in contrast to the earlier, smaller studies that found a benefit of RIPC.

Novel and potential future therapies

Additional therapies that may help prevent AKI are currently being studied. For example, there is some initial evidence that inhaled nitric oxide may reduce perioperative AKI in cardiac surgery, and Berra and colleagues are currently completing a phase 3 trial of this therapy [98,99]. Nitric oxide may affect AKI by eliminating effects of cell-free hemoglobin or enhancing microvascular responses in the kidney. Thielmann and colleagues are studying a small interfering RNA targeting p53 and putatively reducing inflammation. An initial study found that incidence, severity, and duration of early AKI were reduced in high-risk cardiac surgery patients. This finding led to a phase 3 study that has not yet been published but was discontinued due to a lack of efficacy at 3-month follow-up, according to the clinicaltrials.gov registration (NCT03510897) [100].

Care bundles

Implementing KDIGO guidelines as a care bundle has also been a target of investigation. Meersch and colleagues demonstrated that in a single-center trial, a bundle including optimization of volume status, cardiac output, and blood pressure by use of noninvasive cardiac output monitors, avoiding nephrotoxic drugs, and preventing hyperglycemia reduced the rate of AKI compared with controls in cardiac surgery patients [101]. Göcze and colleagues used a urinary biomarker to direct which noncardiac surgery patients should receive the KDIGO care bundle through early identification of AKI risk. With these tools, incidence of AKI (as well as moderate and severe AKI) was decreased, as were postoperative creatinine, length of ICU stay, and length of hospital stay [102]. Therefore, care bundles may be a reasonable approach to help reduce perioperative AKI, but limitations include a true understanding of which interventions in the bundle are beneficial, making further improvements to these protocols difficult.

SUMMARY

Perioperative AKI remains a large burden for patients undergoing major surgery. Further investigations are necessary to help limit the incidence and impact of perioperative AKI. Although perioperative AKI remains an area of intense study, most treatments are supportive in nature. We must improve our understanding of mechanisms contributing to AKI for physicians to prevent and treat AKI more effectively.

CLINICS CARE POINTS

- Perioperative acute kidney injury induces cardiac, pulmonary, and neurologic dysfunction and increases infection in addition to reduced glomerular filtration.
- Hemodynamic and optimizing intravascular fluid are mainstays of the prevention of acute kidney injury.
- Evidence may favor delayed renal replacement therapy compared with early initiation in severe perioperative acute kidney injury.

DISCLOSURES AND FUNDING SOURCES

The authors report no conflicts of interest. M.G. Lopez received funding from NIH (Bethesda, MD, USA) grant K23GM129662 and R01HL164909. F.T. Billings received funding from U.S. NIH grant R35GM145375.

References

[1] Hobson C, Ozrazgat-Baslanti T, Kuxhausen A, et al. Cost and mortality associated with postoperative acute kidney injury. Ann Surg 2015;261(6):1207–14.

[2] Mikkelsen TB, Schack A, Oreskov JO, et al. Acute kidney injury following major emergency abdominal surgery - a retrospective cohort study based on medical records data. BMC Nephrol 2022;23(1):94.

[3] Rosner MH, Okusa MD. Acute kidney injury associated with cardiac surgery. Clin J Am Soc Nephrol 2006;1(1):19–32.

[4] Di Lullo L, Reeves PB, Bellasi A, et al. Cardiorenal syndrome in acute kidney injury. Semin Nephrol 2019;39(1):31–40.

[5] Ng RRG, Tan GHJ, Liu W, et al. The association of acute kidney injury and atrial fibrillation after cardiac surgery in an asian prospective cohort study. Medicine (Baltim) 2016;95(12):e3005.

[6] Cole OM, Tosif S, Shaw M, et al. Acute kidney injury and postoperative atrial fibrillation in patients undergoing cardiac surgery. J Cardiothorac Vasc Anesth 2020;34(7):1783–90.

[7] Ishikawa S, Griesdale DE, Lohser J. Acute kidney injury after lung resection surgery: incidence and perioperative risk factors. Anesth Analg 2012;114(6):1256–62.

[8] Liu X, Zhang J, Yang Y, et al. Analysis of risk factors of acute kidney injury in perioperative patients after lung transplantation. Ann Palliat Med 2021;10(9):9841–7.

[9] Ishikawa S, Griesdale DE, Lohser J. Acute kidney injury within 72 hours after lung transplantation: incidence and perioperative risk factors. J Cardiothorac Vasc Anesth 2014;28(4):931–5.

[10] Deng Y, Yuan J, Chi R, et al. The Incidence, risk factors and outcomes of postoperative acute kidney injury in neurosurgical critically ill patients. Sci Rep 2017;7(1):4245.

[11] Gumus F, Polat A, Yektas A, et al. Prolonged mechanical ventilation after CABG: risk factor analysis. J Cardiothorac Vasc Anesth 2015;29(1):52–8.

[12] Mehta RL, Bouchard J, Soroko SB, et al. Sepsis as a cause and consequence of acute kidney injury: Program to Improve Care in Acute Renal Disease. Intensive Care Med 2011;37(2):241–8.

[13] Rabb H, Griffin MD, McKay DB, et al. Inflammation in AKI: current understanding, key questions, and knowledge gaps. J Am Soc Nephrol 2016;27(2):371–9.

[14] Zhang WR, Garg AX, Coca SG, et al. Plasma IL-6 and IL-10 concentrations predict AKI and long-term mortality in adults after cardiac surgery. J Am Soc Nephrol: JASN (J Am Soc Nephrol) 2015;26(12):3123–32.

[15] Tagawa M, Nishimoto M, Kokubu M, et al. Acute kidney injury as an independent predictor of infection and malignancy: the NARA-AKI cohort study. J Nephrol 2019;32(6): 967–75.

[16] Griffin BR, Teixeira JP, Ambruso S, et al. Stage 1 acute kidney injury is independently associated with infection following cardiac surgery. J Thorac Cardiovasc Surg 2021;161(4): 1346–1355 e1343.

[17] Griffin BR, You Z, Holmen J, et al. Incident infection following acute kidney injury with recovery to baseline creatinine: A propensity score matched analysis. PLoS One 2019;14(6):e0217935.

[18] Kotfis K, Slozowska J, Listewnik M, et al. The impact of acute kidney injury in the perioperative period on the incidence of postoperative delirium in patients undergoing coronary artery bypass grafting-observational cohort study. Int J Environ Res Public Health 2020;17(4):1440.

[19] Baumgaertel MW, Kraemer M, Berlit P. Neurologic complications of acute and chronic renal disease. Handb Clin Neurol 2014;119:383–93.

[20] Kao CC, Wu CH, Lai CF, et al. Long-term risk of dementia following acute kidney injury: A population-based study. Ci Ji Yi Xue Za Zhi 2017;29(4):201–7.

[21] Bihorac A, Yavas S, Subbiah S, et al. Long-term risk of mortality and acute kidney injury during hospitalization after major surgery. Ann Surg 2009;249(5):851–8.

[22] French WB, Shah PR, Fatani YI, et al. Mortality and costs associated with acute kidney injury following major elective, non-cardiac surgery. J Clin Anesth 2022;82:110933.

[23] Siddiqui NF, Coca SG, Devereaux PJ, et al. Secular trends in acute dialysis after elective major surgery–1995 to 2009. CMAJ (Can Med Assoc J) 2012;184(11):1237–45.

[24] Thakar CV, Arrigain S, Worley S, et al. A clinical score to predict acute renal failure after cardiac surgery. J Am Soc Nephrol 2005;16(1):162–8.

[25] Thadhani R, Pascual M, Bonventre JV. Acute renal failure. N Engl J Med 1996;334(22): 1448–60.

[26] Billings FT, Lopez MG, Shaw AD. The incidence, risk, presentation, pathophysiology, treatment, and effects of perioperative acute kidney injury. Can J Anaesth 2021;68(3): 409–22.

[27] Devarajan P. Acute kidney injury: Acute kidney injury: still misunderstood and misdiagnosed. Nat Rev Nephrol 2017;13(3):137–8.

[28] Improving Global Outcomes (KDIGO) Acute Kidney Injury Work Group. KDIGO. Clinical Practice Guideline for Acute Kidney Injury. Kidney inter 2012;2:1–138.

[29] Zarbock A, Koyner JL, Hoste EAJ, et al. Update on perioperative acute kidney injury. Anesth Analg 2018;127(5):1236–45.

[30] Prowle JR, Kirwan CJ, Bellomo R. Fluid management for the prevention and attenuation of acute kidney injury. Nat Rev Nephrol 2014;10(1):37–47.

[31] Lopez MG, Shotwell MS, Morse J, et al. Intraoperative venous congestion and acute kidney injury in cardiac surgery: an observational cohort study. Br J Anaesth 2021;126(3): 599–607.

[32] Patschan D, Patschan S, Buschmann I, et al. Loop diuretics in acute kidney injury prevention, therapy, and risk stratification. Kidney Blood Press Res 2019;44(4):457–64.

[33] Myles PS, Bellomo R, Corcoran T, et al. Restrictive versus liberal fluid therapy for major abdominal surgery. N Engl J Med 2018;378(24):2263–74.

[34] Kellum JA, Romagnani P, Ashuntantang G, et al. Acute kidney injury. Nat Rev Dis Primers 2021;7(1):52.

[35] Xu JY, Ma SQ, Pan C, et al. A high mean arterial pressure target is associated with improved microcirculation in septic shock patients with previous hypertension: a prospective open label study. Crit Care 2015;19(1):130.

[36] Asfar P, Meziani F, Hamel JF, et al. High versus low blood-pressure target in patients with septic shock. N Engl J Med 2014;370(17):1583–93.

[37] Section 3: Prevention and Treatment of AKI. Kidney Int Suppl (2011) 2012;2(1):37–68.

[38] van den Berghe G, Wouters P, Weekers F, et al. Intensive insulin therapy in critically ill patients. N Engl J Med 2001;345(19):1359–67.

[39] Investigators N-SS, Finfer S, Chittock DR, et al. Intensive versus conventional glucose control in critically ill patients. N Engl J Med 2009;360(13):1283–97.

[40] Jacobi J, Bircher N, Krinsley J, et al. Guidelines for the use of an insulin infusion for the management of hyperglycemia in critically ill patients. Crit Care Med 2012;40(12):3251–76.

[41] Qaseem A, Chou R, Humphrey LL, et al. Clinical guidelines committee of the american college of p. inpatient glycemic control: best practice advice from the clinical guidelines committee of the american college of physicians. Am J Med Qual 2014;29(2):95–8.

[42] Fiaccadori V, Ripamonti F, Pochintesta L, et al. Multiple myeloma and severe renal impairment: A safe preparative regimen proposal for autologous stem cell transplant. Bone Marrow Transplant 2011;46:S258–9.

[43] Chawla LS, Davison DL, Brasha-Mitchell E, et al. Development and standardization of a furosemide stress test to predict the severity of acute kidney injury. Crit Care 2013;17(5):R207.

[44] Zarbock A, Kellum JA, Schmidt C, et al. Effect of early vs delayed initiation of renal replacement therapy on mortality in critically ill patients with acute kidney injury: the elain randomized clinical trial. JAMA 2016;315(20):2190–9.

[45] Gaudry S, Hajage D, Schortgen F, et al. Initiation strategies for renal-replacement therapy in the intensive care unit. N Engl J Med 2016;375(2):122–33.

[46] Barbar SD, Clere-Jehl R, Bourredjem A, et al. Timing of renal-replacement therapy in patients with acute kidney injury and sepsis. N Engl J Med 2018;379(15):1431–42.

[47] Investigators S-A. Canadian critical care trials g, australian, et al. timing of initiation of renal-replacement therapy in acute kidney injury. N Engl J Med 2020;383(3):240–51.

[48] Bellomo R, Ronco C, Kellum JA, et al. Acute dialysis quality initiative w. acute renal failure - definition, outcome measures, animal models, fluid therapy and information technology needs: the second international consensus conference of the acute dialysis quality initiative (ADQI) group. Crit Care 2004;8(4):R204–12.

[49] Bhatt GC, Das RR, Satapathy A. Early versus Late initiation of renal replacement therapy: have we reached the consensus? an updated meta-analysis. Nephron 2021;145(4): 371–85.

[50] Karkar A, Ronco C. Prescription of CRRT: a pathway to optimize therapy. Ann Intensive Care 2020;10(1):32.

[51] Carlstrom M, Wilcox CS, Arendshorst WJ. Renal autoregulation in health and disease. Physiol Rev 2015;95(2):405–511.

[52] Walsh M, Devereaux PJ, Garg AX, et al. Relationship between intraoperative mean arterial pressure and clinical outcomes after noncardiac surgery: toward an empirical definition of hypotension. Anesthesiology 2013;119(3):507–15.

[53] Tang Y, Zhu C, Liu J, et al. Association of Intraoperative hypotension with acute kidney injury after noncardiac surgery in patients younger than 60 years old. Kidney Blood Press Res 2019;44(2):211–21.

[54] Sun LY, Wijeysundera DN, Tait GA, et al. Association of intraoperative hypotension with acute kidney injury after elective noncardiac surgery. Anesthesiology 2015;123(3): 515–23.

[55] Futier E, Lefrant JY, Guinot PG, et al. Effect of individualized vs standard blood pressure management strategies on postoperative organ dysfunction among high-risk patients undergoing major surgery: a randomized clinical trial. JAMA 2017;318(14):1346–57.

[56] Salmasi V, Maheshwari K, Yang D, et al. Relationship between intraoperative hypotension, defined by either reduction from baseline or absolute thresholds, and acute kidney and myocardial injury after noncardiac surgery: a retrospective cohort analysis. Anesthesiology 2017;126(1):47–65.

[57] Mathis MR, Naik BI, Freundlich RE, et al. Preoperative risk and the association between hypotension and postoperative acute kidney injury. Anesthesiology 2020;132(3): 461–75.

[58] Gillies MA, Kakar V, Parker RJ, et al. Fenoldopam to prevent acute kidney injury after major surgery-a systematic review and meta-analysis. Crit Care 2015;19:449.

[59] Bove T, Zangrillo A, Guarracino F, et al. Effect of fenoldopam on use of renal replacement therapy among patients with acute kidney injury after cardiac surgery: a randomized clinical trial. JAMA 2014;312(21):2244–53.

[60] Friedrich JO, Adhikari N, Herridge MS, et al. Meta-analysis: low-dose dopamine increases urine output but does not prevent renal dysfunction or death. Ann Intern Med 2005;142(7):510–24.

[61] Kellum JA, J MD. Use of dopamine in acute renal failure: a meta-analysis. Crit Care Med 2001;29(8):1526–31.

[62] Mazer CD, Whitlock RP, Fergusson DA, et al. Restrictive or liberal red-cell transfusion for cardiac surgery. N Engl J Med 2017;377(22):2133–44.

[63] Mazer CD, Whitlock RP, Fergusson DA, et al. Six-Month Outcomes after Restrictive or Liberal Transfusion for Cardiac Surgery. N Engl J Med 2018;379(13):1224–33.

[64] Garg AX, Badner N, Bagshaw SM, et al. Safety of a restrictive versus liberal approach to red blood cell transfusion on the outcome of aki in patients undergoing cardiac surgery: a randomized clinical trial. J Am Soc Nephrol 2019;30(7):1294–304.

[65] Hadimioglu N, Saadawy I, Saglam T, et al. The effect of different crystalloid solutions on acid-base balance and early kidney function after kidney transplantation. Anesth Analg 2008;107(1):264–9.

[66] Khajavi MR, Etezadi F, Moharari RS, et al. Effects of normal saline vs. lactated ringer's during renal transplantation. Ren Fail 2008;30(5):535–9.

[67] Young P, Bailey M, Beasley R, et al. Effect of a buffered crystalloid solution vs saline on acute kidney injury among patients in the intensive care unit: the split randomized clinical trial. JAMA 2015;314(16):1701–10.

[68] Semler MW, Self WH, Rice TW. Balanced crystalloids versus saline in critically ill adults. N Engl J Med 2018;378(20):1951.

[69] Bledsoe J, Peltan ID, Bunnell RJ, et al. Order substitutions and education for balanced crystalloid solution use in an integrated health care system and association with major adverse kidney events. JAMA Netw Open 2022;5(5):e2210046.

[70] Lee EH, Baek SH, Chin JH, et al. Preoperative hypoalbuminemia is a major risk factor for acute kidney injury following off-pump coronary artery bypass surgery. Intensive Care Med 2012;38(9):1478–86.

[71] Lee EH, Kim WJ, Kim JY, et al. Effect of exogenous albumin on the incidence of postoperative acute kidney injury in patients undergoing off-pump coronary artery bypass surgery with a preoperative albumin level of less than 4.0 g/dl. Anesthesiology 2016;124(5): 1001–11.

[72] Lazzareschi DV, Fong N, Mavrothalassitis O, et al. Intraoperative use of albumin in major non-cardiac surgery: incidence, variability, and association with outcomes. Ann Surg 2022; https://doi.org/10.1097/SLA.0000000000005774.

[73] Jacob KA, Leaf DE, Dieleman JM, et al. Intraoperative high-dose dexamethasone and severe aki after cardiac surgery. J Am Soc Nephrol 2015;26(12):2947–51.

[74] Whitlock RP, Devereaux PJ, Teoh KH, et al. Methylprednisolone in patients undergoing cardiopulmonary bypass (SIRS): a randomised, double-blind, placebo-controlled trial. Lancet 2015;386(10000):1243–53.

[75] Ravnskov U. Glomerular, tubular and interstitial nephritis associated with non-steroidal antiinflammatory drugs. Evidence of a common mechanism. Br J Clin Pharmacol 1999;47(2):203–10.

[76] Nussmeier NA, Whelton AA, Brown MT, et al. Complications of the COX-2 inhibitors parecoxib and valdecoxib after cardiac surgery. N Engl J Med 2005;352(11):1081–91.

[77] Devereaux PJ, Mrkobrada M, Sessler DI, et al. Aspirin in patients undergoing noncardiac surgery. N Engl J Med 2014;370(16):1494–503.

[78] Garg AX, Kurz A, Sessler DI, et al. Perioperative aspirin and clonidine and risk of acute kidney injury: a randomized clinical trial. JAMA 2014;312(21):2254–64.

[79] Myles PS, Smith JA, Forbes A, et al. Stopping vs. continuing aspirin before coronary artery surgery. N Engl J Med 2016;374(8):728–37.

[80] Billings FT, Pretorius M, Schildcrout JS, et al. Obesity and oxidative stress predict AKI after cardiac surgery. J Am Soc Nephrol: JASN (J Am Soc Nephrol) 2012;23(7):1221–8.

[81] Burns KE, Chu MW, Novick RJ, et al. Perioperative N-acetylcysteine to prevent renal dysfunction in high-risk patients undergoing cabg surgery: a randomized controlled trial. JAMA 2005;294(3):342–50.

[82] Sisillo E, Ceriani R, Bortone F, et al. N-acetylcysteine for prevention of acute renal failure in patients with chronic renal insufficiency undergoing cardiac surgery: a prospective, randomized, clinical trial. Crit Care Med 2008;36(1):81–6.

[83] Hilmi IA, Peng Z, Planinsic RM, et al. N-acetylcysteine does not prevent hepatorenal ischaemia-reperfusion injury in patients undergoing orthotopic liver transplantation. Nephrol Dial Transplant 2010;25(7):2328–33.

[84] Tian ML, Hu Y, Yuan J, et al. Efficacy and safety of perioperative sodium bicarbonate therapy for cardiac surgery-associated acute kidney injury: a meta-analysis. J Cardiovasc Pharmacol 2015;65(2):130–6.

[85] Billings FT, Hendricks PA, Schildcrout JS, et al. High-dose perioperative atorvastatin and acute kidney injury following cardiac surgery: a randomized clinical trial. JAMA 2016;315(9):877–88.

[86] Zheng Z, Jayaram R, Jiang L, et al. Perioperative rosuvastatin in cardiac surgery. N Engl J Med 2016;374(18):1744–53.

[87] McIlroy DR, Shotwell MS, Lopez MG, et al. Oxygen administration during surgery and postoperative organ injury: observational cohort study. BMJ 2022;379:e070941.

[88] McGuinness SP, Parke RL, Drummond K, et al. A multicenter, randomized, controlled phase iib trial of avoidance of hyperoxemia during cardiopulmonary bypass. Anesthesiology 2016;125(3):465–73.

[89] Holse C, Aasvang EK, Vester-Andersen M, et al. Hyperoxia and antioxidants for myocardial injury in noncardiac surgery: A 2 x 2 factorial, blinded, randomized clinical trial. Anesthesiology 2022;136(3):408–19.

[90] Lopez MG, Pretorius M, Shotwell MS, et al. The risk of oxygen during cardiac surgery (ROCS) trial: study protocol for a randomized clinical trial. Trials 2017;18(1):295.

[91] Tapuria N, Kumar Y, Habib MM, et al. Remote ischemic preconditioning: a novel protective method from ischemia reperfusion injury—a review. J Surg Res 2008;150(2):304–30.

[92] Zarbock A, Kellum JA, Van Aken H, et al. Long-term effects of remote ischemic preconditioning on kidney function in high-risk cardiac surgery patients: follow-up results from the RenalRIP trial. Anesthesiology 2017;126(5):787–98.

[93] Zarbock A, Schmidt C, Van Aken H, et al. Effect of remote ischemic preconditioning on kidney injury among high-risk patients undergoing cardiac surgery: a randomized clinical trial. JAMA 2015;313(21):2133–41.

[94] Zhou H, Yang L, Wang G, et al. Remote ischemic preconditioning prevents postoperative acute kidney injury after open total aortic arch replacement: a double-blind, randomized, sham-controlled trial. Anesth Analg 2019;129(1):287–93.

[95] Song JW, Lee WK, Lee S, et al. Remote ischaemic conditioning for prevention of acute kidney injury after valvular heart surgery: a randomised controlled trial. Br J Anaesth 2018;121(5):1034–40.

[96] Meybohm P, Bein B, Brosteanu O, et al. A multicenter trial of remote ischemic preconditioning for heart surgery. N Engl J Med 2015;373(15):1397–407.

[97] Hausenloy DJ, Candilio L, Evans R, et al. Remote ischemic preconditioning and outcomes of cardiac surgery. N Engl J Med 2015;373(15):1408–17.

[98] Lei C, Berra L, Rezoagli E, et al. Nitric oxide decreases acute kidney injury and stage 3 chronic kidney disease after cardiac surgery. Am J Respir Crit Care Med 2018;198(10):1279–87.

[99] Marrazzo F, Spina S, Zadek F, et al. Protocol of a randomised controlled trial in cardiac surgical patients with endothelial dysfunction aimed to prevent postoperative acute kidney injury by administering nitric oxide gas. BMJ Open 2019;9(7):e026848.

[100] Thielmann M, Corteville D, Szabo G, et al. Teprasiran, a small interfering RNA, for the prevention of acute kidney injury in high-risk patients undergoing cardiac surgery: a randomized clinical study. Circulation 2021;144(14):1133–44.

[101] Meersch M, Schmidt C, Hoffmeier A, et al. Prevention of cardiac surgery-associated AKI by implementing the KDIGO guidelines in high risk patients identified by biomarkers: the PrevAKI randomized controlled trial. Intensive Care Med 2017;43(11):1551–61.

[102] Gocze I, Jauch D, Gotz M, et al. Biomarker-guided intervention to prevent acute kidney injury after major surgery: the prospective randomized BigpAK study. Ann Surg 2018;267(6):1013–20.

Advances in Anesthesia 41 (2023) 225–238

ADVANCES IN ANESTHESIA

Donation After Cardiac Death
Origins, Current State, and New Directions

Nathan E. Ashby, MD

Division of Critical Care Medicine, Department of Anesthesiology, Vanderbilt University Medical Center, 1211 21st Avenue South, MAB Suite 422, Nashville, TN 37212, USA

Keywords

- Donation after cardiac death • Donation after circulatory death
- Organ transplantation • Normothermic regional perfusion

Key points

- Organs for transplantation have been and remain in short supply and represent a significant limiter on the field.
- Early organ donation was limited to donation after cardiac death (DCD) and a few living donors for renal transplantation.
- The development of the concept of brain death dramatically changed the source of organs for transplantation but did not resolve the shortage of organs.
- DCD has come back into increasing use in an effort to increase the available transplantable organs.
- New technology may further increase the ability of DCD to help fill the shortfall of needed organs.

INTRODUCTION

Most anesthesia providers will recognize that drug and equipment shortages have become an increasingly common occurrence in the field and that this has had an impact on the ability to provide safe and effective anesthesia. Although drug shortages have always occurred, the frequency, severity and length of shortages has grown in the past 2 decades [1]. These shortages were exacerbated by the coronavirus disease 2019 pandemic and have continued to interfere with anesthesia provider's ability to provide care for patients [2]. Yet as significant as these recent shortages have been for anesthesiology, one area of medicine has suffered a sustained and severe shortage of needed supplies since its inception—organ transplantation. In 2022, there

E-mail address: Nathan.ashby@vumc.org

https://doi.org/10.1016/j.aan.2023.06.008
0737-6146/23/© 2023 Elsevier Inc. All rights reserved.

were approximately 42,800 organ transplantations in the United States, passing the 1 million all-time transplant mark in the United States that same year [3]. Without question, the number of transplants being performed annually is ever growing. Unfortunately, the waiting list for organs has grown even faster and supply of viable organs for transplant has always outstripped demand. At the time of writing, more than 104,000 individuals were on the wait list in the United States with an estimated 6200 individuals dying annually while waiting on an organ for transplant [4]. Although scientific advances continue to push medicine closer to implantable mechanical replacements, laboratory-grown artificial organs, or xenotransplantation, viable alternatives for the current pattern of organ transplantation are still likely years, if not decades, away. The disparity between available organs and those who need them continue to drive organ donation efforts and advancements. The growing number of transplants as well as organ donations put anesthesia providers in growing contact with the field. It therefore behooves anesthesia practitioners to maintain some level of understanding of the field because there are far fewer places in modern medicine that can be as ethically challenging as organ transplantation.

The majority of donated organs currently come from brain dead donors or living related donors [5]. These are sources that are likely to be familiar to many anesthesia providers because they may have been involved in the process of donation or transplantation from these sources at some point in their training or practice. However, a growing number of donations now come from another source. Donation after cardiac death (alternately termed donation after circulatory death and hereafter noted as DCD) has been one of the most active areas of growth to increase available organs for transplant. Although this is an expanding area of organ donation, it is not a new one because the first transplants were often done from donors that would fit these criteria [6], although it did not carry that name at the time. This article seeks to give some understanding of the history of DCD from its origins in early organ transplantation experiments through to modern activity. This article will touch on how this history affects DCD today as well as potential future advances so that practicing anesthesia providers are familiar with the process.

TRANSPLANT HISTORY

Most practitioners are aware of organ transplantation and likely view it as a well-established part of modern medical practice. However, the science of successful transplantation has a relatively short history. Tissue and organ transplantation was first contemplated as far back as 1550 BCE in the form of skin grafting to heal burns [7]. Reports of successful autogenous skin grafts and plastic reconstructions from transplanted tissue appear from about 600 BCE through the end of the sixteenth century [7,8], although the first verifiable successful skin graft was not documented until 1869 [7]. However, these early grafts focused on transplant of tissue from one part of the patient to another (autografts). Although there were attempts to transfer tissue between individuals (homografts), there was little appreciation of the abject failure of these transfers due to issues with surgical technique and poor scientific method [8]. It was not until the early twentieth century that the futility of homografting was fully appreciated [8] and the effort to understand why grafts failed, how they failed, and how to avoid this came into full focus. Research on understanding the immune response and how to suppress it by researchers through the course of the early twentieth century was key to the development of the transplantation field [8,9]. This research on the immune system was accompanied and fueled by experiments developing the surgical techniques needed to make organ transplantation possible. Although skin grafting provided the foundation on which transplantation was built, the initial target of organ donation research was the kidney and the first half of the twentieth century saw attempts around the world to make kidney transplant a reality. Early renal transplant experiments focused on xenografts attempted between animal species and then later between various animal species and humans [8]. These were all predictable failures but continued to provide small bits of the puzzle to understanding rejection. Although the science of immunosuppression was still lagging, the 1930s saw the first human-to-human transplant attempts by Voronoy in Russia followed by a series of attempts in the 1950s in France and in Boston [9]. Although the last transplant in the French group, from a mother to a son, and one in the Boston group did function for a short time following the procedure, these too eventually failed [8]. The year 1954 saw the first truly successful kidney transplant performed between identical twin brothers in the United States [7]. Although this skirted the problems of immunosuppression and rejection, the success was enough to continue fueling research despite the prior decades of frustration. Finally, in the 1960s, kidney transplantation became a reality. Initial attempts with immunosuppression using irradiation to suppress the immune response gave glimpses of success [7]. However, most point to the development of azathioprine and its combination with high dose prednisone as described by Starzl to suppress the immune system as the true beginning of the transplant era [8,10].

Although the initial work of organ transplantation arose from an interest in kidney transplantation, other organs rapidly became the focus as the science of immunosuppression was further established. To accomplish this, new surgical techniques were developed, first in animal laboratories and later in patients with terminal disease processes. The year 1963 saw the first attempt at lung transplantation by James Hardy with a Mississippi man living for 18 days following the attempt [11]. It would be almost a decade before any significant and sustained success would be made in the area [10]. The first tentative steps at liver transplantation were taken in 1963 by Thomas Starzl, although the first recipient died on the operating room table and the other 2 recipients only lived from 7 to 22 days [12]. It would be 1967 before the field would see the first sustained successes in liver transplant [13]. South Africa would produce the first successes in heart transplant in 1967 [6] by Christiaan Barnard, although these were again limited because the first recipient lived only 18 days. With these first tantalizing steps, organ transplantation became a reality in the 1960s, although the science would require decades more research to achieve the outcomes that modern readers would recognize as success.

EARLY DONORS

The review of the foundation of organ transplantation is relevant to the discussion of DCD for 2 reasons. First, to impress on the reader the immense change in the science of organ donation over a relatively short period and how this rapid change will continue to be seen in the field. Second, to show that what is new was once old. Organ donation has its earliest roots in DCD. Perhaps, the first mention of donating tissues or organs from a dead person to a living one may come from the stories of Saint Cosmas and Damian. These early Christian saints were the frequent subjects of medieval and Renaissance artists who frequently depicted the duo replacing the diseased leg of a Deacon of Rome with that of a recently deceased Moor [14]. The deacon had fallen asleep praying to Cosmas and Damian to cure his leg and had a dream that the duo came to his side in the night and gave him a new limb. When he awoke, he had a strong and healthy leg but the skin was dark. Meanwhile, the body of a Moor who had recently died was found missing a leg. Although this is not a scientific account, it does demonstrate that the idea of transplantation of body parts from a deceased person to a living one originated long before the ability to do so was ever developed.

Those early renal transplant attempts mostly derived donated organs from individuals following cessation of cardiac function. Voronoy's 1933 attempt at kidney transplantation used a kidney taken from a dead donor 6 hours after the patient had been declared, likely contributing to the failure of the graft [8]. The French attempts in the 1950s sped the process up because they initially used kidneys harvested immediately after the donors died from execution by the guillotine [9]. The early Boston attempts obtained some of the kidneys transplanted from donors who died during surgery [8]. Of course, the fact that most healthy humans have 2 kidneys with excess capability allowed for the option of living related donation as well. These early living related donations provided some notable exceptions to organs derived from dead donors including the first successful transplant between the twin brothers in Boston in 1954 [9].

As transplantation advanced, the availability of living donors was not an option with the other organs during these early experimental days. The first attempt at lung transplantation derived the transplanted organ from a patient who presented to the emergency department of the University of Mississippi Hospital and ultimately succumbed to a massive myocardial infarction [15]. It would not be until 1990 that living related lung donation would become a possibility as lobar transplant from adult to child was pioneered at Stanford [16]. The first heart transplant similarly derived the donor graft from a deceased individual. In this case, the donor was a young female who had sustained devastating and nonsurvivable brain injury after being hit by a car. As the concept of brain death was in its infancy at this time, Barnard had to ensure that the donor had succumbed to cardiac arrest before harvesting the organ for transplantation. In order to accomplish this task, he had the State Forensic Pathologist present and declare the patient once she had passed before rapidly opening the chest and starting cardiopulmonary bypass and cooling before removing the donated heart [17]. Early attempts at liver transplantation similarly used organs harvested from patients declared dead following cessation of cardiac function. Due to the technical difficulties of extracting the organ and maintaining graft function, extensive work was required to choose the potential donor and rapid resuscitation of the organ had to be performed after declaration of death [13,18]. It would be 1989 before living donor liver transplantation would become a reality [19].

SEA CHANGE

As noted, early organ transplantation was limited to the use of donors who had suffered cardiac death (with a few cases of living donor in renal transplant) because, at the time, there was no other formal conception of death. As the sciences of immunosuppression, surgical technique, and organ preservation (jump started in the early 1960s [9]) developed through the middle of the twentieth century, the ethics and legal frameworks surrounding transplant were forced to keep up. Regardless of the successes in these areas of transplant research, the difficulty of obtaining viable grafts would make transplantation a fringe field if a larger supply of grafts was not available. The development of the concept of brain death was of major importance in driving the transplant field into the mainstream because more high-quality organs became available for transplantation. Although no formal definition or agreement of brain death existed in the early days of transplantation, many of the early researchers demonstrated a preference for donors who had sustained severe neurological injuries [13,17,18]. This allowed for a level of predictability in the donor suffering cardiac arrest once life support equipment was removed. This might have also been influenced by a growing sense of the incompatibility between recovery or sustained life and the most severe forms of neurological injury. By 1959, authors began to write about irreversible loss of neurological function while maintaining a heartbeat if appropriately supported with mechanical ventilation. This was labeled "coma dépassé" or "death of the nervous system" by these authors [20]. This early discussion of coma dépassé influenced a Belgian surgeon, Guy Alexandre, who developed a series of conditions that he thought were indicative of death by failure of the neurological system. In 1963, he used this list of conditions to justify the first organ transplant from a "beating heart donor" when he removed a kidney from a patient who had suffered a significant neurological injury and who met the parameters of coma dépassé, thus opening the era of brain death donation [7]. This would be followed by a similar event in Sweden in 1964 when a single kidney was removed from a donor with significant neurological injury while awaiting death by cardiovascular criteria. This would trigger an uproar in the Swedish medical and legal communities for a time but prompted formulation of additional criteria for consideration of brain death [21]. Alexandre would go on to repeat the process of harvesting donor kidneys from coma dépassé patients several more times before presenting his study to a group of leading names in the realm of transplantation at the CIBA Symposium on Transplantation in 1966 [20]. Although this meeting did not lead to a definitive publication of the concept of brain death, it did contribute some of the early work on developing the concept. A few years later, the Ad Hoc Committee of the Harvard Medical School published their clinical definition of brain death and the concept rapidly became medically and legally accepted [20]. Concepts of brain death have continued to be refined and clarified up to the present day [22]. A series of legal acts further enshrined brain death and its interface with organ donation, including the establishment of the Uniform Anatomical Gift Act in 1968, the Uniform Definition of Death Act in 1981, and The National Organ Transplant Act of 1984 [10] in the United States. Organs harvested from brain-dead donors rapidly became the norm and DCD became a rare occurrence for several decades [23].

WHAT IS OLD IS NEW

As the science of organ transplantation matured in the 1980s and early 1990s, transplantation became increasingly common and successful. Although the donor pool increased during this time, it did not increase at the same rate as those being listed for transplant [24]. Despite efforts to increase the donor pool through advocacy for living related donors, broader criteria for accepting organs, and improved donation efficiency, gains were well outstripped by increasing demand [25]. This deficit drove interest in going back to the original donor source—postcardiac death donors, often termed "non–heart beating donors" in contrast to the "heart-beating" brain-dead donor. A few transplant centers had maintained formal programs for non–heart beating donors, such as the University of Wisconsin at Madison, although they produced relatively small numbers of organs during several decades and were largely focused on renal transplants [26]. During this time, however, these groups also began to look at the viability of other organs from non–heart beating donors [27]. Other programs with a history of procuring non–heart beating donors in special circumstances began to look at developing new formal programs with standardized criteria and protocols. One of the early centers tackling the question of how to pursue DCD in a more systematic manner in the United States was the University of Pittsburgh. Although initial conversations about how best to create such a program had been ongoing among members of the University staff since 1987, there had been no events to drive the conversations to a conclusion. It was not until a series of requests by 4 patients/families to donate following removal of life support, and the questions/issues those requests raised, that a policy was initially formulated [28]. An internal policy was ultimately produced and published in 1992. It would be disseminated and became a significant focus of the discussion of non–heart beating donation during the next couple of years [29]. Research in the United States was also being mirrored in Europe with the Maastricht group being one of the early leaders in the field. The study from this center set forth the commonly cited Maastricht classification of non–heart beating donors (Table 1 Below) [30], although this would be modified several times during the next several years with some groups adding a category for euthanasia (legal in some European countries) or splitting out the in-hospital unsuccessful resuscitations from the out-of-hospital [31].

The discussion about the legality and ethics of DCD as well as the growing need for donated organs would continue during the next several years. Given the potential for ethical pit falls and the immense need for organs, the topic ultimately prompted the Department of Health and Human Services to instruct the Institute of Medicine to undertake an extensive evaluation of the subject of organ donation following death by cardiac criteria. This identified that DCD was a viable option for organ donation but that there was a need for well thought-out policies and procedures for any hospital or organ procurement organization (OPO) undertaking donation in these circumstances [25]. With the legitimacy of DCD assured, DCD went from less than a hundred donors per year in the 1990s to 4778 by 2022 [5].

TIME OF DEATH

The overriding influence of the Dead Donor Rule has driven organ donation policy and practice for decades. This ethical concept mandates that donors must be dead before the removal of any vital organs and that removal of organs cannot result in the donor's death [32]. Because of this influence, the criteria for diagnosing brain death in the United States has been repeatedly refined with guidelines published by the American Academy of Neurology in 1995 followed by a significant review and revision in 2010 [33]. Brain death was further clarified and expanded in 2020 [22] in an international

Table 1
Original Maastricht classification system for donation after cardiac death donors

Category 1 Dead on arrival	Uncontrolled	Presenting to the health-care system already dead with no resuscitation efforts made
Category 2 Unsuccessful resuscitation	Uncontrolled	Patient arrested inside or outside of the health-care system, unsuccessful resuscitation
Category 3 Awaiting cardiac arrest	Controlled or uncontrolled	Withdrawal of care in the operating room (OR) (controlled) or outside the OR (uncontrolled)
Category 4 Cardiac arrest after brain death	Uncontrolled	Donor who suffers brain death but then suffers cardiac arrest before organ donation

collaboration, although there remains controversy in some of the details. Given the amount of effort put into ensuring that brain death is diagnosed and dealt with in a uniform manner across the country (and the world), it may be surprising that the DCD process is more localized and is affected by local law as well as hospital and OPO policy. Part of this variability develops from the manner in which cardiac death is diagnosed. There had been little debate over the centuries about how to diagnose a patient as having died by cardiopulmonary criteria [34]. As the diagnosis was often made well after the event, death was often obvious with lack of heartbeat or breath during a prolonged period and development of rigor, postmortem livedo, and even putrefaction assisting with recognition. However, as time of death became important in civil law [35] and then even more important in organ donation [34, 36], attempts to develop criteria for determining death were made in legal statues. Although the Uniform Determination of Death Act looked to create a baseline definition of brain death and cardiopulmonary death across all US state law, it provided very little detail [37] and has arguably contributed to the variety in DCD protocols. Because of the need for irreversibility in diagnosing death and the need for donors to be diagnosed as dead, DCD policies vary in the length of time that the patient must be observed to ensure that death has occurred and is irreversible. This ranged from a low of 2 minutes in some protocols to as much 10 minutes [36] with even some outliers to 20 minutes [23] in the 1997 Institute of Medicine review. Given the variability in this area and others noted in the 1997 IOM review, additional work by the Institute of Medicine was undertaken in 2000 and focused on 5 minutes although noted that there were protocols that recommended 2 minutes [38].

ETHICS CONSIDERATIONS

Even in the early days of organ transplantation, there was a recognition of the potential for conflict of interest and violation of basic medical ethics in obtaining organs for transplantation. Starzl wrote about the need to separate the team caring for a patient that was to undergo the removal of life support from the transplanting team in the 1960s [18]. The policy produced out of the work at the University of Pittsburgh further held up this separation of the patient's care team and the transplant team [28,29] and was considered an important part of the policies developed by OPOs and reviewed in the Institute of Medicine study [25]. The Pittsburgh study also placed an emphasis on the separation of the decisions to withdraw life-support from the consideration of organ donation [29]. Although the 1997 Institute of Medicine study noted that there were differences among OPOs in when the discussion of donation might occur between the OPO and the attending physician for the patient, it upheld that the decision of withdrawal of life support was independent of any consideration of donation potential, which was reiterated in the 2000 report [25,38]. Furthermore, the emphasis of using medication only to control symptoms during the dying process and not for the purpose of shortening the dying process was an early theme [29] in policies for DCD.

One area of ethical debate that has persisted through the development of modern DCD protocols has centered on what medications or procedures to preserve organ function are acceptable before the declaration of death. Heparin is generally needed to circulate through the organs to prevent microthrombi damaging the organs during the recovery process. This is done most efficiently by allowing the patient's cardiac function to do this before death occurs, although there have been concerns that this might contribute to the death of the patient in select instances and has been an area of evolution in many protocols [25,38,39]. This concern is typically thought to be manageable and is generally dealt with via the informed consent process [39]. More invasive preparations such as femoral cannulation for postmortem cooling have caused significantly more consternation and vary by hospital and OPO [25]. Regardless, any such procedures should be discussed in the informed consent process and must be explicitly agreed to by the patient or their decision maker if this is to happen [38,39].

MODERN DONATION AFTER CARDIAC DEATH

Given the above areas of influence, it is easy to see how the DCD process has been developed at a more local level than the work governing brain death. Although there are overarching expectations on DCD processes [38,39], there remains local variation in the details due to this history. Therefore, a generalized description of DCD can be given but readers should note that their local protocols may differ in some details. The ASA maintains a well-structured guideline on DCD that is a good starting place for anesthesia providers to reference [39]. Most DCD donations occur under controlled circumstances (Maastricht Category 3 patients) and are the focus of the following. In general, patients who present to the health-care system with illness or injury that is life threatening without the constant intervention of advanced medical therapy will form the pool of potential candidates for DCD. Many of these will have devastating neurological injuries but will fall short of meeting the diagnosis of brain death. Others may have cardiopulmonary disease processes requiring advanced therapies such as extracorporeal membrane oxygenation (ECMO) but for whom there is no exit strategy possible. Regardless of the disease process, care is focused solely on the patient and any conversations about withdrawal of life support and a shift to comfort care are governed only by the patient's wishes and the limits of what the medical team can provide in achieving those goals. Although there are a variety of notification laws and policies that require notice to the OPO of a patient who is unlikely to survive hospitalization, the OPO does not influence the decision to move to comfort or not and only contacts the patient or their decision maker after the decision of withdrawal of life support is made [38]. If the patient's wishes are consistent with organ donation, the OPO may request a delay in withdrawal of life support to allow time for establishing donation potential and matching. Any procedures or laboratories needed to make this assessment are the financial responsibility of the OPO [38,39] and will require informed consent. Once organ donation potential has been established, the DCD process is set in motion. Here is where much of the variation comes into play. Although all centers will initiate comfort medications as needed and prepare to remove life support, the location and timing varies from locale to locale [39]. Some centers will perform the transition off of life support in the intensive care unit (ICU), some in the post-anesthesia care unit (PACU) or other OR adjacent area, and others in the OR itself. Based on local protocol, any meds or procedures agreed to as part of the informed consent designed to improve the function of recovered organs would generally be given or completed at this time. Regardless of location, the organ recovery team is not present in the same location at the time of withdrawal of support. In many centers, arrangements are made for family presence with the patient, even if in the operating room [38]. Due to the need to minimize warm ischemia, the preparation of the operating room for organ recovery is verified. Once all of these arrangements are complete, life support is removed and only comfort medications are continued. These are titrated to treat symptoms only and are governed by the same protocols as patients transitioning to comfort outside of the DCD process [38]. The patient is closely monitored for transition to cardiopulmonary death. If this does not occur within a specified period, the patient should be returned to the ICU or other appropriate location and comfort care continued as it would for a non-DCD patient. The length of time to observe for cardiopulmonary death will vary from institution to institution but is commonly 1 hour although some protocols allow for longer [39]. If death is observed, this is diagnosed by an appropriate member of the patient's care team and the patient is monitored for the recommended period of observation per local protocol (typically 2–5 minutes) [38,39]. Once declared, the patient care providers leave the location and do not participate in the organ recovery. In locations where the DCD process is performed outside of the OR, the donor (patient becomes a donor only at the diagnosis of death) would need to be moved to the operating room. Any additional preparations such as skin prep and final positioning would be completed at this time. The patient's organs are rapidly cooled and examined for any obvious exclusions. Generally, the anesthesia provider's role in the DCD process will be limited. Comfort care administration and pronouncement of death will be commonly be done by ICU personnel or the patient's primary provider, although there may be local protocols that use the local anesthesia services to do so. If this is the case, those individuals are prohibited from participating in the organ recovery or the anesthesia of the transplant recipient [39]. More commonly, although still rare, anesthesia providers may be asked to assist with the recovery procedures, especially if thoracic organs are to be taken. This may entail reintubating the donor to allow inflation of the lungs [39].

ADVANCES
As DCD has gained acceptance, available organs have increased [5]. Early DCD grafts suffered significantly from warm ischemia but as transplantation

science progressed cooling made significant improvements in graft function [9]. Early experiments by Alexis Carrell and Charles Lindbergh in machine perfusion of the kidney resurfaced and were applied to renal grafts obtained from DCD [23]. This perfusion of kidneys on pump has increased the utilization of marginal grafts because they can be conditioned and monitored for signs that they will recover when implanted [23,40]. Liver perfusion has followed and is increasing the number of marginal grafts that can be successfully implanted [23,40]. Additionally, machine perfusion has shown some promise for rehabilitating previously nonviable hepatic grafts and may open the way for longer periods from excision to transplant [40].

Initially DCD was largely viewed as a source of kidney and liver grafts, although the earliest lung and heart transplants were sourced from donors following cardiac death. Concerns over the ischemic time of these organs led many transplant centers to view DCD sourced organs with suspicion. Additionally, these organs have much lower tolerable times of static cold storage in general, which are further decreased when applied to organs subjected to the warm ischemia of DCD [41]. Machine perfusion of these organs has opened new possibilities. By applying machine perfusion, some sense of the organ's function may be possible while also preserving it during the evaluation period [41]. Additionally, machine perfusion has opened the way for longer storage and, perhaps more importantly, transport times of thoracic organs. This has the potential to provide more viable grafts that can be matched to a wider range of recipients leading to better organ utilization patterns [41].

Although the science of organ preservation and rehab has been advanced with developments in ex vivo pump technology, these techniques are not yet widely available for all organs. One of the potentially more useful applications of technology in DCD organ procurement may lie in normothermic regional perfusion (NRP). In this technique, the donor is rapidly cannulated as if for veno-arterial (VA) ECMO following declaration of death. Use of an oxygenator in the circuit allows for the circulation of oxygenated blood to the organs during this period. This minimizes ischemic time while dissection is undertaken and allows flushing of ischemia-induced cellular byproducts. As in machine perfusion, this can rehabilitate a marginal liver [40]. It can similarly benefit the heart and lungs [41,42] minimizing ischemic time and allowing the organs to recover metabolically for a period. Of particular advantage to this technique is that the organs can be monitored for function for a period in situ allowing the transplant surgeon to evaluate the graft before committing a recipient to excision of the native organ. Although this technique holds great promise, it is ethically more challenging because the action of NRP could be seen as undoing the "irreversibility" of death on which DCD is mandated [41]. To avoid violation of the dead donor rule, the great vessels must be ligated before the initiation of flow through the circuit [42]. This prevents the brain from being resuscitated and effectively shifts the DCD donor to a brain-dead donor during the graft harvest [41].

SUMMARY

Organ transplantation is now a well-established therapy that benefits large numbers of patients but is limited by access to scarce resources in the form of donor grafts. Return to the utilization of organs donated following cardiac death has helped to fill the gap, although there is still a significant need. DCD requires careful attention to detail because there are several potential ethical pitfalls. To avoid this, centers must have clear policies and procedures in place if they are to participate in DCD. Although warm ischemia has been a major limiter to the use of these organs, newer technologies and techniques have rapidly improved outcomes and allowed for increasing utilization from the DCD pool. These new techniques and technologies will continue to challenge the ethical framework on which DCD is built. Continued careful thought and discussion is needed to ensure that the balance is maintained.

DISCLOSURE

The author has nothing to disclose.

References

[1] De Oliveira GS Jr, Theilken LS, McCarthy RJ. Shortage of perioperative drugs: implications for anesthesia practice and patient safety. Anesth Analg 2011;113(6):1429–35.

[2] Feinstein DM, Popovich M. Anesthesiologists face increasing, more routine, equipment shortages. ASA Monitor 2023;87:18–9.

[3] Available at: https://unos.org/news/2022-organ-transplants-again-set-annual-records/. Accessed 4/23/2023.

[4] Available at: https://www.organdonor.gov/learn/organ-donation-statistics. Accessed 4/23/2023.

[5] Available at: https://optn.transplant.hrsa.gov/data/view-data-reports/national-data/. Accessed 4/23/2023.

[6] Barnard CN. The operation. A human cardiac transplant: an interim report of a successful operation performed at Groote Schuur Hospital, Cape Town. S Afr Med J 1967;41:1271–4.

[7] Nordham KD, Ninokawa S. The history of organ transplantation. SAVE Proc 2022;35(1):124–8.

[8] Barker CF, Markman JF. Historical overview of transplantation. Cold Springs Harb Perspect Med 2013;3(4):a014977.

[9] Starzl TE. History of clinical transplantation. World J Surg 2000;24(7):759–82.

[10] Available at: https://www.organdonor.gov/learn/history. Accessed 4/23/2023.

[11] Hardy JD. The first lung transplant in man (1963) and the first heart transplant in man (1964). Transplant Proc 1999;31(1–2):25–9.

[12] Starzl TE, Marchioro TL, Von Kaulla KN, et al. Homotransplantation of the liver in humans. Surg Gynecol Obstet 1963;117:659–76.

[13] Starzl TE, Groth CG, Brettschneider L, et al. Orthotopic homotransplantation of the human liver. Ann Surg 1968;168(3):392–415.

[14] Lippi D. The transplant of the white man's leg: a novel representation of cosma and damian's miracle. Int J Immunopathol Pharmacol 2009;22(2):517–20.

[15] Venuta F, Van Raemdonck D. History of lung transplantation. J Thorac Dis 2017;9(12):5458–71.

[16] Starnes VA, Lewiston NJ, Luikart H, et al. Current trends in lung transplantation. Lobar transplantation and expanded use of single lungs. J Thorac Cardiovasc Surg 1992;104:1060–5.

[17] Brink JG, Hassoulas J. The first human heart transplant and further advances in cardiac trans-plantation at Groote Schuur Hospital and the University of Cape Town. Cardiovascular Jour-nal of Africa 2009;20(1):31–5.

[18] Starzl TE, Marchioro TL, Porter KA. Progress in homotransplantation of the liver. Adv Surg 1966;2:295–370.

[19] Chan SC, Fan ST. Historical perspective of living donor liver transplantation. World J Gastro-enterol 2008;14(1):15–21.

[20] Machado C. The first organ transplant from a brain-dead donor. Neurology 2005;64(11):1938–42.

[21] DeVita MA, Snyder JV, Grenvik A. History of organ donation by patients with cardiac death. Kennedy Inst Ethics J 1993;3(2):113–29.

[22] Greer DM, Shermie SD, Lewis A, et al. Determination of brain death/death by neurologic criteria, the world brain death project. JAMA 2020;324(11):1078–97.

[23] Langer RM. Donation after cardiac death – from then to now. Transplantation Report 2023;8(1):100119.

[24] D'Alessandro AM, Hoffman RM, Belzer FO. Non-heart beating donors: one response to the organ shortage. Transplant Rev 1995;9(4):168–76.

[25] Potts JT Jr, Herdman R. Non-heart-beating organ transplantation: medical and ethical issues in procurement. Washington (DC): National Academies Press (US); 1997 PMID: 25101455.

[26] Cooper JT, Chin LT, Krieger NR, et al. Donation after cardiac death: the university of wiscon-sin experience with renal transplantation. Am J Transplant 2004;4:1490–4.

[27] D'Alessandro AM, Hoffman RM, Knechtle SJ, et al. Successful extrarenal transplantation from non-heart beating donors. Transplantation 1995;59:977–82.

[28] DeVita MA, Snyder JV. Development of the university of pittsburgh medical center policy for the care of terminally ill patients who may become organ donors after death following the removal of life support. Kennedy Inst Ethics J 1993;3(2):131–43.

[29] University of pittsburgh medical center policy and procedure manual. Kennedy Inst Ethics J 1993;3(2):A-1-A-15.

[30] Daemon JWUC, deWit RJ, Heineman E, et al. Kidney transplantation from non-heart-beating donors. Transplant Rev 1995;9(4):159–67.

[31] Thuong M, Ruiz A, Evrard P, et al. New classification of donation after circulatory death do-nors definitions and terminology. Transpl Int 2016;29:749–59.

[32] Wijdicks EFM, Varelas PN, Grosneth GS, et al. Evidence-based guideline update: deter-mining brain death in adults. Report of the quality standards subcommittee of the American academy of neurology. Neurology 2010;74(23):1911–8.

[33] Schweikert SJ. Reexamining the flawed legal basis of the "Dead Donor Rule" as a founda-tion for organ donation policy. AMA J Ethics 2020;22(12):E1019–24.

[34] White FJ 3rd. Controversy in the determination of death: the definition and moment of death. Linacre Q 2019;86(4):366–80.

[35] Available at: https://biotech.law.lsu.edu/books/lbb/x553.htm. Accessed 04/23/2023.

[36] Dhanani S, Hornby L, Ward R, et al. Variability in the determination of death after car-diac arrest: a review of guidelines and statements. J Intensive Care Med 2012;27(4):238–52.

[37] Parent B, Turi A. Death's troubled relationship with the law. AMA J Ethics 2020;22(12):E1055–61.

[38] Institute of medicine (US) committee on non-heart-beating transplantation II: the scientific and ethical basis for practice and protocols. non-heart-beating organ transplantation: prac-tice and protocols. Washington (DC): National Academies Press (US); 2000 PMID: 25077239.

[39] Available at: https://www.asahq.org/standards-and-guidelines/statement-on-controlled-organ-donation-after-circulatory-death. Accessed 04/23/2023.

[40] Serifis N, Matheson R, Cloonan D, et al. Machine perfusion of the liver: A review of clinical trials. Front. Surg. 2021;8:625394.

[41] Hatami S, Conway J, Freed DH, et al. Thoracic organ donation after circulatory determination of death. Transplantation Reports 2023;8(1):100125.

[42] Hoffman JRH, McMaster WG, Rali AS, et al. Early US experience with cardiac donation after circulatory death (DCD) using normothermic regional perfusion. J Heart Lung Transplant 2021;40(11):1408–18.

Moving?

Make sure your subscription moves with you!

To notify us of your new address, find your **Clinics Account Number** (located on your mailing label above your name), and contact customer service at:

Email: journalscustomerservice-usa@elsevier.com

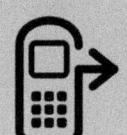

800-654-2452 (subscribers in the U.S. & Canada)
314-447-8871 (subscribers outside of the U.S. & Canada)

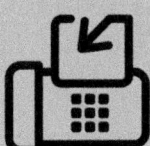

Fax number: 314-447-8029

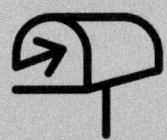

Elsevier Health Sciences Division
Subscription Customer Service
3251 Riverport Lane
Maryland Heights, MO 63043

*To ensure uninterrupted delivery of your subscription, please notify us at least 4 weeks in advance of move.

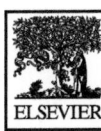

CPI Antony Rowe
Eastbourne, UK
November 13, 2023